PROGRESS IN OBSTETRICS AND GYNAECOLOGY

PROGRESS IN OBSTETRICS AND GYNAECOLOGY

Contents of Volume 5

PROGRESS IN OBSTETRICS AND GYNAECOLOGY
Volume Six

EDITED BY

JOHN STUDD MD FRCOG

Consultant Obstetrician and Gynaecologist
King's College Hospital and Dulwich Hospital;
King's College Hospital Medical School, London

CHURCHILL LIVINGSTONE
EDINBURGH LONDON MELBOURNE AND NEW YORK 1987

CHURCHILL LIVINGSTONE
Medical Division of Longman Group UK Limited

Distributed in the United States of America by
Churchill Livingstone Inc., 1560 Broadway, New York,
N.Y. 10036, and by associated companies, branches and
representatives throughout the world.

First published 1987
  Reprinted 1988
  Reprinted 1989

ISBN   0-443-03572-5

ISSN 0261-0140

British Library Cataloguing in Publication Data
Progress in obstetrics and gynaecology.
  1. Gynaecology—Periodicals   2. Obstetrics
  —Periodicals
  618.05   RG1

**Library of Congress Cataloging in Publication
Data**
Progress in obstetrics and gynaecology.
  Includes indexes.
  1. Obstetrics—Collected works.   2. Gynaecology—
Collected works.   1. Studd, John [DNLM:
1. Gynaecology—Periodicals.   2. Obstetrics—
Periodicals. W1 PR675PJ
RG39.P73   618   81-21699

Produced by Longman Singapore Publishers Pte Ltd
Printed in Singapore

Preface

An objective medical historian would recognise that nearly all advances in our specialty over the last 50 years have been European in origin with a disproportionate number such as antibiotics, the management of labour, prenatal diagnosis and the prevention of rhesus disease being from the British Isles.

By chance Volume 6 of *Progress* contains 3 other subjects of germinal importance in the development of obstetrics and gynaecology which were also initiated in this country. Ultrasound and in-vitro fertilisation have changed the whole practice of our specialty and nuclear magnetic resonance is likely to do the same. Sadly there follows the familiar story of the benefits of scientific invention being lost by the inability or unwillingness to exploit commercial potential.

Research into the application of ultrasound for clinical problems is in a few UK Centres incomparably excellent. However the availability of routine early pregnancy anomaly screening throughout the country is not good. It would be more precise to say that there were areas where it is just not available. These hospitals would be without the equipment, without the trained personnel as too few consultants chase around doing too many things. This staffing deficiency is a result of the chronic and deliberate underfunding of the National Health Service with limitations put on the number of appointments so that we have both the least number of doctors and the least number of consultants per unit of population for any country in the Western world.

Within ten years of the first use of ultrasound in Glasgow the manufacturing ultrasound industry in the UK has collapsed. Our competitors get the kudos, the advanced technology, the sales—and we receive the bill.

The story of NMR is even more tragic because it has been so rapid. Although developed in Nottingham there are but 12 systems operating in Britain, 450 in the USA and 150 in Japan. On a more general level the development of CT scan technology tells the same sad story of lost scientific and commercial opportunities.

Only with in-vitro fertilisation do we see continuing research and practical developments. Significantly this occurs only within the private sector. The inability of the NHS to support even a semblance of a comprehensive service for infertility is an embarrassment to gynaecologists and an utter betrayal of the public's faith in our system.

To add to the misery the Medical Research Council and similar bodies in Britain have virtually stopped funding clinical research particularly in obstetrics and gynaecology. However research has not ground to a halt. The reality is that there is hardly any item of successful clinical research such as infertility, cervical pathology, prenatal diagnosis, ultrasound, menopause or premenstrual syndrome that is not wholly or partly supported by the private sector. Bourn Hall, Cambridge which has supplied two outstanding chapters in this Volume is a perfect example of this scientific and entrepreneurial success. This is yet another reason why British medicine has cause to thank Patrick Steptoe (and another reason for dismay is that he has yet to be honoured by the nation).

The demonstration that brilliant research can emerge from private medicine will not be any surprise to our European and American colleagues. Fortunately we are emerging from the dream world of expecting adequate public funding for our work and relearning our past experience that worthy clinical practice and research can occur outside the State system.

London, 1987   J.S.

Contributors

Sabaratnam Arulkumaran FRCS MRCOG
Senior Lecturer, Department of Obstetrics and Gynaecology, National University of Singapore

Bernard B. Azzan
Senior Lecturer and Consultant Obstetrician and Gynaecologist, Lagos University Teaching Hospital, Nigeria

Norman A. Beischer MD BS MGO FRCS(Ed) FRACS FRCOG FRACOG
Senior Obstetrician and Gynaecologist, Mercy Maternity Hospital; and Professor and Chairman, Department of Obstetrics and Gynaecology, University of Melbourne, Australia

Paul Byrne MRCOG
Clinical Research Fellow, Birmingham and Midlands Hospital for Women, UK

Tim Chard MD FRCOG
Professor of Obstetrics, Gynaecology and Reproductive Physiology, St Bartholomew's Hospital Medical College, London, and the London Hospital Medical College, UK

Jacques Cohen BSc MSc PhD
Scientific Director, Reproductive Biology Associates, Atlanta, Georgia, USA

Edward Daw MB ChB FRCOG
North Manchester General Hospital, UK

Robert Derom MD PhD
Associate Professor, Department of Obstetrics and Gynaecology, State University, Ghent, Belgium

Patrick Duff MD
Colonel, MC, USA, Division of Maternal–Fetal Medicine, Madigan Army Medical Center, Tacoma, Washington, USA

Ian D. Duncan MB ChB FRCOG
Senior Lecturer and Honorary Consultant Obstetrician and Gynaecologist, Ninewells Hospital and Medical School, Dundee, UK

Donald Gibb MRCP MRCOG
Senior Lecturer and Honorary Consultant, Department of Obstetrics and Gynaecology, Kings College School of Medicine and Dentistry, London, UK

Osato F. Giwa-Osagie MA MB MSc MRCOG
Associate Professor, Reproductive Endocrinology and Fertility Regulation, Lagos University Teaching Hospital, Nigeria

R. F. Gledhill BSc MB BS MRCP MD
Chief Specialist and Head of Neurology, Kalafong Hospital; Professor, Department of Internal Medicine, University of Pretoria, South Africa

Victor H. H. Goh BSc(Hons) PhD
Clinical Scientist, Department of Obstetrics and Gynaecology, National University of Singapore

Rajat K. Goswamy MB BS MRCOG
Consultant Gynaecologist, Bourn Hall Clinic, Cambridge, UK

Jonathan Hewitt MB ChB MRCOG
Senior Registrar in Obstetrics and Gynaecology, Liverpool Maternity Hospital, UK

Ian Jacobs MA MB BS
Research Fellow, The London Hospital, UK

Jerome N. Kopelman MD
Major, MC, USA, Division of Maternal–Fetal Medicine, Madigan Army Medical Center, Tacoma, Washington, USA

Elizabeth Letsky FRCP
Queen Charlotte's Hospital, London, UK

Gillian Nava MRCOG
Clinical Research Fellow, Birmingham and Midlands Hospital for Women, UK

Jeremy N. Oats MB BS MRCOG FRACOG
Senior Obstetrician and Gynaecologist, Mercy Maternity Hospital; and First Assistant, Department of Obstetrics and Gynaecology, University of Melbourne, Australia

David Oram MB BS MRCOG
Consultant Gynaecologist, The London Hospital, UK

Naren B. Patel MD MRCOG
Consultant Obstetrician and Honorary Senior Lecturer, Ninewells Hospital and Medical School, Dundee, UK

Martin C. Powell MB ChB FRCS(Ed)
Birthright Research Fellow, Department of Obstetrics and Gynaecology, University Hospital, Nottingham, UK

Shan S. Ratnam AM MB BS FRCS(Ed) FRCSG FACS FRACS FRCOG MD
Professor, National University of Singapore

D. Ian Rushton MB ChB FRCPath
Senior Lecturer in Pathology, University of Birmingham; and Honorary Consultant Pathologist, Birmingham Maternity Hospital, UK

Machelle M. Seibel MD
Associate Professor in Obstetrics and Gynecology, Harvard Medical School; and Director, In Vitro Fertilization Program, Beth Israel Hospital, Boston, USA

Kurt Semm MD
Director, Department of Gynaecology and Obstetrics, Christian-Albrechts University of Kiel and Michaelis Midwifery School, West Germany

Marcus E. Setchell MA FRCS FRCS(Ed) FRCOG
Consultant Obstetrician and Gynaecologist, St Bartholomew's Hospital, London, UK

Patrick C. Steptoe FRCOG DSc
Medical Director, Bourn Hall Clinic, Cambridge, UK

David W. Sturdee MD MRCOG
Consultant Obstetrician and Gynaecologist, Solihull Hospital and East Birmingham Hospital, UK

E. Malcolm Symonds MD FRCOG
Foundation Professor of Obstetrics and Gynaecology, University of Nottingham; and Honorary Consultant, Obstetrics and Gynaecology, Trent Regional Health Authority, Nottingham, UK

Michel Thiery MD PhD
Head, Department of Obstetrics, University of Ghent, Belgium

Mary Warnock MA BPhil
Mistress of Girton College, Cambridge, UK

Robin J. Willcourt MD
Associate Professor, Obstetrics and Gynaecology, University of Hawaii

Ciaran B. J. Woodman MB BCh BAO
Registrar in Obstetrics and Gynaecology, Birmingham Maternity Hospital, UK

Brian S. Worthington BSc LIMA MB BS DMRD FRCR
Professor of Diagnostic Radiology, Queen's Medical Centre, Nottingham, UK

Contents

Obstetrics

Computerisation of obstetric records

INTRODUCTION

Data collection in obstetric practice is at a watershed. The traditional accumulation of clinical information into manually prepared notes will almost certainly be replaced by computerised data collection, and this changeover will be virtually complete by the end of this century. The reasons for this, and the means by which it will be achieved, are the subject of the present review.

Obstetrics (particularly antenatal care) lends itself well to computerised data collection and maternity has traditionally generated better statistics than other medical specialties. In the majority of cases the total number of relevant facts about an individual patient is relatively small, certainly by comparison with the amount and variety of information which must be assembled for most medical and surgical problems. The information tends to be extremely repetitive with a virtually identical structure in all subjects. Much of the important information is negative (e.g. that the patient had a normal previous pregnancy). Errors, when they occur, are more frequently of omission than commission. Failure to act on information simply because that information has not been adequately communicated is one of the main problems of obstetric management and one which lends itself especially well to solution by a computer. Unlike the human attendants, the machine has unfailing vigilance. It is able to capture 100 per cent of the relevant clinical data, and to recall these data with absolute accuracy. The human (or more commonly, a succession of humans) may forget to recheck an alpha fetoprotein level if gestational age is reassigned as a result of ultrasound examination. The computer does not.

Another development with important implications for obstetric data collection is the increasing requirement that antenatal care should be devolved from the hospital into the community. For this process to succeed without a decline in the overall quality of care it is essential that information on a patient should be readily and speedily communicated between all sites at which she may encounter the medical system. The problem of emergency admission of a woman in labour, with no notes on the pregnancy, is well

3

known. More significant if less dramatic is the immense amount of time that may be wasted by skilled professionals in pursuing the results of special investigations or laboriously reacquiring information which is already available on another site. The communication abilities of a computer system become almost mandatory under these circumstances.

This review describes the different types of data collection systems; the criteria for an optimal system; the methods and rules of clinical data entry; and, finally, some of the practical considerations in the computerisation of obstetric records.

PROSPECTIVE VERSUS RETROSPECTIVE SYSTEMS

It is important at an early stage to distinguish between prospective and retrospective systems. A *prospective* system is one in which all or most of the clinical information on a given pregnancy is entered into the computer as it is collected (i.e. at the booking clinic and at all subsequent visits including admissions); under these circumstances the computer terminal becomes effectively the clinical notes, and the system contributes directly to the management of the individual woman in her current pregnancy. A *retrospective* system is one in which the information is collected after the event (i.e. usually at the time the patient is discharged from the post-natal ward); the principal aims are administrative and to provide an on-going audit of obstetric care. There is no direct contribution to the individual patient other than the production of some repetitive paperwork (e.g. birth notification forms, etc.).

The distinction between the two types of system is important because of frequent claims that an obstetric unit has been entirely 'computerised' when in fact a rather simple retrospective system has been introduced as opposed to a far more sophisticated and complex prospective system. It is also important to recognise that prospective systems are far superior to restrospective systems in terms of quality of data, because it is possible to monitor quality at the actual time of data collection: retrospective systems are often no better than manual systems in respect of omission rates (Jelovsek & Hammond, 1978). In addition there are hybrid systems in which some but not all of the clinical data is available via terminals for management of the individual patient; it is increasingly common for laboratory results to be available in this manner (Bleich et al, 1985).

Many of the current well-known obstetric data collection systems are restrospective rather than prospective. This applies to the Korner data set (see below), to the Standard Maternity Information System (SMIS) (Barron et al, 1983), and to many of the published systems (Table 1.1). Many of the published prospective systems are only in prototype form; fully operational prospective systems such as that at King's College Hospital are exceptional at the present time.

A summary of published obstetric data collection systems is given in

Table 1.1 Published descriptions of computerised obstetric data collection systems. Some of these publications are brief and provide only incomplete information on the operation of the system

Author	Equipment	Language	Retro-spective/ prospective	Geographic area	On-line input	No. of cases/ year
Abdella et al, 1982	DEC	BASIC	—	Memphis	—	—
Anderson, 1985	Diacon	DBase II	R	Cleveland	No	1,200
Andersen et al, 1976[1]	—	—	—	—	Yes	—
Davidson et al, 1982	—	—	R	Los Angeles	—	10,000
Davis et al, 1982	Control data	—	R	Georgia	No	2,400
Dunt & Parker, 1973	CDC	—	R	Melbourne	No	—
Eden et al, 1985	—	Informix	P	Chicago	Yes	—
Gibbons et al, 1982	—	—	R	Illinois	Mixed	—
Grover et al, 1982	—	—	R	Illinois	No	—
Hammond et al, 1982	—	—	R/P	North Carolina	Mixed	—
Herbert et al, 1982	IBM	—	R	North Carolina	No	13,000
Houlton et al, 1984	Apple	Pascal	R	Bristol	Yes	—
Jennett et al, 1978	Data General S/2000 Eclipse	MUMPS[2]	R/P	Phoenix	(?)	900
Lilford et al, 1981, 1983a	Commodore	BASIC	P	London	Yes	—
Maresh et al, 1983	Commodore	BASIC	R	London	Yes	—
Merkatz et al, 1982	Time-sharing	—	R	Cleveland	No	—
Michel et al, 1982	Prime 550	P-STAT[3]	R	South Carolina	—	—
Smith et al, 1982	DEC	IDA	R	Montreal	Yes	5,000
Sokol & Chik, 1982	DEC	FORTRAN	P (?)	Cleveland	—	3,200
South & Rhodes, 1971	CDC	FORTRAN	R	London	No	4,500
Studney et al, 1977	—	—	P	Massachusetts	No	700
Thatcher, 1969	—	—	R	Adelaide	No	—
Tuck et al, 1976	UNIVAC	FORTRAN	R	London	No	4,500
Wirtschafter et al, 1982	Data General IBM	—	P	Birmingham	Yes	4,000
Work & Kriewell, 1982	—	—	R	Michigan	No	—
Yamamoto et al, 1985	—	—	R	Japan	—	—
Yeh & Lincoln, 1985	Apple/IBM	—	R	Los Angeles	Yes	3,200

[1] Data collected for a computer-assisted decision-making system.
[2] MUMPS—Massachussets-General-Hospital Utility Multi-Programming System
[3] P-STAT—Princeton STATistical analysis package

Table 1.1. The present review has as its major topic the prospective systems—those used for care of the individual patient. However, many of the observations apply equally well to retrospective systems.

Criteria for a prospective system of obstetric data collection

A perfect and fully integrated system for obstetric data collection probably does not exist at the present time. The criteria which should be met by such a system are summarised in Table 1.2 and can be detailed as follows:

1. Information should be collected *exclusively* at computer terminals. Paper transactions (other than printing by the computer) should be eliminated, in order to ensure that all information is captured within the computer system. In an obstetric system provision must be made

Table 1.2 Operational criteria for a fully computerised prospective obstetric data collection system

---

1. All transactions take place via computer terminals.
2. All information available throughout the system.
3. Response times not more than seconds.
4. Reliability.
5. Confidentiality.
6. 'User-friendly' interface.
7. Full documentation.
9. Preparation of routine paperwork.
10. Transfer of data to other systems.
11. 'Feedback' capability.
12. Flexibility.

No current system meets all these criteria, but systems may be compared by the extent to which they do reach them. The individual items are discussed in more detail in the text.

for entry of data which by definition cannot be entered via a terminal, e.g. information on domiciliary deliveries.

2. Information obtained or entered at one terminal should be immediately available at all other terminals within the system. Printed reports, which almost by definition become out of date as soon as they are produced, will be progressively replaced by data retrieval at terminals which give immediate access to the most up-to-date information.

3. The response time of the system should be rapid. Delays of even a few seconds can be counterproductive to the acceptance by routine users. Within a single building or campus, serviced by dedicated lines, delays should be of the order of milliseconds (i.e. not detectable at all by the user). If the system extends throughout a community via ordinary telephone lines then slightly longer delays may be expected, though even at baud rates as low as 300 information is presented rather faster than it can be read by the human eye. (Baud rate = rate of signal events per second; 300 baud is approximately equal to 30 letters or numerals per second.)

4. The system must be reliable, and anything other than the most dramatic failures should not last for more than a few minutes. Under *no* circumstances should users ever lose data. Even a distant prospect of this is likely to inhibit the essential switchover from manuscript to electronic recording.

5. Confidentiality is obviously a requirement, but its presence must be clearly demonstrated. Given that confidentiality is relatively easy to achieve with staff passwords and other checks (more so than with traditional manuscript notes), it is important that both staff and patients have 'confidence in the confidentiality'. Systems must also conform to data protection regulations. In the U.K. this is the Data Protection Bill (1984) whereby all users of computer systems which hold identifiable information must register their systems and their uses.

6. The computer programs should be 'user-friendly'. This is an over-used term which has often been applied to systems which are remarkably unfriendly. A truly user-friendly program should be usable without any instruction manual, and it should be easier for the obstetrician to obtain a laboratory result from the computer terminal than from a telephone call. Teaching the use of a system should take the form of a simple and enjoyable demonstration rather than hard instruction: if there are rules to memorise, it should be the machine which does it. It should be unnecessary to emphasise that the system must also be 'patient-friendly'—that it should not interfere with the rapport between the woman and her professional attendant (Fawdry, 1985).

7. Complete background documentation is essential for the specialist operator who may need to modify or upgrade existing programs. A transaction log must be maintained for all changes made to the basic structure of the system. At every terminal there should be a procedure list including who to call if there is a breakdown.

8. There must be a common system of registration for all patients so there is only one set of identifying information which covers all possible events, obstetric or otherwise. The data generated by the obstetric system must be easily linked with the district Patient Administration System (PAS), such that there is no need to key-in patient information more than once. Electronic linking of this type sounds straightforward but in practice can be remarkably difficult because of the inability of many computer systems to 'talk' to other systems.

9. The system must be capable of preparing all or most of the repetitive paperwork associated with obstetric cases (Table 1.3). This aspect provides a powerful motive for acceptance of a new system by all members of staff.

10. The system must be able to collect and transfer selected retrospective

Table 1.3 Some of the 'output' documents which should be available from an obstetric computer system (this list does not include the actual case notes).

1. At first visit:	production of 'expected patients' list; letter from GP; production of Sighthill-type risk cards.
2. At admission:	ward lists for social workers, etc.
3. At delivery:	birth notification form; production of notes for child.
4. At admission to neonatal unit:	summary of maternal information; summary of labour ward book.
5. At discharge:	letter to GP; discharge lists for community midwives and administration; discharge summary.

If existing documents are not in a format which can be produced by a computer (e.g. double-sided birth notification cards) then they should be redesigned.

data (the Korner minimum data set) to regional mainframe computers (this is usually performed in batches).

11. The system should have 'feedback' capability, i.e. it should be able to use information collected at different times to flag inconsistent or abnormal findings.

12. The system should be flexible so that it can be readily enhanced (e.g. to include a linked neonatal system) or altered according to local needs. In the latter respect it should be emphasised that some measure of standardisation is essential—especially with the items required by the Korner minimum data set.

THE TECHNOLOGY OF COMPUTERISED OBSTETRIC DATA COLLECTION

Virtually every known means of data collection and analysis have at one time or another been applied to obstetric data collection. Many obstetricians will have personal experience of retrospective systems: for example, preparing handwritten lists from delivery suite record books, or making punched cards and sorting them by mechanical systems of varying degrees of complexity, or filling in printed questionnaires, usually of the 'box and tick' variety, for subsequent transfer to a computer by professional staff (Gledhill, et al, 1970; South & Rhodes, 1971; Dunt & Parker, 1973; Jelovsek & Hammond, 1978; Barron et al,1983). Printed questionnaires are probably the most widely used system at the present time. However, all these systems are likely to be replaced, where this is not happening already, by direct entry of data into a computer via a terminal consisting of a visual display unit and a keyboard. The advantages of this for either prospective or retrospective systems are so obvious once demonstrated that the only restraints to immediate application are some awareness and experience on the art of the potential user, and economic considerations which are minor in the case of restrospective procedures but more substantial for a complete prospective system.

The key practical feature of the present technical revolution is the *immediate availability of information* to users. In principle, systems of the type discussed in this review could have been devised at any time within the past 20 years. In practice, it is the rapid spread of inexpensive microprocessor-based computing power into every facet of professional life which will make this type of development a reality. There is nothing revolutionary about the desirability of complete, error-free information obtained with the minimum of effort; but this was simply not possible with the technology of the 1970s.

Data entry into a computer

Virtually everyone must now be somewhat familiar with the concept of interactive data-entry via a terminal, for example, at any check-in desk at an airport. Briefly, the user is presented with a questionnaire in the form of successive screens of text on a visual display unit. Each screen contains either a single question or a group of questions and the answer (for example a name or a 'Y' or an 'N') is entered via the keyboard. Once the input to each screen is completed and validated the program scrolls automatically to the next screen containing the next question or a group of questions. When the entry is complete, the data are permanently recorded/memorised on a magnetic medium which is usually in the form of a disc. Information can then be recalled from memory and inspected or modified at any time.

In most current systems the screen is set out as a table (Fig. 1.1). The table is 'filled in' and thereafter can be recalled in exactly the same way as a page of manuscript notes. This approach has the great advantage of familiarity: filling in the table on the screen is very comparable to manual entries on a printed questionnaire.

The commonest system for data entry is the traditional 'QWERTY' keyboard. This has been attacked as awkward and outdated but has the supreme advantage of familiarity—not least to junior staff and the patients themselves. Other systems of data-entry have been described including the use of specially designed keyboards (Lilford et al, 1983b; Lucas et al, 1977), light pens, and touch-sensitive screens. The use of a printed questionnaire in which the questions are answered by passing a light pen over a bar-code has been successfully implemented in a prospective system at King's College Hospital. The problem with this approach is that it can be somewhat cumbersome if it has to accommodate extensive branching to ancillary questions.

Hardware—equipment for an obstetric data collection system

Details of the hardware will not be discussed in detail here. Briefly, most units will be likely to operate around a multi-user, multi-tasking system—

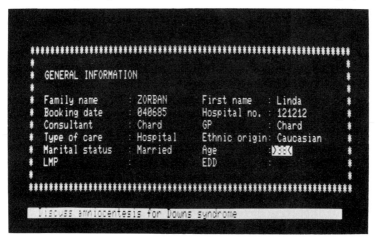

Fig. 1.1 Example of a questionnaire screen laid out as a table. After each response is typed in the cursor moves automatically to the next line. Note also that the computer has 'flagged' the advanced maternal age as a possible indication for amniocentesis.

usually a mini-computer, with terminals at suitable sites inside or outside the hospital. Future planning may incline more towards 'intelligent' terminals (comparable to present-day microcomputers) linked in a network and sharing central memory stores (Chard & Lilford, 1984). Substantial memory stores are essential, together with regular (probably daily) backups to magnetic tape. From the point of view of the practising obstetrician the choice of hardware should be immaterial. It is merely required to perform exactly what he wants, how he wants, and when he wants. The absence of significant restraints on the 'consumer' is part and parcel of the computer revolution.

Some guidance in respect of hardware for obstetric data systems in the U.K. has been provided by the Computer Policy Committee (National Health Service Computer Policy Committee Evaluation of Maternity Pilot Trials, March 1985. Available from the Administrator, NHS-Computer Policy Committee, 19 Calthorpe Rd, Birmingham B15 1RP). They propose that Health Districts should focus on either DEC or ICL equipment, and that with these they should consider using the data collection systems developed at Nottingham City Hospital and St Mary's Hospital, London, respectively. However, at the present time neither of these systems is 'prospective' in the sense that the term is used here, and considerable further development will be needed before they meet all the criteria of Table 1.2. It should also be noted that transfer of files between systems using different communication protocols can be problematic: for example, from a district-based DEC to a regional ICL mainframe.

Software for an obstetric data collection system

As with hardware, hard-and-fast rules cannot be given about software. Packages exist for both ICL and DEC equipment (e.g. 'MUMPS') but usually do not meet all the criteria of Table 1.2. It is also important to emphasise that many current questionnaire/database systems are excellent for 'horizontal' searches, i.e. finding and presenting the facts on an individual patient, but much less effective in 'vertical' searches, e.g. finding all patients who had a Caesarean section during labour. (These data relationships are also often referred to as 'hierarchical' and 'relational' respectively.) 'Vertical' information of this type is essential in practical obstetric management for the recall of patients with high-risk factors, and is also needed for many administrative and research purposes. If not available, a special, separate enquiry package may have to be written (Young, 1985).

The rules of obstetric data collection: analysis of responses and error traps

The overriding advantage of using a computer to collect clinical information (i.e. entry via a screen and keyboard) is the availability of immediate feedback on the validity of an answer. It is a platitude to re-state that the quality of information available from any system is directly related to the quality of the data input (the 'garbage-in, garbage-out' problem). This problem is almost entirely eliminated by data entry through an interactive system in which every answer is examined as soon as it is input and rejected or at least flagged if it does not meet certain predefined criteria. A system of this type should eliminate most major errors—for example, if a patient's age is entered as '72' in error for '27'. It cannot, however, eliminate minor errors such as the inversion of '23' to '32'.

The types of error trap which are incorporated into an interactive questionnaire have been reviewed in detail elsewhere (Cowan & Chard, 1985) and will only be summarised here.

General error traps

General error traps can be divided into 'transparent' and 'message' types. 'Transparent' error traps are those which automatically reject any answer which is not an obvious option displayed on the screen (Table 1.4). 'Message' error traps are those in which the answer is rejected; an explanation of the error is displayed on the screen and the user is invited to repeat the question (Table 1.5). General traps of the latter type are aimed at two mistakes: making an entry of the wrong length; and entering information which is basically impossible. General error traps are always absolute: unlike some of the specific error traps, there is never an option to confirm a response once it has been rejected: it must be repeated in the correct form.

Table 1.4 Examples of general error traps which are 'transparent' to the user, *i.e. there is no response of any kind to pressing the wrong key*

1. Rejection of all keys except 'Y' and 'N' in response to a yes/no question.
2. Rejection of all letter/symbol keys in response to questions calling for a numeric input (or vice-versa).
3. Rejection of all but a defined range in choosing a number from a list.

Table 1.5 Examples of general error traps which give a 'message' to the user. The answer to the question must then be repeated in full.

1. Rejection of entries of the wrong length, e.g. a date of more or less than six digits; a time of more or less than four digits.
2. Rejection of entries which are definitively impossible, e.g. a day greater than 31; a month greater than 12; a time greater than 2400.

Specific error traps

Specific error traps are associated with individual questions and are applied after the general validity checks. They are always of the message type and may be absolute or optional, or even sometimes a combination of the two.

Table 1.6 Examples of specific error traps based on predetermined criteria. The user is asked to confirm the answer or repeat the question

1. Maternal age less than 15 or more than 40 years.
2. More than 10 previous pregnancies; more than 6 livebirths; more than 3 stillbirths, miscarriages or terminations.
3. Systolic blood pressure more than 140 or less than 100; diastolic of more than 80 or less than 60.
4. Haemoglobin of more than 15 or less than 7.
5. Postpartum blood loss of less than 100 or more than 500.
6. Delivered weight of less than 2500 or more than 4200.

These optimal limits can also be expanded to absolute limits if the range is extended. The exact limits can be specified by the individual unit.

They may be based on pre-determined information (Table 1.6; Fig. 1.2) or on information acquired in an earlier section of the questionnaire (Table 1.7) or on earlier occasions. Cross-validation with other data fields is particularly important in antenatal care where by definition data are collected at a number of different points in time and the interpretation of new data is critically related to earlier findings—for example, correction of other information once scan dates are known (Fig. 1.3).

Table 1.7 Examples of specific error traps based on information obtained in an earlier part of the questionnaire. The user is asked to confirm the answer or repeat the question.

1. Total number of previous deliveries does not equal livebirths plus stillbirths.
2. Date of delivery more than 1 month from expected date of delivery.
3. Day and time of delivery more than 24 hours from onset of labour.
4. Complications such as thalassaemia or sickle-cell disease if the patient is not of the appropriate ethnic group.

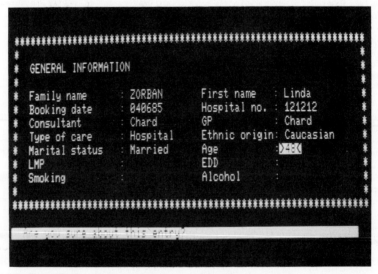

Fig. 1.2 Example of an error trap based on predetermined information. This program requests confirmation of any maternal age greater than 40.

It is worthwhile to emphasize that specific error traps have great flexibility in terms of the limits applied. The staff of an obstetric unit should be able to select the precise figure at which a response is flagged. For example, it might be perfectly reasonable to define any number between 12 and 20 as the lower limit requiring confirmation of maternal age. The essential factor is that the presence of limits should eliminate the more obvious errors which may occur with traditional data collection methods.

An extension of the concept of error traps is the use of 'help' screens which can be deliberately called by the user—for example, defining complications (Fig. 1.4). Training files can also be of great assistance to first-time users: a block of 'artificial' records is created and can be used to learn the operation of the system.

The rules of obstetric data collection: types of questions

Questions may be of four types (Table 1.8). Discursive questions require either a partly structured response (e.g. dates, times) or an unstructured response (e.g. proper names, names of diseases, free text). Questions in

Table 1.8 Types of questions for an obstetric questionnaire

1. Discursive (structured or unstructured)
2. Yes/No
3. Selection of a number (multiple choice)
4. Selection of a number (mutually exclusive)

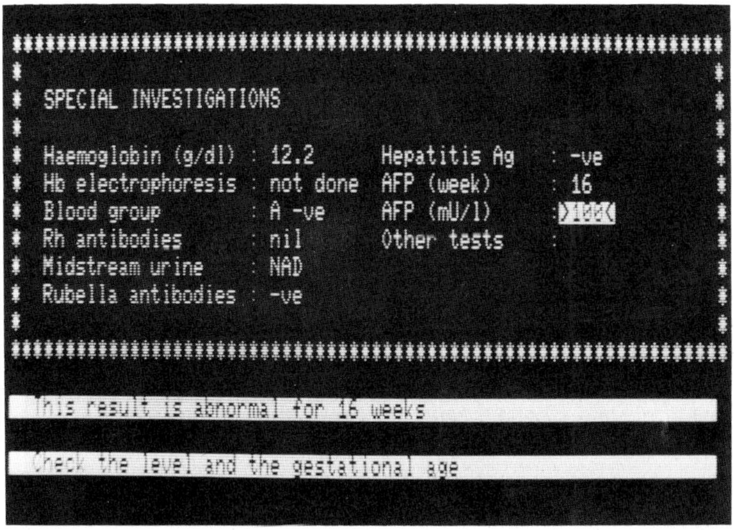

```
*******************************************************************
*                                                                 *
*  SPECIAL INVESTIGATIONS                                          *
*                                                                 *
*  Haemoglobin (g/dl)  : 12.2      Hepatitis Ag    : -ve          *
*  Hb electrophoresis  : not done  AFP (week)       : 16          *
*  Blood group         : A -ve     AFP (mU/l)       : )100(       *
*  Rh antibodies       : nil       Other tests      :             *
*  Midstream urine     : NAD                                      *
*  Rubella antibodies  : -ve                                      *
*                                                                 *
*******************************************************************

  This result is abnormal for 16 weeks

  Check the level and the gestational age
```

Fig. 1.3 Example of cross-validation based on data collected at different points in time. When the AFP result is input the computer looks up the gestational age of the patient as estimated at a previous visit. The two numbers are examined relative to a table held in the computer memory, and the result is flagged if abnormal.

which a number is selected from a menu can be mutually exclusive (i.e. only one number can be chosen, and this excludes all others) or multiple choice (i.e. one or more numbers can be chosen, in virtually any combination). Almost all questions should include some type of 'don't know' escape clause.

A point of good practice in computerised data entry is to minimise the option for input of free test. Most worthwhile questions can be structured in such a way as to require a yes/no response or selection of a number from a menu (Fig. 1.5). The elimination of free text has many advantages. By definition, a much better and more standardised record is produced. Trivia (e.g. 'feels better', 'all well') are avoided. Responses can be cross-validated, which is virtually impossible with unstructured information. Much less memory space is used.

The rules of obstetric data collection: the structure of a questionnaire

Questions must be designed as a logical sequence of sections covering different aspects of a patient's history. In the case of the booking clinic a typical sequence would be general information and history, past obstetric history, past gynaecological history, past medical history, results of examination, and plan of special investigations. The exact order and layout should represent a balance of logic and convenience; the implementation of a new obstetric data collection system should provide some units with a stimulus to revise their clinical records (Fawdry & Mutch, 1985).

Within a given section the order of questions should be arranged so as to minimise the total amount of text required. For example, in the history of a previous pregnancy there should be an enquiry as to whether there were any

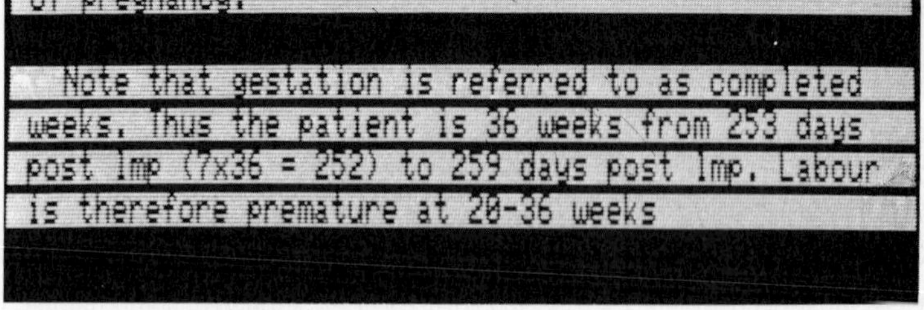

Fig. 1.4 Example of a 'help' screen. The user is uncertain of the exact definition of premature labour and can call up this short explanation from computer memory. Note that this also serves a useful educational function.

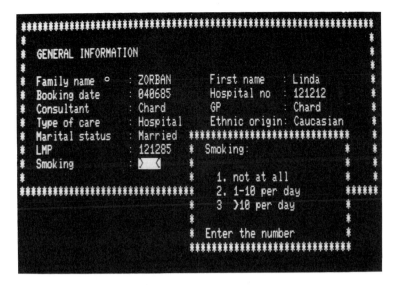

Fig. 1.5 Example of a question requiring the choice of a number from a list—in this case, the patient's smoking habits. Note that the user is forced to be somewhat specific about the response—much better than a simple discursive entry such as 'heavy'.

complications. If the answer is 'No' the program can then branch to bypass a group of redundant questions. If the answer is 'Yes' then a more detailed question is presented to identify the problem more precisely (Fig. 1.6). As a general rule it should never be necessary to repeat a question, nor should any question appear which is irrelevant in the light of a previous answer. Although this rule may appear obvious, it is frequently broken in questionnaire designs.

A question should always ask for exact data rather than a response which depends upon the user's opinion or analysis of the data. This again, would seem obvious, were it not that the rule is so frequently broken. An excellent example is the patient's age, which is recorded at the first antenatal visit. However, this is not necessarily the age at conception or delivery, and it is actually unlikely that the age will be the same at all three times. The rule is to record the mother's date of birth; if this needs to be translated into an age at any other time, the machine can perform the calculation much faster than a human. Another example is the definition of pathology. Pre-eclampsia has so many definitions that the response to a question of the form of 'Pre-eclampsia: yes or no, and if yes gives severity' is likely to be meaningless. It is far more straightforward to note the systolic and diastolic blood pressures since these 'facts' at least do not beg the question as to what constitutes a cut-off point between normal and abnormal.

Another point of good design is the use of ancillary questions to establish the seriousness or otherwise of a given event in the past history.

Several groups have advocated the use of ICD (International Classification

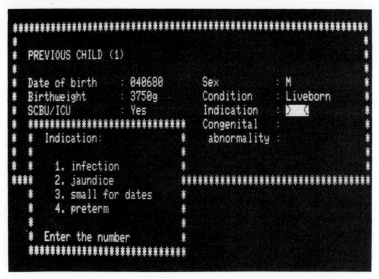

Fig. 1.6 Example of a 'branch'. After a 'yes' response to the question of whether the child was given special care, the computer presents a list of possible indications. The point to emphasise is that this is 'transparent' to the user if the answer is 'No', when the program simply proceeds to the next question. The efficient accumulation of information in this manner is a simple example of the subject known as 'artificial intelligence'.

of Disease) codes to record complications of pregnancy. Though superficially attractive, this approach presents many practical problems, not least that it calls for a level of knowledge and interpretation which may not be possessed by all users. The possibilities of automatic generation of these codes by computer, or the introduction of 'help' screens to permit manual entry by skilled staff are attractive, but not as yet explored within obstetric systems. Some such procedure will be essential because the use of ICD codes is mandated by the Korner Report.

The rules of obstetric data collection: how much information should be collected

The designers of new systems for data collection, especially those involving computer questionnaires, are often tempted to include immense amounts of information, much of which is unnecessary, and not part of the traditional process. The acquisition of superfluous information is particularly likely when questionnaires are designed by a committee.

There is a certain level of information which must be regarded as 'definitive': the retrospective data set recommended by the Korner Committee is a good example of this, since it describes the minimum information required for management of health services (see below). Thereafter the prime criteria for inclusion of an individual item of information are: (1) can it be collected with reasonable accuracy?; and (2) is it likely to be useful? These criteria beg the question of what is meant by 'reasonable' or 'useful' but do at least serve to eliminate some of the more obvious irrelevancies. Another factor is the total amount of information collected. There is a natural temptation to include even the smallest detail because its potential importance cannot be denied. However, there comes a point, difficult to judge objectively, when extra detail becomes counter productive: this is the point at which the sheer quantity of material demanded leads to a degradation in the quality of the response.

It is difficult to provide precise guidelines about the content of an obstetric questionnaire. However, it is not necessary to define a rigid formula as there should be considerable flexibility for individual units to determine what material should be included in their own database. The key point is that such flexibility can be readily accommodated by the current technology.

The Korner Report

This report will have a major impact on health service information systems in general and data collection in obstetrics in particular. The Steering Group on Health Services Information was appointed in 1980 under the chairmanship of Mrs Edith Korner. Since then it has produced four reports to the Secretary of State of which the first (1982) and the fourth (1984) contain material relevant to obstetric practice. The aim of the group was to identify the information needed by a district health authority for the effective management of their health services. To this end the group proposed a 'minimum data set' (Tables 1.9 and 1.10) (collection of which will soon become mandatory) and a small number of optional items ('clinical options')

Table 1.9   The Korner minimum data set

Mother	Each baby
Number/identifier	Number/identifier
—	Sex
Address code	Address code
Date of birth	Date of birth
Marital status	—
Category of patient	—
GP code	GP code
Method of admission	Method of admission
Source of admission	Source of admission
Date of first a/n assessment	—
Intended management	—
Wards occupied	Wards occupied
Operative procedures	Operative procedures
Method of discharge	Method of discharge
Destination on discharge	Destination on discharge
Consultant/GP codes	Consultant/GP codes
ICD diagnoses	BPA diagnoses (ICD compatible)

Note that the generation of ICD codes for specific diagnoses is an ideal indication for a short interactive program (items collected for all patients)

Table 1.10   The Korner minimum data set (items collected by notification and registration of each birth)

Mother	Delivery	Identifiers
Notification		
Parity	Place of delivery	Mother's number/identifier
—	Original intention	Mother's date of birth
Baby	Reason for change	Baby's number/identifier
Birth order	Number of babies	Baby's date of birth
Live-stillbirth	Length of gestation	Baby's time of delivery
Birthweight	Method of labour onset	—
Resuscitation	Method of delivery	
Registration		
—	Parental occupation	Baby's NHS number

(Table 1.11). Obstetrics differs somewhat from other specialities in that the 'maternity' is the unit of statistical account, rather than an individual episode of hospital care. It should be emphasised that the minimum data set is strictly aimed at administration of services. The system is restrospective and its collection has little or nothing to contribute to the management of an individual patient. However, the Korner information will be used as an essential part of financial performance indicators and these, in turn, will determine the resources available to a given specialty.

In 1985 a supplement was published to the first and fourth reports, this time under the chairmanship of M J Fairey. The supplement deals exclusively with maternity services, and provides more detailed definitions of the terms in both the minimum data set and the clinical options.

Table 1.11   The Korner clinical option

Mother	Each baby
Height	Head circumference at birth
Blood group	Birth length
Previous pregnancies	Apgar score
—	Hips examination
Delivery	Jaundice presence
Length of first stage	Type of feeding established
Length of second stage	PKU + BCG performed
Pain relief given	Gestation (paediatric assessment)
Presentation of fetus	Additional diagnoses
—	Follow-up arrangements

Some practical aspects of the implementation of an obstetric data collection system

At the present time there is no complete, working prospective system which meets the criteria set out in Table 1.2 and which can be installed on a 'turnkey' basis in a district which does not have existing skills in this area.

However, it can be virtually guaranteed that such systems will become available in the next 2–4 years, and it is likely that they will evolve from some of the excellent prototypes which have already been described.

Even then it is important to recognise that a fully worked-out prospective data collection system cannot be installed overnight and replace all other procedures on the following day. Detailed advance planning is necessary and pilot-scale studies are a *sine qua non*, even though the latter may call for exceptional commitment because of the need to run duplicate systems. It is essential that three or four members of existing staff be appointed to choose and then supervise the implementation of the system, and even more essential that a *full-time* member of staff be available for at least 1 year from the commencement of the pilot trial. Outside contractors can also be of immense assistance in the earlier phases of implementation. Even then, problems can arise, as seen with some current installations of the Patient Administration System (see *Computing The Newspaper*, 26 September 1985, pp. 22–23).

Failure to recognise that people and expertise are vital for the successful operation of clinical computing systems is likely to generate many problems, however obvious this advice may appear. Furthermore, it is essential that good relations be established with all hospital community staff from the earliest possible stage. 'Good relations', in this context, means communication and education; there are few people who do not respond with enthusiasm to a careful explanation of the operation and potential benefits of computerised data collection.

Another important 'carrot' is to ensure that one of the first functions performed by the system is repetitive form-filling: users can thus obtain some immediate and very tangible benefit.

At an almost trivial, but still important, level thought should be given to the physical location of the system. The central unit and memory stores should be accommodated and managed by existing district computer services (there must be few sites in the U.K. where these are not available). The 'clinical terminals' must obviously be immediately adjacent to the site of patient contact (e.g. desk of interview room, examination cubicle, delivery suite); space is often remarkably difficult to identify but becomes much easier once all staff are motivated towards the use of the system. An annoying feature which has led to the rejection of some prototype systems is the noise made by some dot-matrix printers. However, quieter systems are now available and this should not present a significant problem in the future.

CONCLUSIONS

There can be no doubt that within the next 10 years computers will play an increasing role in the preparation of obstetric patient records. In this review a set of criteria for an optional system are described (Table 1.2); however, despite the obvious desirability of each and every one of these criteria, it will probably be some time before all of them are met simultaneously in a single practical system. Indeed, as with any rapidly developing subject, it is likely and even desirable that there will be a diversity of approach and a number of 'competing systems' (see Table 1.1). Underlying this diversity is a number of fairly basic rules—how best to ask for and classify simple clinical information. These rather obvious and very common-sense rules are worth documenting because of the frequency with which they are broken in many prototype systems.

There are some observers who would regard all attempts at mechanisation of clinical data collection as 'utopian'—and, implicitly, as superfluous. Such critics may well choose to point at the lack of published evidence that the use of computers will reduce perinatal mortality and morbidity, the primary aim of all antenatal care. In reality it is unlikely that such proof will ever be available, any more than it exists for many currently well-accepted aspects of obstetric management. What can and has been proven is that the computer is a more efficient collector of information than a human: if 'good' information is an essential part of 'good' clinical care then it is certain that the machine must sooner or later win. Finally, at a very practical level, the implementation of the Korner proposals will *mandate* a certain level of mechanical data collection as a universal feature of maternity services. The leap from the installation of a sophisticated retrospective system to a prospective system is much smaller than that from no system at all. This, more than any other factor, makes it virtually certain that the keyboard will eventually replace the pen in antenatal care.

REFERENCES

Abdella T N, Ryan G M Jr, Anderson G D, Boswell D K 1982 Development of the Memphis perinatal data project. Acta Obstetrica Gynecologica Scandinavica Supplement 109: 60
Anderson G, Llerena C, Davidson D, Taylor T R 1976 Practical application of computer-assisted decision-making in an antenatal clinic—a feasibility study. Methods of Information in Medicine 15: 224–229
Andersen H F 1985 Developing a perinatal database on a microcomputer. American Journal of Perinatology 2: 148–149
Barron S L, Morris D, Barron W 1983 Standard Maternity Information Systems (SMIS). Personal communication.
Bleich H L, Beckely R F, Horowitz G L, Jackson D J, Moody E S, Goodman C F S R, McKay M W, Pope R A, Walden T, Bloom S M, Slack W V 1985 Clinical computing in a teaching hospital. New England Journal of Medicine 312: 756–764
Chard T, Lilford R 1984 Clinical computing to the end of the decade. British Journal of Healthcare Computing 1: 8–13
Cowan D B, Chard T 1985 The perinatal database. British Journal of Hospital Medicine 34: 37–41.
Davidson E C Jr, Gore J, Umbdenstock L 1982 Different regional users: qualitatively different informational needs for a perinatal database system. Acta Obstetrica Gynecologica Scandinavica Supplement 109: 22–25
Davis H C, Etersque S, Sutherland J G, Fadel H E, Smith C 1982 Computer report generating system for perinatal data in a tertiary hospital. Acta Obstetrica Gynecologica Scandinavica Supplement 109: 45–48
Dunt D R, Parker L M 1973 A computer data processing system for hospital obstetric records.

Obstetric complications in non-English speaking migrants. Medical Journal of Australia 2: 693–698.

Eden R, Winegar A, Stopa W, Vidyasagar D, Work B, Spellacy W N 1985 Computerised provider–linkage system; UNIPEN. Computers in Obstetrics, Gynaecology and Neonatology 4: 2–4

Fawdry R D S 1985 Antenatal history taking: the acceptability of a computer questionnaire requiring simple direct input by the expectant mother. Journal of Obstetrics and Gynaecology 5: 206

Fawdry R D S, Mutch L M M 1985 Antenatal history taking: what are we asking? Journal of Obstetrics and Gynaecology 5: 201–205

Gibbons P S, Pishotta F T, Moawad A H, Lowensohn R I, Woo D 1982 The Obfile^c perinatal database. Acta Obstetrica Gynecologica Scandinavica Supplement 19: 51–52

Gledhill V X, McPherson T A, McKay I R 1970 The application of computers in medical records: a computer system for the storage and retrieval of medical records. Australian Annals of Medicine 19: 16–23

Grover J W, Peterson P Q, Raju T N K, Vidyasagar D, Winegar A 1982 A centralised computer-based perinatal-patient data retrieval system for thirteen metropolitan hospitals. Acta Obstetrica Gynecologica Scandinavica Supplement 109: 37–39

Hammond W E, Stead W W, Straube M J, Jelovsek F R 1982 A perinatal database management system for ambulatory care. Acta Obstetrica Gynecologica Scandinavica Supplement 109: 40–41

Herbert W N P, Burnett J E Jr, Wiegand F G, Easley H A 1982 Development of a multicenter computerized obstetrical record abstract. Acta Obstetrica Gynecologica Supplement 109: 35–36

Houlton M, Austin J, Jenkins D, Turner G M, Wilkins D G 1984 A micro-computer system in the delivery suite. British Journal of Obstetrics and Gynaecology 91: 555–559

Jelovsek F, Hammond W 1978 Formal error rate in a computerized obstetric medical record. Methods of Information in Medicine 17: 151–157

Jennett R J, Gall D, Waterkotte G W, Warford H S 1978 A computerized perinatal data system for a region. American Journal of Obstetrics and Gynecology 131: 157–161

Lilford R J, Chard T 1981 Microcomputers in antenatal care: a feasibility study on the booking interview. British Medical Journal 283: 533–539

Lilford R J, Chard T 1984 The use of a small computer to provide action suggestions in the booking clinic. Acta Obstetrica Japonica 36: 119–125

Lilford R J., Bingham P, Fawdry R, Setchell M, Chard T 1983a The development of on-line history-taking systems in antenatal care. Methods of Information in Medicine 22: 189–197.

Lilford R J, Glyn-Evans D, Chard T 1983b The use of a patient-interactive microcomputer system to obtain histories in an infertility and gynecologic endocrinology clinic. American Journal of Obstetrics and Gynecology 146: 374–379

Lucas R W, Mullin P J, Lun C B X, McInroy D C 1977 Psychiatrists and computers as interrogators of patients with alcohol-related illness—a comparison. British Journal of Psychiatry 131: 160–166

Maresh M, Beard R W, Conbe D, Dawson A M, Gillmer M D G, Smith G, Steer P J 1983 Selection of an obstetric data base for a microcomputer and its use for on-line production of birth notification forms, discharge summaries and perinatal audit. British Journal of Obstetrics and Gynaecology 90: 227–231

Merkatz I R, Stephan P, Dickinson W 1982 The Cleveland regional perinatal network's computerized information system. Acta Obstetrica Gynecologica Scandinavica 109: 17–21

Michel Y, Miller M C III, Levkoff A H 1982 The South Carolina statewide perinatal information system. Acta Obtetrica Gynecologica Scandinavica Supplement 109: 26–28

Smith I P, de Leon A, Funnell W R, Lalonde A B, Mclean F H, Usher H 1982 A research-oriented system for McGill obstetrical and neonatal data (Mond). Acta Obstetrica Gynecologica Scandinavica Supplement 109: 49–50

Sokol R J, Chik L 1982 A perinatal database system for research and clinical care. Acta Obstetrica Gynecologica Scandinavica Supplement 109: 57–59

South J, Rhodes P 1971 Computer services for obstetric records. British Medical Journal 4: 32–34

Studney D R, Adams J B, Gorbach A, Guenthner S, Morgan M W, Barnett G O 1977 A computerised prenatal record. Obstetrics and Gynaecology 50: 82–87

Thatcher R A 1969 A package deal for computer processing in obstetric records. Medical Journal of Australia 2: 766–768

Tuck C S, Cundy A, Wagman H, Usherwood M McD, Thomas M 1976 The use of a computer in an obstetric department. British Journal of Obstetrics and Gynaecology 83: 97–104

Wirtschafter D D, Blackwell W, Goldenberg R, Henderson S, Peake P, Huddleston J F, Howell M 1982 Obstetrical automated medical record system. Acta Obstetrica Gynecologica Scandinavica Supplement 109: 29

Work B A Jr, Kriewell T J 1982 Maternal–perinatal data system. Acta Obstetrica Gynecologica Scandinavica 109: 32–33

Yamamoto K, Ogura H, Furutani H, Kitazoe Y, Takeda Y 1985 Progress report on nationwide networking system of perinatal records. Asia-Oceania Journal of Obstetrics and Gynaecology 11: 99–106

Yeh S-Y, Lincoln T 1985 From micro to mainframe: a practical approach to perinatal data processing. American Journal of Perinatology 2: 158–160.

Young D W 1985 COSTAR and its medical query language In: Bryant J R, Kostrewski B (eds) Current perspectives in health computing. British Journal of Healthcare Computing, pp. 38–46

Anaemia in obstetrics

Healthy pregnancy is associated with marked changes in the circulating blood, which show wide variations. These physiological adjustments include increases in the blood volume and alterations in the interacting factors involved in haemostasis.

It is not possible to assess accurately the haematological status of pregnant women by the criteria used for males and non-pregnant females. In order to understand the haematological problems associated with the obstetric patient a knowledge of the dramatic changes in the blood in normal pregnancy is required. These changes have special relevance to the most important and potentially hazardous haematological problems of pregnancy; namely, anaemia, thromboembolism and haemorrhage.

This chapter will be dealing with the first and most common of these problems—anaemia in pregnancy.

Blood volume

Although the 'plethora' of pregnancy was recognised early in the nineteenth century, and German work as far back as 1854 showed a rise of blood volume in pregnant laboratory animals, the evidence for plethora in pregnant women rested primarily on the demonstration of reduced concentration of solids and cells in the blood until the early twentieth century (Miller et al, 1915). The best estimate of total blood volume is obtained when plasma volume and red cell mass are measured simultaneously, but the majority of published reports of blood volume in pregnancy are based on either measured plasma volume or total red cell mass, the fraction not directly estimated being calculated from body haematocrit.

The plasma volume and total red cell mass are controlled by different mechanisms, and changes during pregnancy provide a dramatic illustration of this point.

Plasma volume

The measurement of plasma volume in pregnancy has a long history which was comprehensively reviewed by Hytten and Leitch in 1971 and more recently by Hytten 1985. Plasma volume rises progressively throughout pregnancy, with a tendency to plateau in the last 8 weeks (Pirani et al, 1973). The terminal fall in plasma volume, described by almost all investigators previously, occurs only when measurements are made in the supine position. The under-estimation in the supine position is due to the bulky uterus obstructing venous return from the lower limbs resulting in incomplete mixing of dye.

There is little doubt that the amount of increase in plasma volume is correlated with clinical performance and the birthweight of the baby. Since second and subsequent pregnancies tend to be more successful than the first, with bigger babies, a larger plasma volume increase in multigravidae would be expected, but the evidence is not entirely satisfactory. Women with multiple pregnancy have proportionately higher increments of plasma volume.

In contrast women with poorly growing fetuses, particularly multigravidae with a history of poor reproductive performance, have a correspondingly poor plasma response.

In summary, healthy women in a normal first pregnancy increase their plasma volume from a non-pregnant level of almost 2600 ml by about 1250 ml. Most of the rise takes place before 32–34 weeks gestation; thereafter there is relatively little change. In subsequent pregnancies the increase is greater. The increase is related to the size of the fetus and there are particularly large increases in association with multiple pregnancy.

The red cell mass in pregnancy

The red cell 'mass' is a confusing term which expresses the total volume of red cells in the circulation. The more logical alternative term 'red cell volume' cannot be used because of its specific meaning in haematology of the volume of a single erythrocyte.

There is less published information on red cell mass than plasma volume and the results are more variable.

There is still disagreement as to how much the red cell mass increases in normal pregnancy. The extent of the increase is considerably influenced by iron medication, which will cause the red cell mass to rise further in apparently healthy women with no clinical evidence of iron deficiency, but who on investigation prove to have depleted iron stores (see below).

A recent overview of the literature is to be found in Hytten (1985). If one accepts a figure of about 1400 ml for the volume of red cells in the average healthy woman before pregnancy, then in round figures the rise in pregnancy for women not given iron supplements is about 240 ml (18 per cent) and for those given iron 400 ml (30 per cent). The increase is probably higher from the end of the first trimester to term. As with plasma volume the extent of the increase is related to the size of the conceptus, particularly large increases being seen in association with multiple pregnancy (Letsky, 1980).

Changes in blood volume at parturition and during the puerperium

Dramatic changes in maternal blood volume occur at delivery whether per vaginem or by Caesarean section due to the acute blood loss. If the blood loss at vaginal delivery is meticulously measured it proves to be slightly more than 500 ml of blood associated with the delivery of one infant and almost 1000 ml on delivery of twins. Caesarean section is associated with an average loss of 1000 ml of whole blood.

The response of the mother to this acute blood loss differs from that of non-pregnant females, in whom a rapid blood loss precipitates an immediate drop in blood volume compensated for by vasoconstriction. Within a few days the blood volume expands to near-normal values because of an increase in plasma volume. This leads to a considerable fall in the haematocrit which is proportional to the amount of blood lost in the non parturient female.

In the normal pregnant female at term the hypervolaemia modifies the response to blood loss considerably. The blood volume drops following the acute loss at delivery but remains relatively stable unless the blood loss exceeds 25 per cent of the pre-delivery volume. There is no compensatory increase in blood volume and there is a gradual fall in plasma volume, due primarily to diuresis. The red cell mass increase during pregnancy not lost at delivery is slowly reduced as the red cells come to the end of their life-span. The overall result is that the haematocrit gradually increases and the blood volume returns to non-pregnant levels.

In the first few days following delivery there are fluctuations in plasma volume and haematocrit due to individual responses to dehydration, pregnancy hypervolaemia and the rapidity of blood loss. The average blood loss which can be tolerated without causing a significant fall in haemoglobin concentration is around 1000 ml, but this depends in turn on a healthy increase in blood volume prior to delivery. Almost all the blood loss occurs within the first hour following delivery under normal circumstances. In the following 72 hours only approximately 80 ml are lost per vaginem. Patients with uterine atony, extended episiotomy or lacerations will, of course, lose much more. If the haematocrit or haemoglobin concentration at 5–7 days post-delivery proves to be significantly less than pre-delivery levels, either there was pathological blood loss at delivery, or there was a poor increase in blood volume during pregnancy or both (Peck and Arias, 1979).

Benefits of hypervolaemia in pregnancy

The widely different responses in plasma volume and red cell mass should have a rational basis and make biological sense.

The hypervolaemia *per se* combats the hazard of haemorrhage for the mother at delivery, as illustrated above. It also protects the mother from hypotension in the last trimester when sequestration occurs in the lower extremities on standing, sitting or lying supine.

The red cell mass should increase in line with the need for extra oxygen. By the end of pregnancy the increase in requirement has been calculated to be around 15–16 per cent more than the average non-pregnant requirement (de Swiet, 1980) and is met adequately by an increase in red cell mass of 18–25 per cent.

The role of the much greater increase in plasma volume becomes clear when the distribution of the raised cardiac output is defined. Most of the extra circulation is directed to the skin and kidneys (de Swiet, 1980). Both serve as organs of excretion during pregnancy. The basal metabolic rate increases by about 20 per cent and the vastly increased blood flow in the skin allows for heat loss. There is also a decrease in viscosity which causes a decreased resistance to blood flow and a decrease in cardiac force required to maintain the circulation. This makes biological sense of what is often seen as a disproportionate increase in plasma volume.

Total haemoglobin

The haemoglobin concentration, haematocrit and red cell count, fall during pregnancy because the expansion of the plasma volume is greater than that of the red cell mass. Paradoxically there is, however, a rise in total circulating haemoglobin directly related to the increase in red cell mass. This in turn is dependent partly on the iron status of the individual. Published evidence for the rise in total haemoglobin is unsatisfactory and confused by the varying iron status of the women studied. It is impossible to give physiological limits for the expected rise in total haemoglobin until better figures are available, and controversies resolved.

The lowest normal haemoglobin in the healthy adult non-pregnant woman living at sea level is 12·0 g/dl (World Health Organisation, 1972).

In most published studies the mean minimum in pregnancy is between 11 and 12 g/dl. The lowest haemoglobin observed in a carefully studied iron supplemented group was 10·44 g/dl (de Leeuw et al, 1966). The mean minimum acceptable to the World Health Organisation is 11·0 g/dl. (World Health Organisation, 1972).

IRON METABOLISM IN PREGNANCY

The commonest haematological problem in pregnancy is anaemia resulting from iron deficiency. As this is such an important and frequent problem during the reproductive years in the female, a brief account of iron metabolism outside pregnancy and the physiological changes which occur to meet the demands of pregnancy and the puerperium is appropriate here.

The bulk of iron in the body is contained in the haemoglobin of circulating and developing red cells and iron exchange is both extremely limited and precisely regulated. The unique feature of iron balance in the human is that the iron content of the body is controlled largely by a limited variation in absorption and not by excretion. A normal mixed diet supplies about 14 mg of iron each day of which only 1–2 mg (5–10 per cent) is absorbed. Iron absorption is increased when iron stores are depleted, e.g. when there is a low ferritin level and a high concentration of unsaturated transferrin (see below) and also when there is erythroid hyperplasia with a rapid iron turnover.

It is during adolescence that the male and female begin to differ in terms of iron balance. Once growth is completed the male is in a comparatively favourable position requiring only 1 mg of iron a day to cover passive losses, the total body iron remaining relatively constant throughout adult life. The female requires another 0·5–1·0 mg per day to meet the requirements resulting from menstrual losses.

During pregnancy there is an average requirement of 4 mg per day, rising from 2·5 mg in early pregnancy to 6·6 mg per day in the last trimester. This demand arises from the increase in red cell mass and the requirements of the developing fetus and placenta. By far the greatest single demand for iron is that for the expansion of the red cell mass. The fetus derives its iron from the maternal serum by active transport across the placenta, mainly in the last 4 weeks of pregnancy. The total extra requirement of iron is of the order of 700–1400 µg. There is evidence that absorption of dietary iron is enhanced in the latter half of pregnancy, but the maximal daily absorption possible is approximately 3·5 mg per day for a *non-anaemic* individual with iron deficiency on an adequate diet, and a reasonable expectation would be an absorption of roughly 2·0 mg per day (Finch and Cook, 1984). It follows then that the daily iron requirements of pregnancy can only be met by maximal absorption of dietary iron and mobilisation of iron stores.

Absorption of dietary iron

In the past the value of a diet in terms of iron nutrition was assessed in terms of the iron content, but we now know that there is extreme variability in the availability of iron in various foods. There are two distinct pathways for iron absorption—one for inorganic and one for haem iron—which accounts for the difference in food iron availability. In most foods inorganic iron is in the 'ferric' form and has to be converted to the ferrous form before absorption can take place. In foods derived from grain, iron often forms a stable complex with phytates and only small amounts can be converted to a soluble form. The iron in eggs is poorly absorbed because of binding with phosphates present in the yolk. Milk, particularly cows' milk, is poor in iron content. Tea inhibits the absorption of iron.

Haem iron derived from the haemoglobin and myoglobin of animal origin is more effectively absorbed than non-haem iron. Factors interfering with or promoting the absorption of inorganic iron have no effect on the absorption of haem iron. Haem iron also promotes the absorption of inorganic iron. This puts vegetarians at a disadvantage in terms of iron sufficiency.

Populations from the underdeveloped parts of the world subsist largely on non-haem iron and its poor availability in the absence of reducing agents or augmentors such as meat goes a long way to explain the world-wide prevalence of iron deficiency with the highest incidence in the third world.

The amount of iron absorbed will depend very much on the extent of iron stores, the content of the diet and whether or not iron supplements are given.

It was found that absorption rates differed markedly, in a carefully controlled study in Sweden (Svanberg, 1975), between those pregnant women receiving 100 mg ferrous iron supplements daily and those receiving a placebo. Iron absorption increased steadily throughout pregnancy in the placebo group. In the supplemented group there was no increase between the 12th and 24th week of gestation and thereafter the increase was only 60 per cent of the placebo group. After delivery the mean absorption in the placebo group was markedly higher. These differences can be explained by the difference in storage iron between the two groups (Svanberg, 1975).

Many women enter pregnancy with already low or depleted iron stores because of demands of previous pregnancies and menstrual losses. They will not be anaemic at this stage, a fall in haemoglobin concentration being a late manifestation of iron depletion, but they will be at risk of developing quite severe anaemia and other metabolic defects of iron deficiency as pregnancy progresses (see below).

Over the years there have been many studies which have proved without doubt that iron supplements prevent the development of anaemia (Lund, 1951; Magee & Milligan, 1951; Gatenby, 1956; Morgan, 1961; Chanarin et al, 1965; Chisholm, 1966) and that in women on a good diet who are not apparently anaemic at booking, the mean haemoglobin level can be raised by oral iron therapy throughout pregnancy. The difference in favour of those so treated is most marked at term when the need for adequate haemoglobin is maximal (Morgan, 1961; de Leeuw et al, 1966; Fenton et al, 1977; Taylor et al, 1982).

Non-haematological effects of iron deficiency

Overt symptoms of iron deficiency are generally not prominent. Defects in oxygen-carrying capacity are compensated for but the health implications of iron deficiency have recently been examined in a more detailed manner. Of particular interest are effects produced by impairment of the function of iron-dependent tissue enzymes. These are not the ultimate manifestation of severe untreated iron deficiency, but develop hand in hand with the fall in haemoglobin concentration.

It has been possible to demonstrate a marked decrease in work capacity in the iron-depleted, but non-anaemic rat, due to impaired mitochondrial function. There is also an impairment in temperature maintenance which has also been shown in human subjects. Studies have suggested behavioural abnormalities in children with iron deficiency related to changes in concentration of chemical mediators in the brain. Iron deficiency in the absence of anaemia is also associated with poor performance on the Bayley Mental Development Index, and this performance can be corrected by the administration of iron (Oski, 1985).

Progress is being made in defining the biochemical abnormalities produced by iron deficiency in the central nervous system. In training we have all been taught that parenteral treatment of megaloblastic anaemia with appropriate haematinics, either folic acid or vitamin B_{12}, results in an immediate subjective feeling of improvement and well-being in the patient long before the haemoglobin starts to rise. This is because of the non-haematologic effects of depletion of these vitamins on various tissues. A similar immediate subjective feeling of well-being is experienced by those few patients under my care who have received a total dose infusion of iron, presumably for similar reasons (Letsky, personal observations). Tissue enzyme malfunction undoubtedly occurs even in the very first stages of iron deficiency and it is obvious that the prevention of nutritional iron deficiency is a desirable objective, especially at times of maximal stress on the haemopoietic system such as during pregnancy.

Diagnosis of iron deficiency in pregnancy

Haemoglobin

A reduction in concentration of circulating haemoglobin is a relatively late development in iron deficiency. This is preceded by a depletion of iron stores and then a reduction in serum iron before there is any detectable change in haemoglobin level. However, this is the simplest non-invasive practical test at our disposal and is the one investigation on which further action is usually taken.

The changes in blood volume and haemodilution are so variable that the normal range of haemoglobin concentration in healthy pregnancy at 30 weeks gestation in women who have received parenteral iron is from 10·0–14·5 g/dl. However, haemoglobin values of less than 10·5 g/dl in the second and third trimesters are probably abnormal and require further investigation.

Red cell indices

The appearance of red cells on a stained film is a relatively insensitive gauge of iron status in pregnancy. Most hospital laboratories now possess electronic counters, using which accurate red cell counts can be performed.

The size of the red cell (MCV), its haemoglobin content (MCH) and haemoglobin concentration (MCHC) can be calculated from the red cell

Table 2.1   Red cell indices in thalassaemia and iron deficiency

		Normal range	Iron deficiency	Thalassaemia
PCV RBC	MCV	75–99 fl	Reduced	Very reduced
Hb RBC	MCH	27–31 pg	Reduced	Very reduced
Hb PCV	MCHC	32–36 g/dl	Reduced	Normal or slightly reduced

PCV: packed cell volume; RBC: red cell count; Hb: haemoglobin; MCV: mean corpuscular volume; MCH: mean corpuscular haemoglobin; MCHC: mean corpuscular haemoglobin concentration

count (RBC), haemoglobin concentration and packed cell volume (PCV) (Table 2.1). A better guide to the diagnosis of iron deficiency in pregnancy is the examination of these red cell indices.

The earliest effect of iron deficiency on the erythrocyte is a reduction in cell size MCV, and in pregnancy with the dramatic changes in red cell mass and plasma volume this appears to be the most sensitive indicator of underlying iron deficiency. Hypochromia and a fall in MCHC only appear with more severe degrees of iron depletion.

Of course some women enter pregnancy with already established anaemia due to iron deficiency, or with grossly depleted iron stores, and they will quickly develop florid anaemia with reduced MCV, MCH and MCHC. These do not present any problems in diagnosis. It is those women who enter pregnancy in precarious iron balance with a normal haemoglobin who present the most difficult diagnostic problems.

The recognition of iron deficiency before a drop in haemoglobin or an effect on indices depends on three non-invasive laboratory tests.

1. Ferritin

This is a high molecular weight glycoprotein which circulates in the plasma of healthy adult females in the range of 15–300 μg/l (Jacobs et al, 1972). A level of 12 μg/l or below is taken to indicate iron deficiency. Ferritin is stable and not affected by recent ingestion of iron, and appears to reflect the iron stores accurately and quantitatively in the absence of inflammation, particularly in the lower range associated with iron deficiency which is so important in pregnancy. In the development of iron deficiency a low serum ferritin is the first abnormal laboratory test.

Serum ferritin is estimated by a sensitive immunoradiometric assay. Not all hospital laboratories can offer this service and if the Supraregional Assay Service is used there is a delay in obtaining results. A number of commercial kits have now become available which will facilitate the test being done on site, but they are still rather expensive. Even if there is a delay in obtaining the result, it is valuable to have an accurate assessment of iron stores before therapy is started.

2. Serum iron and total iron binding capacity (TIBC)

The second measurement is that of serum iron together with the TIBC from which the transferrin saturation can be estimated. A reduced transferrin saturation indicates a deficient iron supply to the tissues and this is the second measurement to be affected in the development of iron deficiency.

At this stage erythropoiesis is impaired and there is an adverse effect on iron-dependent tissue enzymes.

In health the serum iron of adult non-pregnant women lies between 13 and 27 µmol/l. It shows immense individual diurnal variation and fluctuates even from hour to hour. The total iron binding capacity (TIBC) in the non-pregnant state lies in the range of 45–72 µmol/l. It is raised in association with iron deficiency and found to be low in chronic inflammatory states. It is raised in pregnancy because of the increase in plasma volume. In the non-anaemic individual the TIBC is approximately one-third saturated with iron.

In pregnancy most workers report a fall in the serum iron and percentage saturation of the total iron binding capacity; the fall in serum iron can be largely prevented by iron supplements. Serum iron even in combination with TIBC is not a reliable indication of iron stores because it fluctuates widely and is affected by recent ingestion of iron and other factors such an infection not directly involved with iron metabolism. With these reservations a serum iron of less than 12 µmol/l and a TIBC saturation of less than 15 per cent indicate deficiency of iron during pregnancy.

3. Free erythrocyte protoporphyrin (FEP)

This is the third estimation of iron status. Erythroblast protoporphyrin represents the substrate unused for haem synthesis and levels rise when there is defective iron supply to the developing red cell. This test takes 2–3 weeks to become abnormal once iron stores are depleted. Estimation may be of value in patients recently treated with iron because there is also a delay in values returning to normal. However the use of this estimation is limited in that a misleading rise in FEP levels is observed in patients with chronic inflammatory disease, malignancy or infection.

In ideal circumstances these three measurements, together with the haemoglobin concentration, allow classification of iron-deficient individuals—those with depleted stores (decreased ferritin only), those with severe iron deficiency but as yet no anaemia (decreased ferritin and reduced TIBC saturation plus an increased FEP), and those with anaemia due to iron deficiency (reduced haemoglobin concentration and iron-deficient indices in addition to decreased ferritin, reduced TIBC saturation and increased FEP).

Marrow iron

The most rapid and reliable method of assessing iron stores in pregnancy is be examination of an appropriately stained preparation of a bone marrow sample. If properly performed, marrow aspiration need not result in any major discomfort. In skilful hands the procedure takes no more than 10 minutes. The iliac crest (anterior or posterior) as the aspiration site should always be used in preference to the sternum, for the benefit and comfort of the patient. In the absence of iron supplementation there is no detectable stainable iron in over 80 per cent of women at term (de Leeuw et al, 1966). No stainable iron (haemosiderin) may be visible once the serum ferritin has fallen to below 40 μg/l, but other stigmata of iron deficiency in the developing erythroblasts, particularly the late normablasts, will confirm that the anaemia is indeed due to iron deficiency in the absence of stainable iron. The effects of frequently accompanying folate deficiency will also be apparent (see below). A block of incorporation of iron into haemoglobin occurs in the course of chronic inflammation, particularly of the urinary tract, even if iron stores are replete. This problem will be revealed by examination of the marrow aspirate stained for iron.

Management of iron deficiency anaemia

Established iron deficiency

The management of iron deficiency anaemia diagnosed late in pregnancy presents a particular challenge to the obstetrician because a satisfactory response has to be obtained in a limited space of time. It is assumed that the woman has had inadequate antenatal care and failed to take oral supplements. Iron sorbitol citrate can be given as a series of intramuscular injections, but it is associated with toxic reactions such as headache, nausea and vomiting if given simultaneously with oral iron (Scott, 1963). Iron dextrans (Imferon) is an extensively used preparation which can be administered as a series of intramuscular injections or as a total dose infusion, which is the preferred method. Rare anaphylactic reactions do occur in the case of intravenous infusions, but usually during the period when the first few millimetres are being given (Clay et al, 1965). For this reason infusion should always be started slowly and the patient watched carefully for the first few minutes. This preparation does not appear to be associated with toxicity if given simultaneously with oral iron (Scott, 1962).

In the absence of any other abnormality an increase in haemoglobin of 0·8 g/dl per week (1·0 g/dl in the non-pregnant female) can be reasonably expected with adequate treatment. The response is similar whether iron is given orally or parenterally (see below). If there is not enough time to achieve a reasonable haemoglobin for delivery then transfusion with all its hazards is indicated. It is obvious that it would be desirable to avoid this situation, which was not unusual in the United Kingdom in the not-so-distant past.

Prophylaxis

More economical in the long run in terms of investigation and treatment are measures that will prevent the development of severe anaemia.

Supplementation involves the administration of iron salts to those individuals whose physiological needs are greatest. A significant number of women, even in developed countries, have iron stores which are inadequate to meet the requirements of the last trimester. Relatively small supplements of 20–30 mg daily taken between meals are required to prevent iron deficiency in this setting. The amount of iron required may have been overestimated (see below) because iron in multicomponent preparations is often poorly absorbed (Finch and Cook, 1985).

In the United Kingdom the management of iron deficiency in pregnancy has largely become prevention by daily oral supplements. Oral supplementation of 60–80 mg elemental iron per day from early pregnancy maintains the haemoglobin in the recognised normal range for pregnancy but does not maintain or restore the iron stores (Fleming et al, 1974a; de Leeuw et al, 1968). The World Health Organisation (1972) recommends that supplements of 30–60 mg per day be given to those pregnant women with iron stores, and 120–240 mg to those women with none. Whether all pregnant women need iron is controversial, but if it is accepted that iron is necessary a bewildering number of preparations of varying expense are available for use. In those women to whom additional iron cannot be given by the oral route, either because of non-compliance or because of unacceptable side effects, intramuscular injection or iron, 1000 mg, more than assures iron sufficiency for that pregnancy. The injections are painful and can be skin-staining, but there is no extra risk of incurring malignancy at the injection site as once reported.

There is no haematological benefit in giving parenteral as opposed to oral iron, but the failure rate of some women to take oral preparations is high and the sole advantage is that you can be sure they have received adequate supplementation.

The side-effects of oral administration of iron have been shown to be related to the quantity administered (Hallberg et al, 1966). If the daily dose is reduced to 100 mg and introduction is delayed until the 16th week of gestation, they are rare with any preparation. Although some women do have gastric symptoms the most common complaint is constipation, which is usually easily overcome by simple basic measures. Slow-release preparations, which are on the whole more expensive, are said to be relatively free of side-effects. This is because much of the iron is not released at all, is unabsorbed and excreted unchanged. This means that double doses may have to be given to cover requirements, thereby further increasing expense.

The majority of women tolerate the cheaper preparations with no significant side-effects and in the interests of economy these should be tried first.

All of the preparations used in pregnancy routinely are combined now with an appropriate dose of folic acid (see below).

ARE IRON SUPPLEMENTS DURING PREGNANCY NECESSARY?

There is still considerable controversy about whether all women need iron supplements during pregnancy. Many authors are not able to accept that the physiological requirements for iron in pregnancy are considerably higher than the usual intake of most healthy women with apparently good diets in industrial countries. The arguments about policy among nutritionists wishing to prevent iron deficiency are complicated by the varying problems of applying strategies in countries at different stages of development. The greatest experience in prevention comes from those countries where iron deficiency is least common and least severe (Jacobs and Worwood, 1982).

There is no doubt that in the poorly developed countries, or in underpriveleged populations, the incidence of anaemia and iron deficiency is high, and many women enter pregnancy either anaemic or with grossly depleted iron stores. A small but careful study of anaemia in pregnancy from Nigeria (Ogunbode et al, 1979) showed that by having partially solved the problem of the conditions thought to be primarily responsible, malaria and haemoglobinopathies, by giving antimalarials and folic acid routinely throughout pregnancy, iron deficiency was also present in many of the patients with pregnancy anaemia. The conclusion here was that the deficiency was primarily from poor iron content in the diet, and routine iron supplementation was recommended. Another larger controlled trial from the Phillipines (Kuizon et al, 1979) showed clearly that those women with normal haemoglobins given iron throughout pregnancy maintained their haemoglobin, and that anaemic women on a larger dose raised their haemoglobins compared to those taking placebo or ascorbic acid alone.

One of the earliest large studies in this country (Magee & Milligan, 1951) comes from Manchester. Over 2000 women were studied during pregnancy. In those not taking iron a progressive drop in the haemoglobin was observed—the lowest level being reached at 32 weeks gestation—but it took more than a year postpartum before prepregnancy haemoglobin was returned to. Those women taking iron had consistently higher haemoglobins and the effects persisted into the postnatal period—prepregnancy haemoglobin levels being much more rapidly achieved.

However there was no advantage in terms of subjective health conferred by iron treatment in this study or another double-blind study (Paintin et al, 1966) in Aberdeen.

Fairly recently Hemminki & Starfield (1978) reviewed controlled clinical trials of iron administration during pregnancy in developed western countries. Seventeen trials were found which fulfilled their stated criteria. As a result of their analysis they concluded that there was no beneficial effect in terms of birthweight, length of gestation, maternal and infant morbidity and mortality in those women receiving iron compared with controls. They maintain that while age, economic status and poor nutrition affect the outcome, pregnancy anaemia is not related, and is simply associated with other risk factors. They did not take into account the withdrawal of anaemic patients from the trials they reviewed. In statistical terms their analysis may be true, but anaemia remains a potential danger in pregnancy especially in the face of haemorrhage. The majority of women who do not receive iron supplements have no stores at all at the end of pregnancy (Fenton et al, 1977; de Leeuw et al, 1966). Also offspring of non-anaemic women who have not received supplements have lower iron stores than those of iron-replete women (Fenton et al, 1977).

The observations that oral iron supplements may reduce the bioavailability of zinc (Meadows et al, 1983) and maternal zinc levels during pregnancy (Hambridge et al, 1983) has led to speculation about the relationship of these observations and the fact that there have been reports suggesting that maternal tissue zinc depletion is associated with fetal growth retardation (Meadows et al, 1981). The results of a recent study of serial changes in serum zinc and magnesium concentrations before conception, throughout pregnancy to 12 weeks postpartum, indicates that the decrease in concentrations of both elements is a normal physiological adjustment to pregnancy and that oral iron supplementation does not influence these changes (Sheldon et al, 1985).

An analysis of factors leading to a reduction in iron deficiency in Swedish women of childbearing age (Hallberg et al, 1979) in a 10-year period 1965–75 attributed this 20–25 per cent improvement to greater prescribing of iron tablets (10 per cent) and fortification of food (7–8 per cent); oral contraception also played a part (2–3 per cent).

Svanberg (1975) comments that the suggestion that absence of iron stores in women of fertile age is to be considered as physiological and that the increased iron demand during pregnancy may be met by increased absorption, is not borne out by very careful studies. The conclusion is that even with maximum iron content in the diet the immediate demands of pregnancy cannot be covered by an increased absorption from the diet.

From what evidence is available it would appear that a high proportion of women in reproductive years do lack storage iron (Fenton et al, 1977; de Leeuw et al, 1966). The reasons may be different in different populations. Over thousands of years the human race has changed its way of living and eating, from a society based on hunting and fishing to the present one with a lower intake of iron and a lower intake of meat and fish (Finch & Huebers, 1982). Recent dietary changes in industrialised countries have made it difficult for women to build up iron stores so that iron balance can be maintained in pregnancy.

A more recent study from South Africa (Mayet, 1985) reports the findings on Indian and black women attending an antenatal clinic. Anaemia, by WHO standards, was found in 13·2 per cent of the Asian women in the first trimester, increasing to 28·19 per cent and 47·0 per cent in the second and third trimesters respectively, but iron deficiency (serum ferritin less than 12 μg/l) was found to be far greater, i.e. 35 per cent in the first trimester rising to 86 per cent in the third.

The pregnant black women underwent similar investigations. Anaemia was detected in 18.8 per cent rising to 28.6 per cent. However the proportion with iron deficiency was not so dramatically increased as in the Asian counterparts—19 per cent rising to 40 per cent in the last trimester. This probably reflects the greater number of vegetarians among the Asian populations who therefore will not have sufficient reserves of storage iron to meet the needs of pregnancy.

It has been suggested that women at risk from iron deficiency anaemia could be identified by estimating the serum ferritin concentration in the first trimester. A serum ferritin of less than 50μg/l in early pregnancy is an indication for daily iron supplements. Women with serum ferritin concentrations of greater than 80 μg/l are unlikely to require iron supplements. Unnecessary routine supplementation would thus be avoided in women enjoying good nutrition, and any risk to the pregnancy arising from severe maternal anaemia would be avoided by prophylaxis and prompt treatment (Bentley, 1985).

A recent investigation at Queen Charlotte's Maternity Hospital, London, is of interest in this respect. Serum ferritin levels were estimated in 669 consecutive women who booked at 16 weeks gestation or earlier with a haemoglobin concentration of 11·0 g/dl or above. 552 women (82·5 per cent) had serum ferritins of 50 μg/l or below, and would therefore qualify for routine daily iron supplements by the above criteria. These women are drawn from a cosmopolitan, largely well-nourished population; 12 per cent had serum ferritins of less than 12 μg/l and were already iron deficient at booking in spite of having a haemoglobin of 11 g/dl or more. Only 51 (7·6 per cent) had ferritins of 80 μg/l or above (Letsky, 1985, unpublished data).

In summary, negative iron balance throughout pregnancy, particularly in the latter half, may lead to iron deficiency anaemia in the third trimester. This hazard—together with the increasing evidence of non-haematological effects of iron deficiency on exercise tolerance, cerebral function and temperature control—leads me to the conclusion that it is safer; more practical; and in the long term less expensive in terms of investigation, hospital admission and treatment, to give all women iron supplements from 16 weeks gestation—especially as this would appear to do no harm (Kullander & Kallen, 1976; Sheldon et al, 1985).

FOLATE METABOLISM IN PREGNANCY

Folic acid, together with iron, has assumed a central role in the nutrition of pregnancy.

At a cellular level folic acid is reduced first to dihydrofolic acid (DHF) and then to tetrahydrofolic acid (THF) which forms the cornerstone of cellular folate metabolism. It is fundamental through linkage with L-carbon fragments both to cell growth and cell division. The more active a tissue is in reproduction and growth, the more dependent it will be on the efficient turnover and supply of folate co-enzymes. Bone marrow and epithelial linings are therefore particularly at risk.

Requirements for folate are increased in pregnancy, to meet the needs of the fetus, the placenta, uterine hypertrophy and the expanded maternal red cell mass. The placenta transports folate actively to the fetus even in the face of maternal deficiency, but maternal folate metabolism is altered early in pregnancy like many other maternal functions, before fetal demands act directly.

Investigations in pregnancy

Plasma folate

With the exception of haemoglobin concentration and plasma iron, folic acid must be one of the most studied substances in maternal blood, but there are comparatively few serial data available. It is generally agreed, however, that plasma folates fall as pregnancy advances so that at term they are about half the non-pregnant values (Ball & Giles, 1964; Chanarin, 1979; Fleming et al, 1974b; Landon, 1975).

Plasma clearance of folate by the kidneys is more than doubled as early as the 8th week of gestation (Fleming, 1972; Landon and Hytten, 1971). It has been suggested that urinary loss may be a major factor in the fall of serum folate. The glomerular filtration rate is raised and the marked contrast between the comparatively unchanging plasma levels and the wide variation in urinary loss suggest a change in tubular reabsorption, rather than some alteration in folate metabolism. It is unlikely that this is a major drain on maternal resources and it cannot play more than a marginal role (Landon, 1975).

There have been conflicting reports about the part intestinal malabsorption may play in the aetiology of folate deficiency of pregnancy. Traditionally absorption has been assessed from plasma levels following an oral load. Earlier reports of decreased absorption (Chanarin et al, 1959) were probably due to the underestimation of the rapid clearance of folate following an oral dose. Placenta and maternal tissues contribute from an early stage, probably under the influence of oestrogens, as oral contraceptives also increase plasma clearance of folate (Stephens et al, 1972). There is no change in absorption of either folate monoglutamates in healthy pregnancy (Landon and Hytten,

1972; McLean et al, 1970). There is invariably a wide scatter of results. The incidence of abnormally low serum folates in late pregnancy varies with the population studied and presumably, like iron, reflects the local nutritional standards.

Substantial day-to-day variations of plasma folate are possible and postprandial increases have been noted; this will limit its diagnostic value when an occasional sample taken at a casual antenatal clinic visit is considered.

Red cell folate

The estimation of red cell folate may provide more useful information as it does not reflect daily or other short-term variations in plasma folate levels. It is thought to give a better indication of overall body tissue levels, but the turnover of red blood cells is slow and there will be a delay before significant reductions in the folate concentrations of the red cells, due to folate deficiency, are evident.

A number of investigations of erythrocyte folate in pregnancy have shown a slight downward trend even though, as would be expected, the fall is not so marked as that noted for plasma (Avery & Ledger, 1970; Chanarin et al, 1968). There is evidence that patients who have a low red cell folate at the beginning of pregnancy develop megaloblastic anaemia in the third trimester (Chanarin et al, 1968).

Excretion of formiminoglutamic acid (FIGLU)

A loading dose of histidine leads to increased FIGLU excretion in the urine when there is folate deficiency. As a test for folate deficiency in pregnancy it no longer has much to recommend it, primarily because the metabolism of histidine is altered (Chanarin, 1979) and this results in increased FIGLU excretion in normal early pregnancy (Stone et al, 1967).

Postpartum events. In the 6 weeks following delivery there is a tendency for all the parameters discussed to return to non-pregnant values. However, should any deficiency of folate have developed and remained untreated in pregnancy it may present clinically for the first time in the puerperium and its consequences may be detected for many months after delivery. Lactation provides an added folate stress. A folate content of 5 µg per 100 ml of human milk and a yield of 500 ml daily implies a loss of 25 µg folate daily in breast milk. In the Bantu, megaloblastic anaemia appears frequently in the year following pregnancy in association with lactation. Dietary folate intake is poor and it has been shown (Shapiro et al, 1965) that folate deficiency becomes more apparent, as demonstrated by using FIGLU excretion, as lactation continues. Red cell folate levels in lactating mothers are significantly lower than that of their infant during the first year of life (Chanarin, 1979). In this country, as early as 1919, Osler described the severe anaemias of pregnancy with a high colour index and a striking incidence in the postpartum period.

Interpretation of investigations during pregnancy

The value of these various investigations in predicting megaloblastic anaemia and assessing subclinical folate deficiency has been the subject of numerous reports. Using these various test folate 'deficiency' is pregnancy is not invariably accompanied by any significant haematological change (Shapiro et al, 1965; Stone et al, 1967).

In the absence of any changes megaloblastic haemopoiesis should be suspected when the expected response to adequate iron therapy is not achieved. Evidence of megaloblastic haemopoiesis may become apparent only after iron therapy even though the rise in haemoglobin concentration appears adequate. No help can be expected from the use of tests of folate status. Usually abnormal results are obtained with most of the tests but these are not significantly different from results in healthy pregnant women.

The decline of serum folic acid levels from a mean of 6·0 μg/l in the non-pregnant to 3·4 μg/l at term, should be viewed as the physiological consequence of maternal tissue uptake, urinary loss and placental transfer. It is incorrect to talk of levels below 'normal' in pregnancy when below non-pregnant levels are meant.

It could be argued that the changes noted in pregnancy may be positively advantageous. There is no logical reason why reduced plasma levels of nutrients such as folate should indicate deficiency, while others such as glucose and amino acids are disregarded. The reduced levels may aid conservation in the face of a raised glomerular filtration rate. It is possible that the placenta may be able to compete more effectively with maternal tissues for folate supplies at lower maternal plasma levels and compensate for its relatively small receptive area (Landon, 1975).

The delay in fall of red cell folate makes it an impractical test for folate deficiency in pregnancy.

Blood changes

The blood picture is complex and may be difficult to interpret. There is a physiological increase in red cell size in healthy iron-replete pregnancy. The MCV rises on average by 4 fl but may be as much as 20 fl. This increase in red cell size is not prevented by folate supplements.

The physiological macrocytosis may be masked by the effects of iron deficiency which results in the production of small red cells (see above). Outside pregnancy the hallmark of megaloblastic haemopoiesis is macrocytosis, first identified in routine laboratory investigations by a raised MCV. In pregnancy macrocytosis by non-pregnant standards is the norm and in any event may be masked by iron deficiency. Examination of the blood film may be more helpful. There may be occasional oval macrocytes in a sea of iron-deficient microcytic cells. Hypersegmentation of the neutrophil polymorph nucleus is significant because in normal pregnancy there is a shift to the left. If more than five of 100 neutrophils have five or more lobes, hypersegmentation is present, but hypersegmentation is observed in pure iron deficiency, uncomplicated by folate deficiency.

The diagnosis of folate deficiency in pregnancy has to be made ultimately on morphological grounds and usually involves examination of a suitably prepared marrow aspirate (Chanarin, 1985).

MEGALOBLASTIC ANAEMIA AND PREGNANCY

The cause of megaloblastic anaemia in pregnancy is nearly always folate deficiency. Vitamin B_{12} is only very rarely implicated. A survey of reports from the United Kingdom over the past two decades suggest an incidence ranging from 0·2 per cent to 5·0 per cent, but a considerably greater number of women have megaloblastic changes in their marrow which are not suspected on examination of the peripheral blood only (Lowenstein et al, 1966; Chanarin, 1979). The incidence of megaloblastic anaemia in other parts of the world is considerably greater and is thought to reflect the nutritional standards of the population. Several workers have pointed to the poor socio-economic status of their patients as the major aetiological factor contributing to the anaemia (Coyle & Geoghegan, 1962; Chanarin, 1979), which may be further exacerbated by seasonal changes in the availability of staple foodstuffs. Food folates are only partially available and the amount of folate supplied in the diet is difficult to quantify. In Great Britain analysis of daily folate intake in foodstuffs showed a range of 129–300 µg (Chanarin, 1975). The folate content of 24-hour food collections in various studies in Sweden and Canada proved to be round about 200 µg on average, with a range as large as 70 µg to 600 mg (Chanarin, 1979).

Foods that are very rich in folate include broccoli, spinach and brussel sprouts, but up to 90 per cent of their folate content is lost within the first few minutes, by boiling or steaming. These vegetables are unlikely to be eaten raw. Dietary folate deficiency megaloblastic anaemia occurs in about one-third of all pregnant women in the world, despite the fact that folate is found in nearly all natural foods, because folate is rapidly destroyed by cooking, especially in finely divided foods such as beans and rice (Herbert, 1985). Asparagus, avocados, mushrooms and bananas also have a fairly high folate content, which may delight social class I patients in the United Kingdom, but will not help the average working-class mother to improve her dietary intake. Natural folates are protected from oxidation and degradation by the presence of reducing substances such as ascorbate. The analysis of folate content of food will give very low results if ascorbate is not added to the assay system—as evident in the very earliest studies (Chanarin, 1979). Having established the content of folate in foodstuffs there is only indirect evidence about its absorption. Monoglutamates are almost completely absorbed. Polyglutamates from different sources are variable available, but in general are less well absorbed, so that total folate intake should be combined with information about the source of food folate to give a realistic appraisal of the available folate content. In general, dietary intake is likely to be greater, rather than smaller, during pregnancy but obviously in certain areas of the world malnutrition is an essential aetiological factor in determining folate status.

The effects of dietary inadequacy may be further amplified by frequent childbirth and multiple pregnancy. Several reports have shown a markedly increased incidence of megaloblastic anaemia in multiple pregnancy. An incidence of 1 in 11 in twin pregnancies compared with the expected incidence of 1 in 80 was noted in one survey of over 1000 patients (Chanarin, 1979).

The normal dietary folate intake is inadequate to prevent megaloblastic changes in the bone marrow in approximately 25 per cent of pregnant women. The fall in serum and red cell folate could be a physiological phenomenon in pregnancy but the incidence of megaloblastic change in the bone marrow is reduced only when the blood folate levels are maintained in a steady state by adequate oral supplements. There is much controversy at the moment about the requirement for folate, particularly during pregnancy. World Health Organisation recommendations for daily folate intake are as high as 800 μg in the antenatal period and 600 μg during lactation, and 400 μg in the non-pregnant adult (WHO 1972).

There is an increased need for about 100 μg folic acid daily during pregnancy which, without supplements, must be found from natural folates in the diet (Chanarin, 1979). The WHO recommended intakes clearly over-estimate the needs and the Dunn Nutrition Unit has been asked to investigate these questions. The daily amount of folate that has been given prophylactically in pregnancy varies from 30 μg to 500 μg and even pharmacological doses of 5–15 mg (Chanarin, 1979), 30 μg daily, was found to be too small to influence folate status appreciably (Chanarin et al, 1965) but supplements of 100 μg or more all reduced the frequency of megaloblastic changes in the marrow and eliminated megaloblastic changes in the marrow and eliminated megaloblastic anaemia as a clinical entity (Chanarin, 1979).

In order to meet the folate needs of those women with a dietary intake well below average the daily supplement during pregnancy should be of the order of 200–300 μg daily—still very much below the WHO's recommended daily intake.

THE FETUS AND FOLATE DEFICIENCY

There is an increased risk of megaloblastic anaemia occurring in the neonate of a folate-deficient mother, especially if delivery is pre-term.

The young infant's requirement for folate has been estimated at 20–50 μg/

day (4–10 times the adult requirement) on a weight basis. Serum and red cell folates are consistently higher in cord than in maternal blood, but the premature infant is in severe negative folate balance because of high growth rate and reduced intake. The usual fall in serum and red cell folate in the term neonate is yet greater in the premature neonate and even in the absence of other complicating factors may result in megaloblastic anaemia. This can be prevented by giving supplements of 50 μg/day (Haworth & Evans, 1981; Oski, 1979).

Exciting, initial clinical investigations have suggested an association between periconceptional folic acid deficiency and harelip, cleft palate and, most important of all, neural tube defects (Smithells et al, 1980; Laurence et al, 1981; Smithells et al, 1983).

The association between folate deficiency and neural tube defects awaits confirmation in a mass multi-centre controlled trial of *pre*-pregnancy folate supplementation in susceptible women. This subject has been well reviewed (Elwood, 1983).

Prophylaxis of folate deficiency in uncomplicated pregnancy

The case for giving prophylactic folate supplements throughout pregnancy is a strong one (Giles, 1966; Chanarin, 1979) and an example of excellent preventative medicine (Chanarin, 1985), particularly in countries where overt megaloblastic anaemia is frequent.

The main point at issue over recent years, however, is whether the apparently intrinsic folate deficiency of pregnancy can predispose the mother to a wide variety of obstetric abnormalities and complications, in particular abortion, fetal deformity, prematurity and antepartum haemorrhage. The extensive literature would appear to be almost equally divided in its opinion, but there is no evidence that the routine use of folic acid supplements *during*, not before, pregnancy has reduced the incidence of anything but megaloblastic anaemia (Chanarin, 1979) except in cases of malnutrition where an increase in birthweight has been noted (Baumslag et al, 1970; Iyengar, 1971). The amount of folate needed to maintain the red cell folate levels in a well-nourished population is about 100 μg daily, but in order to meet the needs of all women, including those with poor dietary intake, the supplement needs to be of the order of 200–300 μg pteroylglutamic acid daily. This should be given in combination with iron supplements (see above) and there are several suitable combined preparations available (Chanarin, 1985).

The risk of adverse effects from folate supplements in a pregnant woman suffering from B_{12} deficiency is very small (see below). Patients with that degree of B_{12} deficiency are usually infertile and pernicious anaemia is generally a disease of older people. More important than this, there is not one report of subacute combined degeneration of the spinal cord occurring among the thousands of women who have received folate supplements during pregnancy. 'It is a hypothetical situation which should not detract from the vast benefit provided by routine use of folate supplements in pregnancy' (Chanarin, 1985).

Management of established folate deficiency

Severe megaloblastic anaemia is now uncommon in the United Kingdom, largely as a result of prophylaxis and prompt treatment.

Once megaloblastic haematopoiesis is established treatment of folic acid deficiency becomes more difficult, presumably due to megaloblastic changes in the gastro-intestinal tract resulting in impaired absorption. Treatment initially, if the diagnosis is made in the antenatal period, should be pteroylglutamic acid 5 mg daily, continued for several weeks after delivery or for 4 weeks for those women diagnosed in the puerperium. If there is no response to this therapy parenteral folic acid can be tried. There are a small number of patients who fail to respond to parenteral folate therapy (Giles, 1966) and recover in the puerperium. It is far better to intervene before these difficulties arise and give routine propylaxis throughout pregnancy.

Pregnancy, anticonvulsants and folic acid

Folate status is even further compromised in pregnancy if a woman is on anticonvulsants, in particular phenytoin and phenobarbitone. Although earlier studies suggested that the control of epilepsy became more difficult in pregnancy with folate supplements approaching $5 \cdot 0$ mg daily (Reynolds, 1973), more recent studies with supplements between 100 and 1000 µg daily have not substantiated these findings (Hiilesmaa et al, 1983).

It would appear that the risk of interfering with the control of epilepsy by regular iron/folate supplements during pregnancy have been over-emphasised.

Anticonvulsant therapy is associated with an increased incidence of congenital abnormality, prematurity and low birthweight, therefore folate supplements should, in my opinion, be given to all epileptic women taking anticonvulsants.

Control of epilepsy in pregnancy remains controversial but the best approach would appear to be to try to continue the non-pregnant control regime using one drug alone, monitor blood levels and keep the anti-convulsant at the lowest effective level, and to give appropriate folate supplementation.

Disorders which may affect folate requirement in pregnancy

Problems may be caused in pregnancy by disorders which are associated with an increased folate requirement in the non-pregnant state. Women with haemolytic anaemia, particularly hereditary haemolytic conditions such as haemoglobinopathies and hereditary spherocytosis, require extra supplements from early pregnancy if development of megaloblastic anaemia is to be avoided. The recommended supplement in this situation is 5–10 mg orally daily. The anaemia associated with thalassaemia trait is not strictly due to haemolysis but due to ineffective erythropoiesis (see below). However the increased, though abortive, marrow turnover still results in folate depletion and such women would probably benefit from the routine administration of oral folic acid 5·0 mg daily from early pregnancy.

Folate supplements are of particular importance in the management of sickle cell syndromes during pregnancy if aplastic crises and megaloblastic anaemia are to be avoided.

VITAMIN B_{12} IN PREGNANCY

Muscle, red cell and serum vitamin B_{12} concentrations fall during pregnancy (Ball & Giles, 1964; Chanarin, 1979; Edelstein & Metz, 1969; Temperley et al, 1968). Non-pregnant levels of 205–1025 µg/l fall to 20–510 µg/l at term, with low levels in multiple pregnancy (Temperley et al, 1968). Women who smoke tend to have lower serum B_{12} levels (McGarry & Andrews, 1972), which may account for the positive correlation between birthweight and serum levels in non-deficient mothers.

Vitamin B_{12} absorption is unaltered in pregnancy (Chanarin, 1979; Cooper, 1973). It is probable that tissue uptake is increased by the action of oestrogens as oral contraceptives cause a fall in serum vitamin B_{12} (Briggs & Briggs, 1972). Cord blood serum vitamin B_{12} is higher than that of maternal blood. The fall in serum vitamin B_{12} in the mother is related to preferential transfer of absorbed B_{12} to the fetus at the expense of maintaining the maternal serum concentration (Chanarin, 1979), but the placenta does not transfer vitamin B_{12} with the same efficiency as it does folate. Low serum vitamin B_{12} levels in early pregnancy in vegetarian Hindus do not fall further, while their infants often have subnormal concentrations (Roberts et al, 1973). The vitamin B_{12} binding capacity of plasma increases in pregnancy analogous to the rise in transferrin. The rise is confined to the liver-derived transcobalamin II concerned with transport rather than the leucocyte-derived transcobalamin I which is raised in other myeloproliferative conditions (Fleming, 1975).

Pregnancy does not make a vast impact on maternal vitamin B_{12} stores. Adult stores are of the order of 3000 µg or more, and vitamin B_{12} stores in the newborn infant are about 50 µg (Chanarin, 1979; Roberts et al, 1973).

Addisonian pernicious anaemia does not usually occur during the reproductive years. Vitamin B_{12} deficiency is associated with infertility, and pregnancy is likely only if the deficiency is remedied (Jackson et al, 1967). However, severe vitamin B_{12} deficiency may be present without morphological changes in haemopoietic and other tissues. Pregnancy in such patients may be followed by death *in utero* or proceed uneventfully (Chanarin, 1985).

Vitamin B_{12} deficiency in pregnancy may be associated with chronic tropical sprue.

The megaloblastic anaemia which develops is due to long-standing vitamin B_{12} deficiency and superadded folate deficiency, the result of both demands of pregnancy and poor folate intake. The cord vitamin B_{12} levels remain above the maternal levels in these cases, but the concentration in the breast milk follows the maternal serum levels (Chanarin, 1979).

The recommended intake of vitamin B_{12} is $2 \cdot 0\,\mu g$ per day in the non-pregnant and $3 \cdot 0\,\mu g$ per day during pregnancy (World Health Organisation, 1972). This will be met by almost any diet which contains animal products, however deficient in other essential substances. However, in these days of processed foods certain animal products may lose their B_{12} content in preparation. It has been reported (Herbert, 1985) that a surprising number of underprivileged young adults were suffering from B_{12} deficiency in Mexico City. Their sole source of dietary B_{12} was in processed milks which, on investigation, were found to have very little B_{12} content indeed. Strict Vegans, who will not eat any animal-derived substances, may have a deficient intake of vitamin B_{12} and their diet should be supplemented during pregnancy.

HAEMOGLOBINOPATHIES AND PREGNANCY

Following the influx of immigrants from all parts of the world, obstetricians in Britain frequently encounter women with genetic defects of haemoglobin that are seldom seen in the indigenous population. Although many of these conditions are associated with anaemia, it is more important to recognise the specific defects early in pregnancy, or before conception, because:

1. other clinical effects may complicate obstetric management and appropriate precautions can be taken; and
2. it is now possible to offer prenatal diagnosis to those women carrying a fetus at risk of a serious defect of haemoglobin synthesis or structure at a time when termination of pregnancy is feasible (Weatherall, 1985; Nicolaides et al, 1985)

The haemoglobinopathies are inherited defects of haemoglobin, resulting from impaired globin synthesis (thalassaemia syndromes) or from structural abnormality of globin (haemoglobin variants).

A proper appreciation of these defects requires some understanding of the structure of normal haemoglobin. The haemoglobin molecule consists of four globin chains each of which is associated with a haem complex. There are three normal haemoglobins in man, Hb.A, $Hb.A_2$ and Hb.F, each of which contains two pairs of polypeptide globin chains. The synthesis and structure of the four globin chains, alpha, beta, gamma and delta, are under separate control (Fig. 2.1). The adult levels shown are those achieved by 6 months of age. It is obvious that only those conditions affecting the synthesis

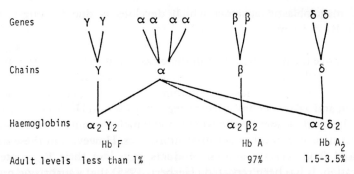

Fig. 2.1   Genetic control of globin chain synthesis. Adult levels achieved by 6 months of age.

or structure of Hb.A ($\alpha_2 \beta_2$) which should comprise over 95 per cent of the total circulating haemoglobin in the adult will be of significance for the mother during pregnancy. Alpha chain production is under the control of four genes, two inherited from each parent, and as can be seen (Fig. 2.1) the alpha chains are common to all three haemoglobins. Beta chain production, on the other hand, is under the control of only two genes, one inherited from each parent.

THE THALASSAEMIA SYNDROMES

The thalassaemia syndromes are the commonest genetic disorders of the blood and constitute a vast public health problem in many parts of the world. The basic defect is a reduced rate of globin chain synthesis resulting in red cells being formed with an inadequate haemoglobin content. They are divided into two main groups, the alpha and beta thalassaemias, depending on whether the alpha or beta globin chain synthesis of adult haemoglobin (Hb.A $\alpha_2 \beta_2$) is depressed.

Beta thalassaemia

Thalassaemia major, homozygous thalassaemia resulting from the inheritance of a defective beta globin gene from each parent, was the first identified form of the thalassaemia syndromes. It was described in the 1920s by Cooley, a physician in practice in the United States. The first few cases were found in the children of Greek and Italian immigrants. The name thalassaemia was derived from the Greek *thalassa* meaning the sea or in the classical sense the Mediterannean, because it was thought to be confined to individuals of Mediterannean origin, but we know now that the distribution is virtually world-wide, although the defect is concentrated in a broad band which does include the Mediterannean and the Middle and Far East. It does not constitute a major health problem in Great Britain, but there are a fair number of heterozygotes, particularly in our immigrant Cypriot and Asian populations. The child of parents who are both carriers of beta thalassaemia has a 1 in 4 chance of inheriting thalassaemia major. The carrier rate in Great Britain is thought to be around 1 in 10 000 compared with 1 in 7 in Cyprus. There are between 300 and 400 patients with thalassaemia major in Britain today, most of them concentrated round the Greater London area, but there are over 100 000 babies born world-wide, with the condition, each year.

Before the days of regular transfusion, a child born with homozygous beta thalassaemia would die in the first few years of life from anaemia, congestive cardiac failure and intercurrent infection. Now that regular transfusion is routine, where blood is freely available, survival is prolonged into the teens and early 20s. The management problem becomes one of iron overload derived mainly from the transfused red cells. This results in hepatic and endocrine dysfunction, but most important of all, myocardial damage, the cause of death being cardiac failure in the vast majority of cases. Puberty is delayed or incomplete and there has only been a very rare case report of successful pregnancy in a truly transfusion-dependent thalassaemic girl (Goldfarb et al, 1982). It remains to be seen how effective recently instituted intensive iron chelation programmes will be.

Diagnosis and management of β thalassaemia in pregnancy

Sometimes survival is possible without regular transfusion in thalassaemia major—but this usually results in severe bone deformities due to massive expansion of marrow tissue, the site of largely ineffective erythropoiesis. Although iron loading still occurs from excessive gastro-intestinal absorption, stimulated by the accelerated marrow turnover, it is much slower than in those who are transfused, and pregnancy may occur in this situation. Extra daily folate supplements should be given but iron in any form is contraindicated. The anaemia should be treated by transfusion during the antenatal period.

Perhaps the commonest problem associated with haemoglobinopathies and pregnancy, in this country today, is the anaemia developing in the antenatal period in women who have thalassaemia minor, heterozygous beta thalassaemia. They can be identified for further examination of the booking blood by finding, as in alpha thalassaemia, low MCV and MCH together with a relatively normal MCHC (Table 2.1). The level of haemoglobin at booking may be normal or slightly below the normal range. The diagnosis will be confirmed by finding a raised concentration of Hb.A$_2$ ($\alpha_2\delta_2$) with or without a raised Hb.F ($\alpha_2\gamma_2$) excess alpha chains combining with delta and gamma chains because of the relative lack of beta chains (Fig. 2.2).

Women with beta thalassaemia minor require the usual *oral* iron and folate supplements in the antenatal period. Oral iron for a limited period will not result in significant iron loading, even in the presence of replete iron

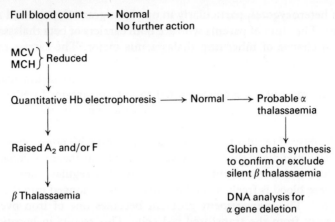

Fig. 2.2 Scheme for identifying individuals who are thalassaemia carriers.

stores, but parenteral iron should *never* be given. A serum ferritin estimation would be advisable early in pregnancy, and if iron stores are found to be high, iron supplements can be withheld. Many women with thalassaemia minor enter pregnancy with depleted iron stores, as do many women with normal haemoglobin synthesis. Iron deficiency has been shown in women in this country with thalassaemia minor (Hussein et al, 1975) by estimation of serum ferritin levels. To cover the requirements of ineffective erythropoiesis folic acid 5·0 mg daily is recommended (see above). If the anaemia does not respond to oral iron and folate, and intramuscular folic acid has been tried, transfusion is indicated to achieve an adequate haemoglobin for delivery at term.

Alpha thalassaemia

Normal individuals have four functional alpha globin genes. Alpha thalassaemia, unlike beta thalassaemia, is often, but not always, a gene deletion defect. There are two forms of alpha thalassaemia trait, the result of inheriting two or three normal alpha genes instead of the usual four. They are called α^0 and α^+ thalassaemia (Fig. 2.3). Hb.H disease is an intermediate form of alpha thalassaemia in which there is only one functional alpha gene. Hb.H is the name given to the unstable haemoglobin formed by tetramers of the beta chain (β_4), when there is a relative lack of alpha chains. Alpha thalassaemia major, in which there are no functional alpha genes (both parents having transmitted α^0 thalassaemia), is incompatible with life and pregnancy ends usually prematurely in a hydrops which will only survive a matter of hours if born alive. The condition is common in South-East Asia. The name Hb.Barts was given to tetramers of the gamma chain of fetal haemoglobin. The tetramer (γ_4) forms *in utero* when no alpha chains are made, and was first identified in a Chinese baby born at St Bartholomews Hospital.

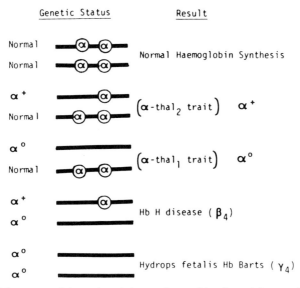

Fig. 2.3   Alpha genes and the various thalassaemias resulting from alpha gene deletion.

Diagnosis and management of alpha thalassaemia in pregnancy

During pregnancy, with its stress on the haemopoietic system, carriers of alpha thalassaemia, particularly those with α^0 thalassaemia (two defective genes) may become very anaemic. They can be identified for further tests at booking, by finding abnormal red cell indices (Table 2.1). They have a reduction in the size of their red cells (MCV) and the individual cell content of haemoglobin (MCH), although the mean cell haemoglobin concentration (MCHC) is usually within the normal range (Table 2.1). These changes are often minimal in α^+ thalassaemia (Fig. 2.2) but this condition is not so important as α^0 thalassaemia in terms of maternal anaemia, genetic counselling and prenatal diagnosis. The diagnosis can only be confirmed by globin chain synthesis studies or, in the case of gene deletion, by DNA analysis of nucleated cells. There is no abnormal haemoglobin made, or excess or lack of one or other of the normal haemoglobins (cf beta thalassaemia) (Fig. 2.2). These individual need iron and folate supplements throughout the antenatal period. Sometimes intramuscular folic acid is helpful but parenteral iron should *never* be given. If the haemoglobin is not thought to be adequate for delivery at term, transfusion is indicated.

Patients with Hb.H disease have a chronic haemolytic anaemia and have 5–30 per cent Hb.H in their peripheral blood. This can be identified on haemoglobin electrophoresis. They have a normal life expectancy but do require daily oral folate supplements to cover the demands of increased marrow turnover. During pregnancy it is recommended to give women with Hb.H disease 5·0 mg folate daily. They will transmit either α^0 or α^+ thalassaemia to their offspring.

Pregnancy with an alpha thalassaemia hydrops is associated with severe, sometimes life-threatening, pre-eclampsia in the mother (cf. severe rhesus haemolytic disease). Vaginal deliveries are associated with obstetric complication, due to the large fetus and very bulky placenta. If routine screening of the parents (see below) indicates that the mother is at risk of carrying such a child, both parents having α^0 thalassaemia, she should be referred, as early as possible in pregnancy, for prenatal diagnosis so that termination of an affected fetus can be carried out before these severe obstetric complications associated with a non-viable child develop.

HAEMOGLOBIN VARIANTS

Over 250 structural variants of the globin chains of normal human haemoglobins have been described but the most important by far, both numerically and clinically, is sickle cell haemoglobin (Hb.S).

Sickle cell syndromes

The sickling disorders include the heterozygous state for sickle cell haemoglobin—sickle cell trait (Hb.AS), homozygous sickle cell disease (Hb.SS)—compound heterozygotes for Hb variants, the most important of which is sickle cell/Hb.C disease (Hb.SC), and sickle cell thalassaemia.

Although these disorders are most commonly seen in black people of African origin, they can be seen in Saudi Arabian, Indian and even white Mediterraneans.

The characteristic feature of homozygous sickle cell anaemia (Hb.SS) is the occurrence of periods of well-being punctuated by period of crisis.

Between 3 and 6 months of age, when normal Hb.A production usually becomes predominant, a chronic haemolytic anaemia develops—the haemoglobin level lying between 6 and 9 g/dl. Even if the haemoglobin is in the lower part of the range, symptoms due to anaemia are surprisingly few because of the low affinity of Hb.S for oxygen; oxygen delivery to the tissues being facilitated. The acute episodes due to intravascular sickling are of far greater partical importance.

There have been articles devoted to sickle cell syndrome previously in this series (Tuck & White, 1981; Tuck & Studd, 1983). Suffice it to say that a prospective multicentre study of routine regular transfusion versus supportive medical care alone is now in progress in this country, and the current approach to management and the controversies involved have been reviewed (Charache & Niebyl, 1985).

Screening for haemoglobinopathies in pregnancy

Selection for screening in a busy antenatal clinic may be more time-consuming than it is worth, and to be efficient should involve detailed documentation of a woman's heritage before excluding her from testing. For this reason, and because of the remote possibility of missing such a defect in the non-immigrant population, general screening for haemoglobinopathies is carried out on every woman's blood during pregnancy at Queen Charlotte's Maternity Hospital, which serves a cosmopolitan population. This involves examination of red cell indices (Table 2.1), haemoglobin electrophoresis and, where indicated, quantitation of Hb.A$_2$ and Hb.F on every sample of blood taken at booking. If a haemoglobin variant or thalassaemia is found (Fig. 2.2), the partner is requested to attend so that his blood can also be examined. By this means we are able to assess the chances of a serious haemoglobin defect in the baby early in pregnancy, and to advise the parents of the potential hazard and offer them parental diagnosis if they so desire.

With the advent of DNA analysis an increasing number of these defects can be prenatally diagnosed on analysis of fetal material obtained as early as 8 weeks gestation, by chorion biopsy techniques (Nicolaides et al, 1985). It is therefore desirable that the parents at risk of producing a child with a serious haemoglobinopathy should be identified before conception, so that advantage can be taken of these intricate and time-consuming, but much more acceptable, methods of prenatal diagnosis should they prove feasible (Weatherall, 1985, Letsky, 1986).

MISCELLANEOUS ANAEMIAS

Many forms of anaemia, in particular the anaemia of renal failure, are made worse by pregnancy. However, supportive and prophylactic therapy for the various medical conditions concerned is improving, and maternal risks for the most part have been reduced, as have the risks to the fetus. Each case has to be considered individually. There are no general rules that can be applied in terms of management.

Aplastic anaemia

There have been sporadic case reports of refractory hypoplastic anaemia, sometimes recurrent, developing in pregnancy and appearing to be related in some way to the pregnancy (Taylor et al, 1968). Occasionally pregnancy occurs when chronic acquired aplastic anaemia is present as an underlying disease. It has been generally considered that in both these situations pregnancy exacerbates the marrow depression, results in rapid deterioration, and should be terminated. It is true that many cases do remit spontaneously after termination (Evans, 1968), but there is no record of excessive haemorrhage at delivery in spite of profound thrombocytopenia. Supportive measures in this situation are improving all the time, and pregnancy should be maintained as long as the health of the mother is not seriously impaired (Lewis, 1982).

Auto-immune haemolytic anaemia and disseminated lupus erythematosus

The rare combination of auto-immune haemolytic anaemia (AIHA) and pregnancy carries great risks both to the woman herself and the fetus. Very careful antenatal supervision and adjustment of steroid therapy is required (Chaplin et al, 1973).

Although pregnancy may result in exacerbations of disseminated lupus erythematosus (DLE) up to 50 per cent of women with this condition are reported to improve during pregnancy, especially in the third trimester (Dubois, 1966).

Haemolytic anaemia, leukopenia and thrombocytopenia have all been observed in infants of women with active disease, presumably due to IgG antibody involved in the disease process crossing the placenta. There have been a number of reports in which women have been treated with steroids and other immune suppressives throughout pregnancy for a variety of conditions including ITP, DLE, AIHA and some forms of malignancy. These drugs would not appear to be teratogenic, and pregnancy has ended in the delivery of a normal infant. The problems of their use are essentially the same as those outside pregnancy, but more frequent monitoring and adjustment is required due to the rapidly changing blood volume and changes in the circulating hormones during the antenatal and postnatal periods.

Leukaemia

In normal pregnancy the total leukocyte count start to rise during the first trimester and reaches a peak by 30 weeks gestation. In the final trimester counts as high as $16 \times 10^9/l$ may be normal, but only about 20 per cent of females will have counts of more than $10 \times 10^9/l$. During labour there is a further rise and counts of $25–30 \times 10^9/l$ are not unusual. A return to normal non-pregnant levels usually occurs by the 6th post-partum day. The increase in leukocyte count reflects a selective hyperactivity of granulopoiesis in the bone marrow, leading to proportional increase in neutrophil count while the lymphocyte and monocyte numbers remain unaltered. Immature granulocytes are released into the circulation and an increasing number of myelocytes and metamyelocytes are to be found as pregnancy progresses. This will become exaggerated dramatically in the presence of infection (Peck & Arias, 1979) and may create diagnostic confusion and investigations for myeloproliferative disease unless this physiological response to pregnancy is appreciated.

Another situation which may cause confusion is that of severe megaloblastic anaemia, now uncommon in this country during pregnancy (see above). As recently as May 1980 two case histories of severe macrocytic anaemia presenting in the puerperium with pancytopenia were published

(McCann et al, 1980). In both cases leukaemia was considered because of the combination of anaemia, profound thrombocytopenia, an increase in promyelocytes in the bone marrow, as well as florid megaloblastic change. Both responded completely to therapy with folic acid.

One in 1000 pregnancies is complicated by malignant disease (Rothman et al, 1973). The incidence of leukaemia in pregnancy would not be expected to exceed 1 in 75 000 pregnancies, but the information used to calculate this incidence is obtained from cases recorded in the literature, which has serious limitations. The peak incidence years for cancer do not coincide with the peak reproductive years. Nevertheless leukaemia was reported in 1969 as the second most common cause of death from malignant disease in females aged 15–34 in the United States (Vital Statistics of the United States, 1969). Several hundred cases of leukaemia in association with pregnancy have now been reported. Most papers give an account of a specific case or cases, and include a review of the published literature (e.g. Ewing and Whittaker, 1973; Gokal et al, 1976; Nicholson, 1968) and some give an overview (e.g. McLain, 1974).

Adult leukaemia is almost invariably fatal, and one of the reasons why acute leukaemia is seen so rarely in association with pregnancy is that without the aggressive treatment with cytotoxic drugs instituted in the last decade the disease is characterised by rapid deterioration and death within weeks of diagnosis.

There is no objective evidence that pregnancy has a deleterious effect on leukaemia (McLain, 1974; Ewing & Whittaker, 1973). Survival times in pregnant women with leukaemia do not differ statistically from those of non-pregnant women. The application of modern treatment can result in remission of the disease sometimes repeated, and more affected women may now have the opportunity to conceive or to survive till the fetus is viable.

The diagnosis during pregnancy is made most frequently in the second and third trimesters although the disease may have been present earlier. This is because the early symptoms are non-specific, the most common being fatigue, which is often attributed by the woman and her obstetrician to the pregnancy itself. This emphasises the importance of carrying out proper investigations, including bone marrow examination of unexplained anaemia in pregnancy. The occurrence of pregnancy in a woman suffering from, or who develops, acute leukaemia creates special clinical problems which fall into two main groups—those arising from the malignant process and those arising from its treatment.

There is an increased risk of infection, haemorrhage and abortion arising from the disease process itself. Fetal loss occurs in approximately 14 per cent of women with chronic myeloid leukaemia and approximately 33 per cent of women with acute leukaemia. Haemorrhage may result from thrombocytopenia due to bone marrow infiltration or from a consumptive coagulopathy which is a particularly common problem in acute myelomonocytic leukaemia.

The powerful cytotoxic drugs which are often used to achieve remission in acute adult leukaemia include cytosine arabinoside, daunorubicin, thioguanine and more recent derivatives. Such agents have been shown to be toxic to fetal tissue in experimental animals. Malformations have occurred after treatment with cytotoxic drugs in the first trimester (Nicholson, 1968). Methotrexate, a folic acid antagonist, is the most teratogenic drug known to man. Its administration early in pregnancy always results in either abortion or congenital malformation. Other published data have indicated that cytotoxic drugs can be given with safety in the second and third trimesters (Nicholson, 1968; Gokal et al, 1976).

It has been suggested (Gokal et al, 1976) that a pregnant leukaemic woman should be treated with aggressive chemotherapy until a remission is achieved. The risk of a malformed fetus in a woman so treated in the first trimester is high, and termination should be considered once she is in remission and this can be performed with safety. Termination of pregnancy when therapy is started in the second or third trimester has to be carried out on moral and medico-social grounds, as the fetus is likely to develop normally. Examination of chromosomes of fetal amniotic fluid cells and of fetal hair under the scanning electron microscope may provide evidence of fetal damage in those cases where treatment is started early in the second trimester (Gokal et al, 1976).

Not one case has been reported of leukaemia in the newborn infant of a mother suffering from the disease, but long-term follow-up should be carried out on the offspring of mothers treated with cytotoxic drugs for late development of neoplasm and possible adverse drug effects such as daunorubicin-induced cardiotoxicity.

Splenic irradiation alone, with careful shielding of the uterus, has been used with success to manage chronic myeloid laukaemia during pregnancy (McLain, 1974; Richards & Spiers, 1974). The late carcinogenic effects of a fetus exposed to irradiation *in utero* have to be borne in mind. Treatment with drugs such as busulfan, thioguanine, 6-mercaptopurine, etc, should be held in reserve until the third trimester or, if possible, until after safe delivery of the infant.

REFERENCES

Avery B, Ledger W J 1970 Folic acid metabolism in well nourished pregnant women. Obstetrics and Gynecology 35: 616–624

Ball E W, Giles C 1964 Folic acid and vitamin B_{12} levels in pregnancy and their relation to megaloblastic anaemia. Journal of Clinical Pathology 17: 165–174

Baumslag N, Edelstein T, Metz J 1970 Reduction of Incidence of prematurity of folic acid supplementation in pregnancy. British Medical Journal 1: 16–17

Bentley D P 1985 Iron metabolism and anaemia in pregnancy. In: Letsky E A (ed) Haematological disorders in pregnancy. Clinics in haematology 14: Saunders, Eastbourne, pp 613–628

Briggs M, Briggs M 1972 Endocrine effects on serum vitamin B_{12}. Lancet ii: 1037

Chanarin I 1975 The folate content of foodstuffs and the availability of different folate analogues for absorption. In: Getting the most out of food. Van den Bergh and Jurgens, London, p 41

Chanarin I 1979 Megaloblastic anaemia of pregnancy. In: The megaloblastic anaemias, 2nd edn. Blackwell Scientific Publications, Oxford

Chanarin I 1985 Folate and cobalamin. In: Letsky E A (ed) Haematological disorders in pregnancy. Clinics in haematology 14: Saunders, Eastbourne, pp 629–641

Chanarin I, MacGibbon B M, O'Sullivan W J, Mollin D L 1959 Folic acid deficiency in pregnancy; the pathogenesis of megaloblastic anaemia in pregnancy. Lancet ii: 634–639

Chanarin I, Rothman D, Berry V 1965 Iron deficiency and its relation to folic acid status in pregnancy: results of a clinical trial. British Medical Journal i: 480–485

Chanarin I, Rothman D, Ward A, Perry J 1968 Folate status and requirement in pregnancy. British Medical Journal ii: 390–394

Chaplin H, Cohen R, Bloomberg G, Kaplan H J, Moore J A, Dorner I 1973 Pregnancy and idiopathic auto-immune haemolytic anaemia. A prospective study during 6 months gestation and 3 months post-partum. British Journal of Haematology 24: 219–229

Charache S, Niebyl O R 1985 Pregnancy in sickle cell disease. In: Letsky E A (ed.) Haematological disorders in pregnancy. Clinics in haematology 14: Saunders, Eastbourne, pp 729–746

Chisholm J 1966 A controlled clinical trial of prophylactic folic acid and iron in pregnancy. Journal of Obstetrics and Gynaecology of the British Commonwealth 73: 191–196

Clay B, Rosenburg B, Sampson N, Samuels S I 1965: Reactions to total dose intravenous infusion of iron dextran (Imferon). British Medical Journal i: 29–31

Cooper B A 1973 Folate and vitamin B_{12} in pregnancy. Clinics in Haematology 2: 461–476

Coyle C, Geoghegan F 1962 The problem of anaemia in a Dublin maternity hospital. Proceedings of the Royal Society of Medicine 55: 764–766

de Leeuw N K M, Lowenstein L, Hsieh Y S 1966 Iron deficiency and hydremia in normal pregnancy. Medicine, Baltimore 45: 291–315

de Leeuw N K M, Lowenstein L, Tucker E C, Dayal S 1968 Correlation of red cell loss at delivery with changes in red cell mass. American Journal of Obstetrics and Gynaecology 100: 1092–1101

de Swiet M 1980 The respiratory system. In: Hytten F E, Chamberlain G V P (eds) Clinical physiology in obstetrics. Blackwell Scientific Publications, Oxford, pp 289–327

Dubois E L 1966 Lupus erythematosus. McGraw Hill, New York

Edelstein T, Metz J 1969 The correlation between vitamin B_{12} concentration in serum and muscle in late pregnancy. Journal of Obstetrics and Gynaecology of the British Commonwealth 76: 545–548

Elwood J M 1983 Can vitamins prevent neural tube defects? Canadian Medical Association Journal 129: 1088–1092

Evans I L 1968 Aplastic anaemia in pregnancy remitting after abortion. British Medical Journal 3: 166–167

Ewing P A, Whittaker J A 1973 Acute leukaemia in pregnancy. Obstetrics and Gynecology 42: 245–251

Fenton V, Cavill I, Fisher J 1977 Iron stores in pregnancy. British Journal of Haematology 37: 145–149

Finch C A, Cook J D 1984 Iron deficiency. American Journal of Clinical Nutrition 39: 471–477

Finch C A, Huebers H 1982 Perspectives in iron metabolism. New England Journal of Medicine 306: 1520–1528

Fleming A F 1972 Urinary excretion of folate in pregnancy. Journal of Obstetrics and Gynecology of the British Commonwealth 79: 916–920

Fleming A F 1975 Haematological changes in pregnancy. Clinics in Obstetrics and Gynaecology 2: 269–283

Fleming A F, Martin J D, Hahnell R, Westlake A J 1974a Effects of iron and folic acid antenatal supplements on maternal haematology and fetal well-being. Medical Journal of Australia ii: 429–436

Fleming A F, Martin J D, Stonehouse N S 1947b Pregnancy anaemia, iron and folate deficiency in Western Australia. Medical Journal of Australia ii: 479–484

Gatenby P B B 1956 The anaemias of pregnancy in Dublin. Proceedings of the Nutrition Society. 15: 115–119

Gatenby P B B, Little E W 1960 Clinical analysis of 100 cases of severe megaloblastic anaemia of pregnancy. British Medical Journal ii: 1111–1114

Giles C 1966 An account of 335 cases of megaloblastic anaemia of pregnancy and the puerperium. Journal of Clinical Pathology 19 : 1–11

Gokal R, Durrant J, Baum J D, Bennett M J 1976 Successful pregnancy in acute monocytic leukaemia. British Journal of Cancer 34 : 299–302

Goldfarb A W, Hochner-Celnikier D, Beller U, Menashe M, Dagan I, Palti Z 1982 A successful pregnancy in transfusion dependent homozygous β-thalassaemia : a case report. International Journal of Gynaecology and Obstetrics 20 : 319–322

Hallberg I, Ryttinger L, Solvell L 1966 Side effects of oral iron therapy. Acta Medica Scandinavica, 459 : Supplement 3–10

Hallberg L, Bengtsson C, Garby L, Lennartsson J, Rossander L, Tibblin E 1979 An analysis of factors leading to a reduction in iron deficiency in Swedish women. Bulletin of the World Health Organisation 57 : 947–954

Hambridge K M, Krebs N F, Jacobs M A, Guyette L, Ikle D N 1983 Zinc nutritional status during pregnancy : a longitudinal study. American Journal of Clinical Nutrition 37 : 429–442

Haworth C, Evans D I K 1981 Nutritional aspects of blood disorders in the new-born. Journal of Human Nutrition 35 : 323–334

Hemminki E, Starfield B 1978 Routine administration of iron and vitamins during pregnancy : review of controlled clinical trials. British Journal of Obstetrics and Gynaecology 85 : 404–410

Herbert V 1985 Biology of disease—megaloblastic anaemias. Laboratory Investigation 52 : 3–19

Hiilesmaa V K, Teramo K, Granstrom M-L, Bardy A H 1983 Serum folate concentrations during pregnancy in women with epilepsy : relation to anti-epileptic drug concentrations, number of seizures and fetal outcome. British Medical Journal 287 : 577–579

Hussein S S, Hoffbrand A V, Laulicht M, Attock B, Letsky E A 1975 Serum ferritin levels in beta thalassaemia trait. British Medical Journal ii : 920

Hytten F 1985 Blood volume changes in normal pregnancy. In : Letsky E A (ed) Haematological disorders in pregnancy. Clinics in haematology 14 : Saunders, Eastbourne, pp 601–612

Hytten F E, Leitch I 1971 The volume and composition of the blood. In : The physiology of human pregnancy, 2nd edn. Blackwell Scientific Publications, Oxford, pp 1–68

Iyengar L 1971 Folic acid requirements of Indian pregnant women. American Journal of Obstetrics and Gynecology 111 : 13–16

Jackson I M D, Doig W B, McDonald G 1967 Pernicious anaemia as a cause of infertility. Lancet ii : 1159

Jacobs A, Worwood M 1982 Iron metabolism, iron deficiency and iron overload. In : Hardisty R M, Weatherall D J (eds) Blood and its disorders, 2nd edn. Blackwell Scientific Publications, Oxford, pp 173–180

Jacobs A, Miller F, Worwood M, Beamish M R, Wardrop C A 1972 Ferritin in serum of normal subjects and patients with iron deficiency and iron overload. British Medical Journal 4 : 206–208

Kuizon M D, Platon T P, Ancheta L P, Angeles J C, Nunez C B, Macapinlac M P 1979 Iron supplementation among pregnant women. South East Asian Journal of Tropical Medicine 10 : 520–527

Kullander S, Kallen B 1976 A prospective study of drugs and pregnancy. Acta Obstetrica Gynecologica Scandinavica 55 : 287–295

Landon M J 1975 Folate metabolism in pregnancy. Clinics in Obstetrics and Gynaecology 2 : 413–430

Landon M J, Hytten F E 1971 The excretion of folate in pregnancy. Journal of Obstetrics and Gynaecology of the British Commonwealth 78 : 769–775

Landon M J, Hytten F E 1972 Plasma folate levels following an oral load of folic acid during pregnancy. Journal of Obstetrics and Gynaecology of the British Commonwealth 79 : 577–583

Laurence K M, James N, Miller M H, Tennant G B, Campbell H 1981 Double-blind randomised controlled trial of folate treatment before conception to prevent recurrence of neural tube defects. British Medical Journal 282 : 1509–1511

Letsky E A 1980 The haematological system. In : Hytten F E, Chamberlain G V P (eds) Clinical physiology in obstetrics. Blackwell Scientific Publications, Oxford, pp 43–78

Letsky E A 1986 Haemoglobinopathies. In: Chamberlain G, Lumley J (eds) Pregnancy care. John Wiley, Chichester, pp 223–243.

Lewis S M 1982 Aplastic anaemia in pregnancy. In: Hardisty R M, Weatherall D J (eds) Blood and its disorders, 2nd edn. Blackwell Scientific Publications, Oxford, pp 1239–1240

Lowenstein L, Brunton L, Hsieh Y-S 1966 Nutritional anemia and megaloblastics in pregnancy. Canadian Medical Association Journal 94: 636–645

Lund C J 1951 Studies on the iron deficiency anaemia of pregnancy including plasma volume, total haemoglobin, erythrocyte protoporphyrin in treated and untreated normal and anemic patients. American Journal of Obstetrics and Gynecology 62: 947–961

McCann S R, Lawlor E, McGovern M, Temperley I J 1980 Severe megaloblastic anaemia of pregnancy. Journal of the Irish Medical Association 73: 197–198

McGarry J M, Andrews J 1972 Smoking in pregnancy and vitamin B_{12} metabolism. British Medical Journal ii: 74–77

McLain C R 1974 Leukemia in pregnancy. Clinical Obstetrics and Gynecology 17(4): 185–194

McLean F W, Heine M W, Held B, Streiff R R 1970 Folic acid absorption in pregnancy: comparison òf the pteroylpolyglutamate and pteroylmonoglutamate. Blood 36: 628–631

Magee H E, Milligan E H M 1951 Haemoglobin levels before and after labour. British Medical Journal ii: 1307–1310

Mayet F G H 1985 Anaemia of pregnancy. South African Medical Journal 67: 804–809

Miller J R, Keith N M, Rowntree L G 1915 Plasma and blood volume in pregnancy. Journal of the American Medical Association 65: 779–782

Meadows N J, Ruse W, Smith M F et al 1981 Zinc and small babies. Lancet ii: 1135–1137

Meadows N J, Grainger S L, Warwick Ruse, Keeling P W N, Thompson R P H 1983 Oral iron and the bioavailability of zinc. British Medical Journal 287: 1013–1014

Morgan E H 1961 Plasma iron and haemoglobin levels in pregnancy. The effect of oral iron. Lancet i: 9–12

Nicholson H O 1968 Leukaemia and pregnancy. Journal of Obstetrics and Gynaecology of the British Commonwealth 75: 517–520

Nicolaides K H, Rodeck C H, Mibashan R S 1985 Obstetric management and diagnosis of haematological disease in the fetus. Clinics in Haematology 14: 775–805

Ogunbode O, Akinyele I O, Hussain M A 1979 Dietary iron intake of pregnant Nigerian women with anaemia. International Journal of Gynaecology and Obstetrics 17: 290–293

Oski F A 1979 Nutritional anemias. Seminars in Perinatology 3: 381–395

Oski F A 1985 Iron deficiency—facts and fallacies. Paediatric Clinics of North America 32: 493–497

Osler W 1919 Observations on the severe anaemias of pregnancy and the post-partum state. British Medical Journal 1: 1–3

Paintin D B, Thomson A M, Hytten F E 1966 Iron and the haemoglobin level in pregnancy. Journal of Obstetrics and Gynaecology of the British Commonwealth 73: 181–190

Peck T M, Arias F 1979 Hematologic changes associated with pregnancy. Clinical Obstetrics and Gynecology 22: 785–798

Pirani B B K, Campbell D M, MacGillivray I 1973 Plasma volume in normal first pregnancy. Journal of Obstetrics and Gynaecology of the British Commonwealth 80: 884–887

Reynolds E H 1973 Anticonvulsants, folic acid and epilepsy. Lancet i: 1376–1378

Richards H G, Spiers A S 1974 Chronic granulocytic leukaemia in pregnancy. Journal of Clinical Pathology 27: 927

Roberts P D, James H, Petrie A, Morgan J O, Hoffbrand A V 1973 Vitamin B_{12} status in pregnancy among immigrants to Britain. British Medical Journal iii: 67–72

Rothman L A, Cohen C J, Astarloa J 1973 Placental and fetal involvement by maternal malignancy: a report of rectal carcinoma and review of the literature. American Journal of Obstetrics and Gynecology 116: 1023–1033

Scott J M 1962 Toxicity of iron sorbitol citrate. British Medical Journal ii: 480–481

Scott J M 1963 Iron sorbitol citrate in pregnancy anaemia. British Medical Journal 2: 354–357

Shapiro J, Alberts H W, Welch P, Metz J 1965 Folate and vitamin B_{12} deficiency associated with lactation. British Journal of Haematology 11: 498–504

Sheldon W L, Aspillaga M O, Smith P A, Lind T 1985 The effects of oral iron supplementation on zinc and magnesium levels during pregnancy. British Journal of Obstetrics and Gynaecology 92: 892–898

Smithells R W, Sheppard S, Schorah C J et al 1980 Possible prevention of neural-tube defects by periconceptional vitamin supplementation. Lancet i: 339–340

Smithells R W, Nevin N C, Seller M J et al 1983 Further experience of vitamin supplementation for prevention of neural tube defect recurrences. Lancet i: 1027–1031

Stephens H E M, Craft I, Peters T J, Hoffbrand A V 1972 Oral contraceptives and folate metabolism. Clinical Science 42: 405–414

Stone M L, Luhby A L, Feldman R, Gordon M, Cooperman J M 1967 Folic acid metabolism in pregnancy. American Journal of Obstetrics and Gynecology 90: 638–648

Svanberg B 1975 Absorption of iron in pregnancy. Acta Obstetrica et Gynecologica Scandinavica. Supplement 48: 7–108

Taylor D J, Mallen C, McDougall N, Lind T 1982 Effect of iron supplementation on serum ferritin levels during and after pregnancy. British Journal of Obstetrics and Gynaecology 89: 1011–1017

Taylor J J, Studd J W W, Green I D 1968 Primary refractory anaemia and pregnancy. Journal of Obstetrics and Gynaecology of the British Commonwealth 75: 963–968

Temperley I J, Meehan M J M, Gattenby P B B 1968 Serum vitamin B_{12} levels in pregnant women. Journal of Obstetrics and Gynaecology of the British Commonwealth 75: 511–516

Tuck S, Studd J W N 1983 Obstetric problems in the black community. In: Studd J (ed.) Progress in obstetrics and gynaecology, vol. 3. Churchill Livingstone, London, pp 17–34

Tuck S, White J M 1981 Sickle cell disease. In: Studd J (ed.) Progress in obstetrics and gynaecology, vol. 3. Churchill Livingstone, London, pp 70–80

Weatherall D J 1985 Prenatal Diagnosis of Inherited Blood Diseases. In: Leksky E A (ed) Haematological Disorders in Pregnancy. Clinics in Haematology 14: Saunders, Eastbourne. p 747–774

World Health Organisation 1972 Nutritional anaemias. Technical Report Series No. 503.

Neurological disorders and pregnancy

Between 1977 and 1982 there were at least five authoritative publications on the subject of neurological disorders and pregnancy (Hopkins, 1977; Aminoff, 1978; Donaldson, 1978; Dalessio, 1982; Graham, 1982). All are broad in their scope; those by Donaldson (1978) and Dalessio (1982) also cover the subject in considerable depth. This presentation will therefore concentrate on those disorders that have featured in the literature more recently. Inevitably, not all such disorders can be included. The criteria used for selection were clinical importance and/or scientific interest for students of obstetrics or neurology. (To limit any further personal bias, they are considered in alphabetical order!). In addition, there are sections dealing with special investigations and certain drugs used in the treatment of neurological disorders.

BENIGN INTRACRANIAL HYPERTENSION (PSEUDOTUMOUR CEREBRI)

Though the association is well known, the occurrence of benign intracranial hypertension (BIH) in pregnancy is uncommon. Indeed, Palop et al (1979) were able to locate only 29 case reports to 1979. Moreover, the association may be no more than fortuitous. Using age- and parity-matched controls, Digre et al (1984) concluded from their study of 109 female patients with BIH that its occurrence in pregnancy is probably only a reflection of the fact that it is particularly common in women of childbearing age. Kassam et al (1983) go further, believing the incidence in pregnancy is less than would be expected in a disorder with a preponderance of females aged 20 to 30. Whatever relationship pregnancy may have to its onset, BIH invariably resolves rapidly after termination or parturition (Palop et al, 1979; Dalessio, 1982; Koontz et al, 1983). All nine of Koontz et al's (1983) patients were symptom-free within 72 hours of delivery and none required medication beyond 3 months postpartum.

When developing in pregnancy, BIH tends to present in the first two trimesters, particularly the first (Digre et al, 1984). Presentation in the third trimester is so unusual that Caroscio & Pelimar (1978) claimed their case report was the first such example. A recurrence in subsequent pregnancies is rare (Koontz et al, 1983), the risk being no greater than for its occurrence in pregnancy in a patient who was not pregnant when BIH first developed (Digre et al, 1984).

Most pregnancies with BIH result in good maternal and neonatal outcomes (Koontz et al, 1983; Digre et al, 1984), though patients should avoid becoming pregnant until in remission (Koontz et al, 1983). In general the prognosis for vision is no different in the pregnant than the non-pregnant patient (Digre et al, 1984). If vision is threatened despite vigorous medical treatment, optic nerve decompression may allow the pregnancy to continue without further visual damage (Shekleton et al, 1980). No diagnostic procedure for BIH, and none of the other standard therapies, including CSF shunting, is contraindicated in pregnancy (Koontz et al, 1983; Digre et al, 1984). Nonetheless, Digre et al (1984) emphasise the need to be cautious in calorie restriction, while at the same time limiting weight gain to 9 kg, and to check for evidence of reduced maternal blood volume if diuretics are used.

Though rapid resolution of BIH may follow termination it should seldom be necessary (Koontz et al, 1983; Digre et al, 1984) and delivery should be based on obstetric indications (Kassam et al, 1983). However, intracranial pressure is normally increased in labour, as a result of both uterine contractions and pain (Kassam et al, 1983; Koontz et al, 1983), and since similar changes occur with general anaesthesia, continuous regional anaesthesia is the treatment of choice for the management of labour in these patients (Palop et al, 1979; Kassam et al, 1983).

CEREBROVASCULAR DISEASE

Occlusion

A number of unresolved and controversial issues concerning cerebrovascular occlusion in pregnancy and the puerperium are highlighted in the study reported recently by Srinivasan (1983). Of the 135 patients seen over 8 years, the majority developed stroke in the puerperium, particularly in the first 10 days after delivery. The process responsible was judged to be venous occlusion in 129; arterial occlusion was demonstrated in the remaining six. Whereas the high incidence in the puerperium of stroke in general, and of venous occlusion in particular, is typical (Aminoff, 1978; Lavin et al, 1978; Donaldson, 1981; Fehr, 1982; Graham, 1982), the much greater number of venous compared to arterial lesions overall is in striking contrast to the pattern described by Aminoff (1978), Donaldson (1981) and Dalessio (1982). One explanation for this discrepancy may be that the patients in Srinivasan's (1983) study were Indian. Hopkins (1977) and Dalessio (1982) have stressed that, in the past, cerebral venous thrombosis (CVT) has been diagnosed in many instances on the basis of probabilities rather than documental proof. (This, in fact, continues to be the case (Beal & Chapman, 1980; Monteiro et al, 1984).) With this in mind, it is noteworthy that in only 64 of Srinavasan's (1983) patients was angiography ($n=60$) or sinography ($n=4$) performed, and that venous occlusion was proven in just 13 of them. In the remainder, as in Beal & Chapman's (1980) three patients, the diagnosis was made on the grounds of clinical features and CSF findings.

Though computed tomography (CT) may be useful (Kelton & Hirsh, 1982), angiography is the definitive antemortem investigation for the diagnosis of CVT (Donaldson, 1978; Rocco et al, 1981; Graham, 1982; Kelton & Hirsh, 1982). This point is well illustrated by the patient reported by Fehr (1982), in whom CT brain scan was normal while angiography revealed extensive thrombosis of dural sinuses and deep veins. For the diagnosis of superior sagittal sinus thrombosis, digital subtraction angiography may now be the procedure of choice (Savoiardo & Bracchi, 1984). In certain circumstances, though, angiography may yield false-negative results. For example, occluded cortical veins may not be easy to visualise in the absence of dural sinus involvement, or recanalisation may have occurred (Beal & Chapman, 1980). Also, appropraite techniques may not have been employed to clearly visualise the venous phase (Srinivasan, 1983).

Pregnancy and the puerperium are accompanied by haemostatic, rheological and haemodynamic changes which may predispose to thrombosis, especially in the venous system (Laros & Alger, 1979; Beal & Chapman, 1980; Tooke & McNicol, 1981). The cerebral cortical veins may be additionally predisposed by virtue of having no valves, low pressure and fibrous septae (Lavin et al, 1978). Among haemostatic changes, platelet count, fibrinogen and factor VIII may have particular relevance to the development of CVT as all are notably increased in the puerperium (Tooke & McNicol, 1981), and at the time when deep vein thrombosis is most common (Laros & Alger, 1979; Tooke & McNicol, 1981). In addition, patients with puerperal venous thrombosis have been reported to have a notable reduction in fibrinolytic activity (see Beal & Chapman, 1980). In Srinivasan's (1983) series overall, platelet count was more than $500 \times 10^3/$ mm^3 in 8 of 32 patients. Elevated fibrinogen was present in 104 of 120 patients, a finding Srinivasan (1983) considered may portend the development of CVT, especially if a serial increase is demonstrated.

Whereas the use of anticonvulsants and agents to reduce cerebral oedema (other than mannitol) is widely recommended and not in dispute, the employment of anticoagulants in the treatment of CVT is controversial, both as to their value (Graham, 1982) and the risks involved (see Rocco et al, 1980). Notwithstanding the almost constant pathological finding of haemorrhagic infarction in such cases (Lavin et al, 1979), a number of circumstances have been proposed to justify their use. These include coincident pelvic or deep leg vein thrombosis (Donaldson, 1978) and when the patient is deteriorating, provided haemorrhage is not visualised on CT brain scan (Beal & Chapman, 1980). Heparin was used in a selected number of Srinivasan's (1980) patients, the criteria for selection including a fibrinogen level greater than 400 mg/dl, the presence of deep vein thrombosis and confinement to bed for longer than 1 week. The mortality of the treated group was much less than the untreated group, an outcome that Srinivasan (1983) felt could be ascribed to the use of heparin.

Rocco et al (1980) reported encouraging results in treating dural sinus thrombosis with a combination of anticoagulant and fibrinolytic agents. All their five patients, including the single case of puerperal thrombosis, showed complete clinical recovery and radiological resolution following early intervention with heparin and urokinase. In spite of the hazards of such combined therapy, further trials seem warranted on the basis of these results.

Subarachnoid haemorrhage

There are no specific contraindications, maternal or fetal, to the use of routine neuroimaging studies and conventional neurosurgical procedures in the investigation and treatment of the pregnant patient with subarachnoid haemorrhage (SAH) (Donaldson, 1981; Tuttleman & Gleicher, 1981).

Demonstration of a structural lesion is more likely in the pregnant than nonpregnant female (see Dalessio, 1982) and is important for optimum patient management. In the case of ruptured aneurysm, standard indications for neurosurgery apply—i.e. operation should be undertaken as soon as the mother's clinical condition allows (Briani et al, 1980). Arteriovenous malformations (AVM) tend to rebleed in the peripartum period (Tuttleman & Gleicher, 1981; Graham, 1982) and the fetal prognosis is especially poor (Dalessio, 1982); early neurosurgical intervention is therefore indicated where possible.

If the lesion responsible, either aneurysm or AVM, has been successfully treated, the goal of obstetric management is a full-term vaginal delivery. The second stage of labour may be modified with extradural anaesthesia and outlet forceps to avoid unneccessary cardiovascular stress; oxytocin can be used for induction (Tuttleman & Gleicher, 1981). If the lesion is inoperable, obstetric management depends on whether an aneurysm or AVM is responsible. (If no lesion is demonstrated, management should probably be as for inoperable aneurysm.)

A patient in whom SAH due to an inoperable aneurysm occurs in the third trimester, or a patient with an inoperable AVM, should have an elective Caesarean section shortly before term (Donaldson, 1981; Tuttleman & Gleicher, 1981). If the patient with an inoperable aneurysm sustained SAH before the third trimester, vaginal delivery, as for operated lesions, is permitted.

CHOREA GRAVIDARUM

Since increased striatal dopaminergic activity is thought to underlie chorea, experimental evidence that female sex hormones may enhance central dopaminergic sensitivity (see Nausieda et al, 1979) could provide an explanation for its occurrence in pregnancy. This evidence could also explain its remission shortly after delivery and its recurrence in subsequent pregnancies (Donaldson, 1978; Dalessio, 1982; Yiannikas, 1984). However, additional factors must be operative that predispose a minority of pregnant woman only to develop chorea. One such factor is thought to be pre-existing basal ganglia pathology (Nausieda et al, 1979). Ichikawa et al (1980) reported the eleventh case of chorea gravidarum with a 'valid' neuropathological examination and reviewed the 10 previously published accounts. These authors concluded that the striatum was indeed the major site of nervous system pathology. Of these 10 patients, three had a past history of rheumatic fever and/or Sydenham chorea. For such reasons these disorders have been strongly linked to the development of chorea in pregnancy (Donaldson, 1978; Patterson, 1979), and the dramatic decline in their incidence and that of chorea gravidarum in the past 50 years has been held to support this linkage (Agrawal & Foa, 1982). Whereas it might be anticipated neuropathological accounts of Sydenham chorea would yield additional information on this matter, Ichikawa et al (1980), consider the reports are too scanty and too difficult to interpret in modern terms.

Donaldson (1978), has emphasised the term chorea gravidarum does not imply a particular cause. Systemic lupus erythematosus (SLE), for example, may present as chorea during gestation (Agrawal & Foa, 1982) or the puerperium (Thomas et al, 1979). Agrawal & Foa's (1982) patient responded to corticosteroids and delivered a normal infant, and these authors advocate treating such patients to suppress SLE rather than the chorea *per se*. Corticosteroids were also used successfully in treating a pregnant patient who developed chorea in association with lupus anticoagulant (Lubbe & Walker, 1983). Noting the rarity of chorea among groups in whom rheumatic fever is still prevalent, Lubbe & Walker (1983) questioned whether chorea may be an autoimmune cerebral disorder of pregnancy and not a sequel to rheumatic fever. This is an intriguing suggestion, as pregnant women seem particularly vulnerable to the adverse effects of lupus anticoagulant (*Lancet*, 1984). Also, there is no adequate explanation for the development of chorea without a history of rheumatic fever or for its non-recurrence in subsequent pregnancies.

In circumstances where no underlying process is established, haloperidol has been advocated as the drug of choice for treating chorea (Donaldson, 1982). However, Patterson (1979) cautions against its use unless the patient is physically disabled, citing reports of teratogenic effects. Chlorpromazine and diazepam were used with success by Ramsay (1984), both patients delivering healthy infants. In neither case, though, was therapy initiated before the third trimester.

EPILEPSY

(The pharmacokinetics and teratogenicity of anticonvulsant drugs are considered elsewhere in this chapter.) There is an almost equal chance that the epileptic patient will experience a change or no change in the frequency of seizures during pregnancy and the puerperium. A review of retrospective studies published between 1884 and 1980, and encompassing 2165 pregnancies, revealed that the frequency of seizures was unchanged in 53 per cent, increased in 24 per cent and decreased in 23 per cent (Janz, 1982). While noting that a similar average percentage of pregnancies with increased seizure frequency had been found in prospective studies also, Janz (1982) pointed out that in these studies the range was between 8 and 46 per cent. In a carefully controlled prospective study, Schmidt et al (1983) compared the frequency of seizures in the 9 months before pregnancy with that in the 12 months of gestation and the puerperium in 139 pregnancies of 122 epileptic patients. Siezure frequency was unchanged in 50 per cent, increased in 37 per cent and decreased in 13 per cent. These authors could not identify any clinical feature(s) in their patients that predicted the course of epilepsy in pregnancy. This finding accords with the view expressed by Philbert & Dam (1982), that those with frequent pregestational seizures are no more likely to deteriorate in pregnancy than those whose seizures are infrequent. Of the 50 patients in Schmidt et al's (1983) study who experienced an increase in seizure frequency, the increase occurred in the first trimester in 29 and was smallest in the third trimester. Relevant to this could be the finding of a subtherapeutic plasma anticonvulsant level at the first antenatal visit in 63 per cent of their patients overall.

Montouris et al (1979) considered that a fall in blood levels of anticonvulsants is the critical factor underlying loss of seizure control in pregnancy. Janz (1982) also comments on the close relationship between increased seizures and low plasma concentrations of these drugs. In addition to altered pharmacokinetics (Boobis & Lewis, 1982; Philbert & Dam, 1982), low blood levels may be due to reduced drug ingestion as a result of nausea or fear of teratogenic effects (Donaldson, 1978; Bruni & Willmore, 1979; *British Medical Journal*, 1980; Schmidt et al, 1983). In 34 of the 50 patients in the study of Schmidt et al (1983) there was a temporal relationship between seizure relapse and non-compliance or sleep deprivation. The detrimental effect of loss of sleep has been emphasised by Janz (1982) and may be of special relevance. In Schmidt et al's (1983) study, eight of the 23 pregnancies in which patients did not take anticonvulsants were accompanied by an increase in seizures, and sleep deprivation was judged to be responsible for this increase in six of them. Other possible explanations for seizure relapse include sodium and water retention (Philbert & Dam, 1982) and respiratory alkalosis (Bruni & Willmore, 1979; Janz, 1982; Philbert & Dam, 1982). Owing to their convulsive properties in experimental animals, oestrogens, too, have been implicated (Bruni & Willmore, 1979; see Philbert & Dam, 1982; see Magos & Studd, 1985). Schmidt et al (1983) were able to account for an increase in seizures in all but six pregnancies, and concluded there was little evidence that pregnancy *per se* affects the course of epilepsy. Perhaps in these six pregnancies mechanisms were operative similar to those underlying 'gestational epilepsy' and seizures occurring for the first time in pregnancy (Montouris et al, 1979).

Donaldson (1978) and Montouris et al (1979) suggested a decrease in seizure frequency in pregnancy may be the result of better compliance; this, as well as improved therapy or correct sleep, was felt to be responsible in 11 of the 18 such pregnancies in Schmidt et al's (1983) study.

Counselling is an essential part of the management of the epileptic patient who becomes, or plans to become, pregnant (Donaldson, 1978; So & Perry, 1981; Dalessio, 1985). The most appropriate setting may be a combined clinic staffed by an obstetrician and a neurologist (Espir & Hytten, 1983). From a compilation of the cited and reported data in the publications by Hopkins (1977), Donaldson (1978), Bruni & Willmore (1979), Montouris et al (1979), *British Medical Journal* (1980), Cohlan (1980), So & Penry (1981), Graham (1982), Nelson & Ellenberg (1982), Philbert & Dam (1982), and Dalessio (1985), the patient may be advised as follows. First, there is 90 per cent chance overall that the child will be normal, particularly if the patient is not diabetic, her epilepsy is not severe, she is aged under 35 and the family history is negative for congental malformations. Second, the chance of the child developing epilepsy is greater (2–5 per cent) than normal (0.5 per cent) and increases considerably if both parents are epileptic (15 per cent). Third, epileptic mothers may have an excess of complications of pregnancy and there is an increased chance the pregnancy will have an unfavourable outcome. Fourth, an unfavourable outcome may be more likely if seizures occur during the pregnancy; and the risk of an unfavourable outcome from seizures may be greater than the risk of teratogenesis from anticonvulsant drugs. Fifth, the risk of congenital malformations in the child is increased approximately two-fold by the disease and its treatment.

For the pregnant patient with established epilepsy the goal of therapy is optimum seizure control using the least number of drugs with the minimum of side-effects (Montouris et al, 1979). In order to achieve this goal the patient will need to be educated regarding compliance and the need for adequate sleep (Dalessio, 1985). Montouris et al (1979), So & Penry (1981), Philbert & Dam (1982) and Dalessio (1985) advocate therapy in amounts sufficient to achieve therapeutic plasma levels, with monthly monitoring and adjustment of doses accordingly. Others, noting the pharmacokinetics of pregnancy are such that plasma concentrations may not reflect the level of unbound, active drug, recommend the clinical picture be used to guide therapy (*British Medical Journal*, 1980; Janz, 1982). Such factors also underlie the need to observe the patient closely for signs of toxicity postpartum, particularly if dosages have been increased during pregnancy to achieve and maintain therapeutic levels (Janz, 1982); for phenytoin this can be as much as 1.2 g/day (Ramsay et al, 1978). Doses should be reduced after delivery and adjusted in accordance with plasma levels (Montouris et al, 1979). These should be monitored regularly and frequently—Philbert & Dam (1982) and Dalessio (1985) recommend weekly—for 6 months postpartum (So & Penry, 1981) or until dosages have returned to preconception levels (So & Penry, 1981; Philbert & Dam, 1982).

Status epilepticus is no more common in the pregnant than the non-pregnant epileptic (Philbert & Dam, 1982). When it does develop, it tends to do so in the latter half of pregnancy and the maternal and fetal mortality is high (Philbert & Dam, 1982). Treatment should be along conventional lines (Montouris et al, 1979; see Dalessio, 1985 for details); only if drug therapy fails should the pregnancy be terminated as a means to control seizures (Philbert & Dam, 1982).

Seizures occurring for the first time in pregnancy are apt to be accompanied by focal features, both clinically and on EEG. (Montouris et al, 1979; *British Medical Journal*, 1980; Philbert & Dam, 1982). Such patients tend to have structural lesions (Montouris et al, 1979) and should be treated with anticonvulsants (*British Medical Journal*, 1980) and further investigated (Donaldson, 1978; *British Medical Journal*, 1980). For those without such focal features, therapy and investigation should be withheld unless more than one seizure occurs (*British Medical Journal*, 1980). Less than 25 per cent of patients in whom seizures first occur in pregnancy will have recurrent seizures only in subsequent pregnancies; for these patients the term 'gestational epilepsy' is applicable (Montouris et al, 1979).

MULTIPLE SCLEROSIS

The puerperium appears to carry a special risk for both the onset of multiple sclerosis (MS) and the development of relapses (Donaldson, 1978; Poser & Poser, 1983; Korn-Lubetzki et al, 1984). Based on 512 replies to a questionnaire circularised to 639 women with MS, Poser & Poser (1983) reported that onset or deterioration occurred two to three times more often in the 6 months after childbirth than in the 9 months of gestation. Korn-Lubetzki et al (1984) evaluated the number of relapses and relapse rate (number of relapses per person per year) in relation to each trimester of pregnancy and the postpartum period in 66 women with clinically definite or probable MS. Relapses occurred in 85 of the 199 pregnancies, 20 during pregnancy and 65 in the 6 months following delivery. Eleven of the relapses during pregnancy occurred in the first trimester and 32 of the 65 in the postpartum period occurred in the first 3 months. Compared to the relapse rate among age- and sex-matched controls, relapses in MS patients were significantly more frequent in the puerperium (especially the first 3 months) frequent in the puerperium (especially the first 3 months) and significantly less frequent in the third trimester. Relapses were also less frequent in the second trimester but the difference from controls was not statistically significant. When the 15 months of pregnancy and the puerperium were considered together, there was no statistical difference between the observed number of relapses and the expected total number of relapses for that period of time (see Korn-Lubetzki, 1984).

Remission in the latter half of pregnancy and exacerbation postpartum is similar to the pattern seen in a number of other diseases in which autoimmunity is believed to have a pathogenetic role (Froelich et al, 1980; Poser & Poser, 1983; Korn-Lubetzki, 1984). In these diseases, such a pattern may have a mutual relation to the several immunological phenomena that have been described in pregnancy, (Froelich et al, 1980; Abramsky et al, 1984) some of which have been attributed to sex hormones or pregnancy-related proteins. Using experimental allergic encephalomyelitis (EAE) as a model, studies have been undertaken for evidence of possible pregnancy-related immunosuppressive substances that may play a role in MS. Poser et al (1979), Poser & Poser (1983) and Korn-Lubetzki et al (1984) cite accounts of the suppressive influence of sex hormones and pregnancy on EAE, including its deterioration following abortion. In considering what mechanisms may be involved, Poser et al (1979) refer to evidence that oral contraceptives may influence the cellular limb of the immune system. In addition, Abramsky et al (1984) have shown that human alpha-fetoprotein from fetal serum has a suppressive effect on EAE in pregnant animals. This effect may be mediated through the ability of alpha-fetoprotein to activate suppressor cells (Froelich et al, 1980). The possible implications of Abramsky et al's (1984) finding could be far-reaching, since alpha-fetoprotein is found in maternal serum in the second and third trimesters of pregnancy (Abramsky et al, 1979), and suppressor T lymphocytes in the peripheral blood fall before, or during, an attack of MS and reappear when the disease is quiescent (see Behan, 1984).

The use of epidural anaesthesia in labour may also be responsible for relapses of MS in the puerperium (Warren et al, 1982). Discounting any contribution from lumbar puncture *per se*, Warren et al (1982) emphasise that local anaesthetic administered extradurally can penetrate the spinal cord (Bromage, 1975) and that a total of 562·5 mg of bupivacaine was used on the second of the two occasions in which their patient developed a relapse following extradural anaesthesia. It is of interest that this patient developed sensory symptoms each time as Bromage's (1975) studies implied that afferent pathways were the more likely to be effected. Warren et al (1982) conclude, nevertheless, that MS should not be a contraindication to extradural analgesia, particularly in circumstances of a high-risk pregnancy.

On the basis of their study through questionnaire, Poser & Poser (1983) found no evidence of an increased frequency of congenital malformations in the offspring of patients with MS—the three patients treated with steroids or azathioprine included. Their study led them to conclude that pregnancy had no deleterious influence on the overall prognosis of MS. This opinion was stated also by Dalessio (1982). However, both Donaldson (1978) and Dalessio (1982) suggested that MS patients with active disease should perhaps be dissuaded from becoming pregnant.

MYASTHENIA GRAVIS

Pregnancy and the puerperium confer an increased chance of change in a patient with usually stable myasthenia gravis (MG) (Plauché, 1983). Based on a personal series of 314 pregnancies in 217 myasthenia mothers, Plauché (1983) recorded exacerbation in 41 per cent (of which 85 per cent were puerperal), remission in 29 per cent and no change in 31 per cent. These findings are similar to those quoted from earlier studies (see Aminoff, 1978; see Dalessio, 1982). In some patients, changes may be due to factors peculiar to pregnancy itself. For example, exacerbations could result from irregular medication (through nausea or fear of teratogenic effects), the physical stress and demands on the perinatal period and diminished respiratory reserve due to uterine enlargement (Plauché, 1983). Also, exacerbations have been reported in gestational hypertension (Duff, 1979). A further factor was proposed by Abramsky et al (1979), namely, an immunosuppressive effect of amniotic fluid (AF). A brief account of the background to this proposal is indicated.

The cause of neonatal MG is well explained by placental transmission of maternal anti-acetylcholine receptor (AChR) antibodies (see Abramsky et al, 1979). Explanations such as a very high maternal antibody titre (Keesey et al, 1977), heterogeneity of antibody specificity or differences between maternal and fetal AChR (Aarli et al, 1984), have been proposed to account for an incidence of only 10–20 per cent (Plauché, 1983) in infants of myasthenic mothers in whom elevated titres of anti-AChR antibodies occur in over 70 per cent (Newsom-Davies, 1984). Abramsky et al (1979), however, showed that human AF inhibits significantly the reaction between anti-AChR antibodies from patients with MG and the receptor antigen. This inhibitory effect was present in AF in the second trimester and tended to increase from week 16 to week 24 and decline thereafter. In addition to possibly explaining some of the events in neonatal MG, Abramsky et al (1979) suggested that such inhibitory factors, if transferred to maternal serum, could explain remission in the second half of pregnancy and relapse in the puerperium. Citing the work of others, Abramsky et al (1979) reasoned that alpha-fetoprotein (a major component in AF) may be the responsible factor as it has immunosuppressive properties; its maximum output is in the second trimester; it is present in maternal serum in the second and third trimesters; and concentrations fall rapidly in the newborn infant. Varying levels of alpha-fetoprotein in maternal serum might also explain the discrepancy between antibody titres and muscle weakness (Plauché, 1983).

In reporting a maternal and fetal mortality rate of 4·2 per cent and 8·2 per cent, respectively, Plauché (1983) remarked that 'the myasthenic woman who chooses to become pregnant puts herself and child at increased risk'. Measures that might reduce maternal mortality have been identified. They include the substitution of parenteral for oral administration of anticholinesterases at the onset of labour (Plauché, 1979)—using, perhaps, the intravenous route if large volumes and frequent injections are required (Coaldrake & Livingstone, 1983)—and avoiding the use of drugs with effects on the neuromuscular junction (Graham, 1982). Notable in this regard are aminoglycoside antibiotics, procaine and magnesium sulphate (Duff, 1979; Plauché, 1979; Graham, 1982). At the same time as advising that Caesarean section be performed under general anaesthesia, and only for obstetric indications, and that pregnancy be avoided if myasthenia is unstable or yet to be controlled, Plauché (1983) found no evidence in favour of offering abortion to those with exacerbation in the first trimester. This latter view is shared by Coaldrake & Livingstone (1983), who believe also that there is a place for regional anaesthesia in delivery by Caesarean section.

Neonatal MG was present in at least 17·6 per cent of infants in Plauché's (1983) series. In an effort to reduce any added risk to the infant, Plauché (1983) advised that breast feeding be avoided if the mother has high titres of anti-AChR antibodies, citing evidence that titres in the newborn tend to reflect those of the mother, and that neonatal MG tends to develop in infants of mothers with the highest titres. For this reason also, plasmapheresis has been proposed in such mothers (see Plauché, 1983). Whereas anticholinesterases are used in the treatment of neonatal MG—and may be needed in 80 per cent of cases (Donaldson, 1978)—breast feeding should be avoided by mothers taking large doses of these drugs to diminish the chances of producing a 'cholinergic crisis' (Plauché, 1983).

Neonatal mortality—though not the incidence of neonatal MG—may be less in women having undergone thymectomy prior to pregnancy (Eden & Gall, 1983). These authors reported the outcome of 12 pregnancies in eight patients with MG in whom thymectomy had been performed 2 to 25 years prior to conception. Four infants had neonatal MG, one of whom died. From a review of the literature, Eden & Gall (1983) concluded that, although less, the incidence of perinatal mortality in the thymectomy group ($n=18$) was not statistically different from that of the non-thymectomy group ($n=27$). While their series is small, the high incidence (33 per cent) of neonatal MG in Eden & Gall's (1983) own study is noteworthy.

Eden & Gall's (1983) literature review, together with their own experience, led them to conclude that patients with MG who have undergone thymectomy and then become pregnant are more likely than non-thymectomised patients to have no change in their myasthenia during pregnancy. Overall, they believe the case for thymectomy as initial treatment for females in their reproductive years with MG is supported but not proven. In stating this view, however, they stress that thymectomy does carry an operative morbidity and mortality risk.

Premature labour may be more frequent in MG, possibly due to increased amounts of circulating acetylcholine (from anticholinesterase therapy) acting on uterine cholinergic receptors (Coaldrake & Livingstone, 1983). However, apart from closer supervision (Dalessio, 1982) and thymectomy reserved for thymoma only, therapeutic management of the pregnant myasthenic differs in no essential way from the non-pregnant, including the continuation of steroids at the lowest controlling dosage (Plauché, 1983). Whether plasmapheresis has a place in the treatment of MG in pregnancy remains to be determined.

NUTRITIONAL AND METABOLIC DISORDERS

There is probably an increased requirement for thiamin in pregnancy (Vir et al, 1980; Moghissi, 1981) and, in all trimesters, pregnant women may be thiamin-depleted (Kübler, 1981). Neurological complications of thiamin deficiency tend to become manifest, however, when additional factors co-exist. Of these, perhaps the most germane is vomiting in early pregnancy. This may also lead to severe dehydration and the recent literature is notable for accounts of Wernicke encephalopathy (WE) developing or progressing when such patients have been resuscitated with parenteral fluids (Nightingale et al, 1982; Lavin et al, 1983; Watanabe et al, 1983; Wood et al, 1983; Nel et al, 1985). Four of these reports (Nightingale et al, 1982; Lavin et al, 1983; Wood et al, 1983; Nel et al, 1985) record the administration of parenteral glucose without thiamin, reiterating the hazards of such therapy (Victor, 1976). In three of the five reports there is clinical evidence that the patients also had a peripheral neuropathy and that thiamin deficiency was the most probable cause. The patient reported by Nel et al (1985) and Case 1 of Lavin et al (1983) are noteworthy for evidence that the neuropathy was axonal in type, as the majority of cases to date were reported (see McGoogan, 1942) before the development of modern neuro-physiological techniques. Little is known about the effects of thiamin deficiency on the human fetus (Nel et al, 1985). However, Vir et al (1980) found no relationship between biochemical status and fetal dimensions, and both Wood et al (1983) and Nel et al (1985) record that their patients were delivered of a normal or healthy infant. In Nightingale et al's (1982) patient, fetal death occurred *in utero* in week 21; the fetus and placenta were macroscopically normal.

A further factor that may have relevance to the occurrence of WE in pregnancy is hypomagnesaemia. In addition to thiamin, magnesium is a cofactor for transketolase, and dysfunction of this enzyme system is believed to have an aetiological role in WE (Traviesa, 1974). Furthermore, there is clinical and experimental evidence to suggest that, in the presence of thiamin deficiency, lack of magnesium may contribute to the development of WE (see Flink, 1978). Finally, serum magnesium tends to fall progressively during pregnancy (De Flamingh & Van der Merwe, 1984) and may reach 10 per cent below non-pregnant values (see Lind, 1980). With this in mind it is of interest that the patient of Nel et al (1985) had a serum magnesium below normal. This patient's encephalopathy was reversed within 48 hours; there is no record that magnesium was given in addition to thiamin. In Traviesa's (1974) patient with WE and hypomagnesaemia, however, both erythrocyte transketolase activity and ophthalmoplegia became normal only following supplementation of thiamin with magnesium.

In addition to WE, parenteral resuscitation may be complicated by the development of central pontine myelinolysis (CPM) (Goebel & Zur, 1976). Clinically characterised by rapidly envolving paraparesis or quadriparesis with supranuclear bulbar palsy, CPM is currently believed to result from the rapid correction of severe electrolyte derangements, in particular that of plasma sodium (Norenberg et al, 1982). To the author's knowledge, there is only one report of CPM occurring in pregnancy (Kusuyama et al, 1982). A further case was observed personally (Thompson et al, 1986). This patient developed CPM following parenteral resuscitation for consequences of hyperemesis gravidarum that included hyponatraemia and azotaemia. Metabolic abnormalities comprising hypernatraemia and, later, hyperglycaemia were present in Kusuyama et al's (1982) patient, but no details concerning resuscitation are recorded. Both these patients with CPM also manifested features of WE, the co-existence of these two disorders being well recognised (Goebel & Zur, 1976).

PERIPHERAL NEUROPATHY

Pollock et al (1982) reported the subacute development of severe sensory and motor deficits in pregnancy in a patient with hereditary motor and sensory neuropathy type I (Dyck, 1975). Caesarean section was occasioned by increasing weakness and pain. Within 12 hours of delivery the patient was pain-free and by 3 months was symptomatically normal. Mild to moderate sensorimotor deficits were elicited at this time, however, and these persisted unchanged during the subsequent 3 years. A sural nerve biopsy undertaken before delivery showed resolving endoneurial oedema which Pollock et al (1982) suggest may have been causally related to the patient's pregnant state. Emphasising that pregnancy is associated with a substantial decrease in colloid pressure and with water storage in connective tissue ground substance, they cite evidence of median nerve oedema in pregnant patients undergoing carpal tunnel surgery. They point out, furthermore, that the estimated 2·6 litre loss of interstitial fluid after delivery could explain the abrupt improvement in their patient's neuropathic symptoms; and that persistence of increased total body water up to 4 months postpartum could explain the delay in return to the prepregnant state.

Because of the subclinical nature of many inherited neuropathies, Pollock et al (1982) suggested that the kinships of women developing an apparently 'new' polyneuropathy in pregnancy should be evaluated. The possibility of a previously unrecognised inherited demyelinating neuropathy, together with the development of nerve oedema as found by Pollock et al (1982), could provide an explanation for recurrent attacks of idiopathic polyneuropathy in pregnancy (see Novak & Johnson, 1973; Jones & Berry, 1981).

The occurrence of acute idiopathic polyneuritis (Guillain–Barré syndrome) in pregnancy is very uncommon. Bravo et al (1982) were able to locate reports of only 28 cases between 1912 and 1982. These authors noted, however, that such pregnancies were accompanied by a high maternal and perinatal mortality rate. This was attributed to respiratory complications in the mother and the hazards of preterm labour and delivery, respectively. They emphasise that, because of the physiologic changes in respiratory function in pregnancy, it is imperative such patients are carefully evaluated and receive prompt intervention.

PREGNANCY-INDUCED HYPERTENSION AND ECLAMPSIA

Computed tomography of the brain (CT scan) has provided further insight into the mechanisms underlying the neurological symptoms and signs and CSF abnormalities (Fish et al, 1972; Morrison et al, 1972) that occur in eclampsia.

In addition to affirming the presence of cerebral oedema—described in autopsy reports (Chapman & Karimi, 1973; Jewett, 1973), but disputed by some (see Donaldson, 1978)—CT scans have shown areas of hypodensity in cerebral hemisphere white matter (see Kirby & Jaindl, 1984; Gaitz & Bamford, 1982). At the time of manifesting a severe quadriparesis, Gaitz & Bamford's (1982) patient had CT scan hypodensities in the internal and external capsules. The authors attributed the neurological deficit to these findings as the CT scan 10 days later was normal when considerable functional recovery had occurred. Limb hyperreflexia is characteristic of eclampsia (Hibbard & Rosen, 1982) and could be adequately explained by pathological changes in the corpus striatum. It is of interest, therefore, that low density was present in the internal capsule in Case 1 of Kirby & Jaindl (1984) and in the basal ganglia of Liebowitz & Hall's (1984) patient whose signs included hyperreflexia.

The published accounts of CT scan appearances in eclampsia resemble those found in hypertensive encephalopathy (Rail & Perkin, 1981), supporting the notion that the pathophysiology of the cerebral manifestations of these two conditions is similar (Donaldson, 1978). It is therefore possible that the areas of low density described in eclampsia represent infarction or oedema of cerebral tissue as a result of vasospasm. Spasm is held to account for the typical appearances of narrowed retinal arterioles in pre-eclampsia (Kline, 1981) and for their rapid reversion and the usually good prognosis for vision following appropriate treatment (Donaldson, 1978; Gandhi et al,

1978). However, disseminated intravascular coagulation (DIC) is a well-recognised complication of eclampsia (Hibbard & Rosen, 1982) and merits consideration as an alternative mechanism. The case report by McNamee et al (1982) is of particular interest in this regard. Their patient developed postpartum DIC and, 3 days later, blindness accompanied by marked elevation in blood pressure. Within 48 hours of successful antihypertensive therapy the patient's vision was normal. The authors consider a 'vasomotor disturbance' could explain these events. Blindness in eclampsia recovering shortly after delivery and due to cortical dysfunction was reported by Nishimura & Koller (1982) and Liebowitz and Hall (1984); neither of these accounts recorded the development of DIC in their patients. Though smaller in area, the CT scan occipital lobe hypodensities in Liebowitz & Hall's (1984) patient were still present 3 days postpartum. These authors consider the visual disturbance in their patient could be explained on the basis of the vascular changes of hypertensive encephalopathy. In both of Nishmura & Koller's (1982) patients the CT scan was normal, and they postulate that vasospasm was the responsible mechanism.

Whereas the clinical manifestations of PIH normally resolve with delivery, abnormalities in the EEG may persist for some time. Novikov & Palinka (1980) studied 140 patients with 'late toxaemia' and undertook a repeat EEG in 69 of them, 2 months to 4 years after parturition. All 140 patients had an abnormal EEG at the time of 'toxaemia' and abnormalities were present in many of the 69 studied postpartum. The abnormalities were most marked 2–4 days after delivery, but the EEG was not completely restored to normal up to 4 years later. These findings suggest that, where appropriate, a history of hypertension in a recent pregnancy should be sought routinely from patients undergoing EEG studies in the investigation of CNS disorders.

PROLACTINOMA

Patients with prolactin-secreting tumours may become pregnant spontaneously, especially if the degree of hyperprolactinaemia is mild to moderate (i.e. up to approx 70 ng/ml), or following bromocriptine therapy (Crosignani et al, 1984). Such patients pose particular problems of management, since prolactin-secreting tumours may enlarge during pregnancy (Bergh et al, 1978; see Crosignani et al, 1984; Goodman & Chang, 1984) consequent to oestrogen-induced hypertrophy or hyperplasia of lactotrophic cells (Bergh et al, 1978). Crisignani et al (1984) believe that the risks surrounding such enlargement are small unless the tumour is a macroadenoma. Nevertheless, these risks have led to the proposal that such tumours should be ablated, either by irradiation or surgery, before conception (Dalessio, 1982; see Crosignani et al, 1984). Further experience with the use of bromocriptine (Crosignani et al, 1984; Goodman & Chang, 1984), however, lends support to the suggestion that tumour removal may not be necessary in the first instance (Bergh et al, 1978; Hancock et al, 1978).

The two patients reported by Crosignani et al (1984) conceived after treatment with bromocriptine, following which the drug was withdrawn. In the third trimester both of them developed signs of extrasellar extension (in the form of visual deficits), as a result of which bromocriptine was reintroduced. In each case, vision returned to normal within 5 weeks and the pregnancy had a normal outcome. Crosignani et al (1984) emphasise that the rapid and marked resolution of visual deficits in their two patients is similar to the experience of others who have adopted this approach. Goodman & Chang's (1984) patient also conceived after therapy with bromocriptine, but in this case there was radiological evidence of extrasellar extension of the tumour prior to treatment. Moreover, bromocriptine was continued throughout pregnancy. As judged by visual field testing and CT brain scan, there was no evidence of enlargement of the tumour during this time and the patient underwent a normal delivery at term with the birth of a healthy infant. This successful outcome provides additional evidence for the safety of bromocriptine in pregnancy (Turkalj et al, 1982).

The use of bromocriptine in the management of the pregnant patient with a prolactin-secreting pituitary adenoma demands careful monitoring of tumour size. This entails regular and frequent assessments of visual fields and visual acuity. The results of endocrinological tests should not be used alone as criteria for tumour growth, for they may be misleading (Goodman & Chang, 1984). So too may the size of the pituitary fossa as judged by skull X-ray, since considerable extrasellar extension can occur if there is a large diaphragma opening (Burry et al, 1978). At present, CT brain scan is the definitive imaging study for assessment of tumour size.

If complications due to extrasellar extension are not controlled by bromocriptine, the stage of gestation determines whether the tumour should be ablated or labour induced (Hancock et al, 1978).

DRUGS USED IN NEUROLOGICAL DISORDERS

Two essential considerations regulate drug therapy in pregnancy. First, adverse effects on the fetus (Ellis & Fidler, 1982); and second, altered pharmacokinetics (Boobis & Lewis, 1982). Virtually all drugs are able to transfer to the embryo and fetus from fertilisation to term (Hollingsworth, 1977), with teratogenic effects characterising the first trimester and defects of growth and development thereafter (Ellis & Fidler, 1982; McEwan, 1982). In addition, the physiological consequences of pregnancy result in diminished absorption, altered distribution and increased metabolism and excretion of drugs (Bruni & Willmore, 1979; Boobis & Lewis, 1982). These pharmacokinetic changes may be influenced by iron and folic acid intake (Philbert & Dam, 1982).

Anticoagulants

'A fully satisfactory anticoagulant regime for pregnant women does not exist at present' (Tooke & McNicol, 1981). Warfarin readily crosses the placenta and may be teratogenic (*British Medical Journal*, 1979; Cohlan, 1980; Stevenson et al, 1980; Kort & Cassel, 1981; Ellis & Fidler, 1982). Also, it is associated with a high incidence of haemorrhagic complications (Ellis & Fidler, 1982), Indeed, Laros & Alger (1979) believe the hazards are such as to contraindicate the use of coumarin agents in pregnancy. Because placental transfer does not occur (*British Medical Journal*, 1979), heparin is the preferred alternative for those requiring long-term anticoagulants. If, however, such patients are unable to tolerate repeated injections, the use of herparin may be confined to the first trimester and from week 36 to term, with warfarin prescribed in the intervening period (*British Medical Journal*, 1979; Kort & Cassel, 1981; Ellis & Fidler, 1982). Altered drug distribution and variations in clotting factors (Boobis & Lewis, 1982; Whitfield et al, 1983) demand close monitoring of anticoagulant activity.

Anticonvulsants

There is an approximately two-fold increased risk for the development of congenital malformations in the offspring of epileptic mothers taking anticonvulsants in pregnancy (Donaldson, 1978; Bruni & Willmore, 1979; Montouris et al, 1979; Cohlan, 1980; So & Penry, 1981; Ellis & Fidler, 1982; Janz, 1982; Philbert & Dam, 1982; Dalessio, 1985). It has yet to be established that anticonvulsants *per se* are wholly responsible, however (Bruni & Willmore, 1979; Montouris et al, 1979; So & Penry, 1981; Graham, 1982; Janz, 1982). The evidence for teratogenic effects is strongest in the case of trimethadione; highly suspect for phenytoin; and suggestive for phenobarbitone, primidone, carbamazepine and sodium valproate (Montouris et al, 1979; *British Medical Journal*, 1980; Cohlan, 1980; So & Penry, 1981; *Lancet*, 1982; Ellis & Fidler, 1982; Graham, 1982; Janz, 1982; Philbert & Dam, 1982; Robert et al, 1984; Dalessio, 1985). Reports of pregnant epileptics treated exclusively with clonazepam (Kriel & Cloyd, 1982) are too few for its evaluation in this context.

While epileptic women should be advised about these increased risks, beyond withdrawing trimethadione (So & Penry, 1981) and avoiding sodium valproate (*Lancet*, 1982; Dalessio, 1985), there may be no justification for altering therapy (Dalessio, 1982; Janz, 1982). As a result of reports linking sodium valproate to neural tube defects, it has been proposed that pregnant epileptics known to have taken this drug in the first trimester should be offered amniocentesis with a view to therapeutic abortion if levels of alpha-fetoprotein are markedly elevated (*Lancet*, 1982; Dalessio, 1985). In the context of possible teratogenic effects, it is of interest that total sodium valproate levels were higher in umbilical cord than maternal serum in all 118 cases studied by Froescher et al (1984). Noting this finding has been recorded in most other studies, these authors believe the lower maternal levels can be explained, at least in part, by lower serum protein binding.

Maternal anticonvulsant therapy, including phenytoin and barbiturates, may be associated with a neonatal haemorrhagic diathesis (Bruni & Willmore, 1979; Montouris et al, 1979; So & Penry, 1981; Deblay et al, 1982; Ellis & Fidler, 1982; Philbert & Dam, 1982). This is related to a decrease in vitamin K-dependent coagulation factors (Bruni & Willmore, 1979; Montouris et al, 1979; So & Penry, 1981) and is due to the anticonvulsants *per se* (Davies et al, 1985), probably as a result of fetal hepatic microsomal enzyme induction (Bruni & Willmore, 1979; Philbert & Dam, 1982). A low neonatal prothrombin can be prevented with maternal oral vitamin K_1 20 mg/day for 2 weeks prior to delivery (Deblay et al, 1982). Alternatively, the infant may be given 1 mg vitamin K_1 parenterally at birth and repeated as necessary to normalise coagulation tests which should be performed every 2–4 hours (Montouris et al, 1979; So & Penry, 1981; Dalessio, 1982).

Neonatal metabolism and elimination of benzodiazepines and barbiturates is such that a risk exists of intoxication in the first few days, especially if the infant is preterm (Philbert & Dam, 1982). Also, infants breast-fed by mothers taking more than 90 mg phenobarbitone per day should be monitored for signs of intoxication in the first week (So & Penry, 1981; Philbert & Dam, 1982). A syndrome characterised by hypothermia, hypotonia and reluctance to feed may occur when (in treating status epilepticus, for example) the mother is prescribed more than 30 mg diazepam (So & Penry, 1981; Ellis & Fidler, 1982; McEwan, 1982). In addition, neonates exposed to barbiturates in late pregnancy may develop features of withdrawal such as restlessness, tremors, hyperreflexia and vasomotor instability 6–7 days after birth (So & Penry, 1981).

As a result of altered pharmacokinetics, plasma levels of several anticonvulsants tend to fall in pregnancy (Janz, 1982; Philbert & Dam, 1982) and increase in the puerperium (Janz, 1982). These changes are reported most marked for phenytoin, less so for phenobarbitone and least for primidone and carbamazepine (Janz, 1982). The limited published data suggest plasma levels of sodium valproate may fall (Froescher et al, 1984) whereas, despite evidence of accelerated metabolism and clearance (Philbert & Dam, 1982), those of clonazepam may rise (Kriel & Cloyd, 1982). However, plasma levels do not indicate the free, biologically active, drug concentration; this may remain unaltered or be increased, as in the case of sodium valproate (Froescher et al, 1984) and highly protein-bound drugs such as phenytoin (Boobis & Lewis, 1982; Janz, 1982).

Antimicrobial agents

The treatment of CNS tuberculosis in pregnancy poses special problems. Streptomycin is ototoxic to the fetus (Boobis & Lewis, 1982; Ellis & Fidler, 1982), the risk being approximately 15 per cent and present throughout pregnancy (Snider et al, 1980), and rifampicin is potentially hazardous as it crosses the placenta, interferes with nucleic acid synthesis and may increase the risk of hypoprothrombinaemia (Donaldson, 1978; Ellis & Fidler, 1982). From an analysis of the outcome of pregnancies of women taking antituberculous therapy, Snider et al (1980) concluded there was no proof that isoniazid, ethambutol or rifampicin were teratogenetic to the human fetus. These authors recommend that isoniazid and ethambutol are the drugs of first choice; that rifampicin be used if a third drug is indicated; and that streptomycin should not be used unless the others are contraindicated.

The optimum therapy for cryptococcal infection of the CNS is a combination of amphotericin B and 5-fluorocytosine (Curole, 1981). Both drugs cross the placenta (Stafford et al, 1983) and, owing to its metabolism to 5-fluorouracil, 5-fluorocytosine has a particular teratogenic potential (Curole, 1981). Fetal toxic effects remain to be determined, however, and on the basis of their experiences and published reports, Stafford et al (1983) recommended that cryptococcal meningitis in pregnancy should be treated with standard therapy. More experience with the use of 5-fluorocytosine and of both drugs in the first trimester (see Curole, 1981) is needed to qualify this advice.

Chloramphenicol should not be used in late pregnancy as it may give rise to the 'grey syndrome' (McEwan, 1982), a neotal disorder with a high mortality rate.

Antipsychotics

Phenothiazines readily cross the placenta, but Dalessio (1982) noted that there were no descriptions of congenital anomalies associated with their use. Though tricyclics also are not contraindicated in pregnancy, lithium should be prescribed with caution in view of the risks of cardiac malformations (see Dalessio, 1982).

Benzodiazepines

Donaldson (1978) cites evidence associating orofacial clefts in the offspring of pregnant women taking benzodiazepines in the first trimester and these drugs, particularly diazepam, are categorised by Cohlan (1980) and Ellis & Fidler (1982) as possible teratogens.

Corticosteroids

While classified as 'suspect' teratogens and therefore to be prescribed judiciously (Cohlan, 1980), corticosteroids are not contraindicated for treating neurological disorders in pregnancy (McEwan, 1982).

Mannitol

The use of mannitol in pregnancy is dangerous (Donaldson, 1978). Experimental studies in which plasma osmolarity was increased by 25 per cent produced fetal dehydration, cyanosis and bradycardia as a result of passage of water and amniotic fluid to the mother (Briani et al, 1980).

Penicillamine

Though a fetal connective tissue defect has been ascribed to the use of D-penicillamine for maternal cystinuria (Mjolnerod et al, 1971) and for rheumatoid arthritis (Solomon et al, 1977), Lyle (1978) concluded from the published accounts there was no evidence this drug was teratogenic when taken throughout pregnancy for Wilson disease, nor were there any contraindications for its use in the pregnant patient with the disorder. Solomon et al (1977) suggested the absence of serious side-effects in such circumstances may be due to chelation of penicillamine with copper, thereby effectively reducing the drug level.

Salicylates

The use of salicylates should be avoided in late pregnancy. As a result of their antiprostaglandin effects, there is an increased risk of postpartum haemorrhage and an association with premature closure of the ductus arteriosus and neonatal haemorrhage (McEwan, 1982).

SPECIAL INVESTIGATIONS

Laboratory studies

(To preserve authenticity, the units of measurement used in the original articles have been maintained.)

Haematology and blood chemistry

Normal haematological and biochemical parameters in pregnancy have been detailed in reviews by Lind (1980) and Tooke & McNicol (1981) and in studies by Davison et al (1981), Olsson (1982) and De Flamingh & Van der Merwe (1984). The general trends and certain pertinent values will be considered here.

In subjects not taking haematinics there is an increase in total red cell volume and a fall in packed cell volume (PCV), haemoglobin, total serum iron, red cell folate (to 150 mg/ml) and serum B_{12} (to 240 pg/ml) (Lind, 1980). An increased plasma volume explains the fall in PCV and probably underlies (Tooke & McNicol, 1981) reports (Olsson, 1982) of a fall in platelet count. The total white cell count may increase to 10 000/mm^3 and the (whole blood) ESR to a mean of 78 mm in 1 hour (range, 44 to 144) (Lind, 1980).

Though concentrations of sodium and potassium fall, they remain within the non-pregnant range (Lind, 1980; De Flamingh & Van der Merwe, 1984). These changes are nevertheless sufficient to reduce plasma osmolality by 10 m Osmol/kg (Lind, 1980; Davison et al, 1981), the lower level being maintained by a reset osmoregulatory system (Davison et al, 1981; *British Medical Journal*, 1978). A similar mechanism involving the respiratory centre has been invoked to explain overbreathing from early pregnancy (*British Medical Journal*, 1978). This may produce a fall in $Paco_2$ to 30 mmHg or less; a compensatory decrease in bicarbonate and an elevation in pH follow (Lim et al, 1976).

There are appreciable decreases in calcium and magnesium (both by approximately 10 per cent), phosphate, albumin (by 7·5 g/ℓ) and IgG (by 1 g/ℓ) (Lind, 1980; De Flamingh & Van der Merwe, 1984). Similar changes in urea (by approximately 25 per cent) and creatinine (to 0·5 mg/dℓ) necessitate the use of revised criteria for diagnosing early renal damage in pregnancy (Lind, 1980, De Flamingh & Van der Merwe, 1984). The level of uric acid falls in the first trimester and that of creatinine phosphokinase (CPK) in the first 20 weeks (to 21 IU/ml), both thereafter rising to non-pregnant levels at term. Suspected Duchenne muscular dystrophy carriers should therefore not have CPK estimations during the first half of pregnancy (Lind, 1980). There are no noteworthy changes in transaminases, dehydrogenases, amylase or acid phosphatase, but levels of alkaline phosphatase increase markedly due to a placenta-derived fraction (Lind, 1980; De Flamingh & Van der Merwe, 1984). All blood lipid fractions are elevated at term and, apart from cholesterol which falls in the first trimester, rise progressively throughout gestation (Lind, 1980). An increase in alpha-2-globulin explains the increase in caeruloplasmin (to 48 mg/dl) (Lind, 1980), but pregnancy produces no consistent changes of copper metabolism in Wilson disease (see Donaldson, 1978).

Serological test for syphilis

Pregnancy is one of a number of conditions in which blood tests for syphilis may yield false-positive results (Morton & Gollow, 1978; Holmes, 1983). Such results are found with non-treponemal and treponemal tests (Morton & Gollow, 1978; Holmes, 1983; Naicker et al, 1983). The latter include the *Treponema pallidum* haemagglutination (TPHA) and fluorescent treponemal antibody absorption (FTA-ABS) tests. Only a positive *T. pallidum* immobilisation (TPI) test provides conclusive proof of past or present treponemal infection (Holmes, 1983). Owing to the care and skill required— as well as its expense—the TPI test is reserved for the resolution of problem cases (Morton & Gollow, 1978). That said, it should be noted that past infection with other treponemes, such as those producing yaws or pinta, can cause a positive TPI test result (Holmes, 1983).

Using a positive FTA-ABS test result as the reference standard for the diagnosis of syphilis, Naicker et al (1983) found false-positive results for the non-treponemal rapid plasma reagent (RPR) test in 11·8 per cent, and for the TPHA test in 15·8 per cent, of 500 antenatal subjects. The RPR and TPHA tests correlated well for these results. As judged by a positive IgM FTA-ABS test result, the RPR test failed to detect active syphilis in 18·9 per cent; there were no false-negative results for the TPHA test. Naicker et al (1983) therefore recommend that the TPHA test, and not the RPR test, should be used for screening pregnant subjects; and that the FTA-ABS test should be used if the TPHA test result is positive.

Urine microscopy and chemistry

Marchant (1978) emphasised the paucity of information available concerning the normal urinary sediment in pregnancy. The mean excretion of red cells and white cells may be greater than normal—i.e. any red cells and more than five white cells per high-power field. Compared to non-pregnant female values of 40–120 mg, urine protein excretion in pregnancy may reach 250–300 mg in 24 hours; the excretion of creatinine and urea are not altered (Marchant, 1978). Pregnancy does not affect the ability either to concentrate or to dilute urine (Marchant, 1978; Davison et al, 1981).

Electrocardiogram

The electrocardiograms of 120 healthy pregnant subjects were studied by Carruth et al (1981). They found the heart rate increased throughout pregnancy, being faster by up to 20 beats per minute in the third trimester. The axis of the QRS complex showed a small rightward deviation in the first trimester and a small leftward deviation in the third. Overall, there was a leftward deviation of the mean T wave axis. There were no significant changes in the cardiac rhythm or ECG intervals.

Electroencephalogram

It remains to be established whether changes in the encephalogram occur during uncomplicated pregnancy. Abnormalities consisting of high-amplitude theta waves and generalised sharp waves have been reported in 10–30 per cent of healthy pregnant women (see Novikov & Palinka, 1980). In their own study, Novikov & Palinka (1980) found no significant changes in 15 pregnant subjects before parturition. However, moderate changes, including excess theta activity, were found during the first 6 days thereafter. These authors believe studies recording abnormalities during gestation may have included subjects with past cerebral disorders, or the EEG findings may have reflected the effects of hypertension in a previous pregnancy. Alternatively, they could have been an early sign of preclinical PIH in the current pregnancy.

Lumbar cerebrospinal fluid

Lumbar puncture should not be withheld because the patient is pregnant (Dalessio, 1982). Davis (1979) reported the results of cerebrospinal fluid studies in 44 pregnant subjects at term. In all of them, opening pressure, white cell count, total protein and protein electrophoresis were normal. Normal results were also found in 21 patients 1–4 days postpartum.

Neuroimaging

Though pregnancy is not a contraindication to neuroimaging studies (Dalessio, 1982), any study should if possible be delayed until after the first trimester (Moseley, in press). Subsequently, plain radiographs of the skull and cervical spine, CT brain scanning (including the use of contrast) and angiography may be undertaken as necessary with as effective shielding of the abdomen as possible (Dalessio, 1982; Moseley, in press). In general, fluoroscopy should be limited and the number of exposures kept to a minimum (Moseley, in press). X-rays of the chest and thoracic and lumbar spines should be undertaken only with the most compelling indications (Dalessio, 1982; Moseley, in press). Myelography poses the most serious problem as it involves fluoroscopy; cervical studies may be performed provided there is adequate shielding, but studies of the thoracic and lumbar regions should be avoided (Dalessio, 1982).

Certain intravascular radionuclides cross the placenta and therefore isotope encephalograms should be postponed until at least the second half of pregnancy. Though the reasoning is arbitrary, it has been recommended that magnetic resonance imaging should not be performed in the first trimester (Moseley, in press).

ACKNOWLEDGEMENTS

I wish to thank Professor Jan Van der Merwe, Dr Marina Greyling and Dr Philip Thompson for their valuable comments, Miss A C Venter and the Medical Library, University of Pretoria for bibliographic assistance, and Mrs J J Edwards for typing the manuscript.

REFERENCES

Aarli J A, Gilhus N E, Hofstad H, Thunold S 1984 Immunology of myasthenia gravis. In: Callaghan N, Galvin R (eds) Recent research in neurology. Pitman, London, ch 14, pp 146–156

Abramsky O, Brenner T, Lisak R P, Zeidman A, Beyth Y 1979 Significance in neonatal myasthenia gravis of inhibitory effect of amniotic fluid on binding of antibodies to acetylcholine receptor. Lancet 2: 1333–1335

Abramsky O, Lubetzki-Korn I, Evron S, Brenner T 1984 Suppressive effect of pregnancy on MS and EAE. Progress in Clinical and Biological Research 146: 399–406

Agrawal B L, Foa R P 1982 Collagen vascular disease appearing as chorea gravidarum. Archives of Neurology 39: 192–193

Aminoff M J 1978 Neurological disorders and pregnancy. American Journal of Obstetrics and Gynecology 132: 325–335

Beal M F, Chapman P H 1980 Cortical blindness and homonymous hemianopia in the postpartum period. Journal of the American Medical Association 244: 2085–2087

Behan W M H 1984 Laboratory tests in neuroimmunological disorders. In: Callaghan N, Galvin R (eds) Recent research in neurology. Pitman, London, ch 12, pp 117–131

Bergh T, Nillius S J, Wide L 1978 Clinical course and outcome of pregnancies in amenorrhoeic women with hyperprolactinaemia and pituitary tumours. British Medical Journal 1: 875–880

Boobis A R, Lewis P 1982 Drugs in pregnancy. Altered pharmacokinetics. British Journal of Hospital Medicine 28: 566–573

Bravo R H, Katz M, Inturrisi M, Cohen N H 1982 Obstetric management of Landry-Guillain Barré Syndrome: A case report. American Journal of Obstetrics and Gynecology 142: 714–715

Briani S, Cagnoni G, Benvenuti L, Guizzardi G, Morichi R 1980 Neurosurgical indications during pregnancy. Clinical and Experimental Obstetrics and Gynecology 7: 13–16

British Medical Journal Editorial 1978 Dyspnoea in normal pregnancy. British Medical Journal 2: 380–381

British Medical Journal Editorial 1979 Thromboembolism in pregnancy. British Medical Journal 1: 1661

British Medical Journal Editorial 1980 Epilepsy and pregnancy. British Medical Journal 2: 1087–1088

Bromage P R 1975 Mechanism of action of extradural analgesia. British Journal of Anaesthesia 47: suppl 199–211

Bruni J, Willmore L J 1979 Epilepsy and pregnancy. Canadian Journal of Neurological Sciences 6: 345–349

Burry K A, Schiller H S, Mills R, Harris B, Heinrichs L 1978 Acute visual loss during pregnancy after bromocriptine-induced ovulation. The elusive tumor. Obstetrics and Gynecology 52: (1 suppl) 19S–22S

Caroscio J T, Pelimar M 1978 Pseudotumor cerebri: Occurrence during the third trimester of pregnancy. Mount Sinai Journal of Medicine 45: 539–541

Carruth J E, Mirvis S B, Brogan D R, Wenger N K 1981 The electrocardiogram in normal pregnancy. American Heart Journal 102: 1075–1078

Chapman K, Karimi R 1973 A case of postpartum eclampsia of late onset confirmed by autopsy. American Journal of Obstetrics and Gynecology 117: 858–861

Coaldrake L A, Livingstone P 1983 Myasthenia gravis in pregnancy. Anaesthesia and Intensive Care 11: 254–257

Cohlan S Q 1980 Drugs and pregnancy. Progess in Clinical and Biological Research 44: 77–96

Crosignani P, Ferrari C, Mattei A M 1984 Visual field defects and reduced visual acuity during pregnancy in two patients with prolactinoma: rapid regression of symptoms under bromocriptine. Case reports. British Journal of Obstetrics and Gynaecology 91: 821–823

Curole D N 1981 Cryptococcal meningitis in pregnancy. Journal of Reproductive Medicine 26: 317–319

Dalessio D J 1982 Neurologic diseases. In: Burrow G N, Ferris T F (eds) Medical complications during pregnancy, 2nd edn. Saunders, Philadelphia, ch 18, p 435–473

Dalessio D J 1985 Seizure disorders and pregnancy. New England Journal of Medicine 312: 559–563

Davies V A, Argent A C, Staub H, Rothberg A D, Atkinson P M, Pienaar N L 1985 Precursor prothrombin status in patients receiving anticonvulsant drugs. Lancet i: 126–128

Davis L E 1979 Normal laboratory values of CSF during pregnancy. Archives of Neurology 36: 443

Davison J M, Vallotton M B, Lindheimer M D 1981 Plasma osmolality and urinary concentration and dilution during and after pregnancy: Evidence that lateral recumbency inhibits maximal urinary concentrating ability. British Journal of Obstetrics and Gynaecology 88: 472–479

Deblay M F, Vert P, Andre M, Marchal F 1982 Transplacental vitamin K prevents haemorrhagic disease of infant of epileptic mother. Lancet 1: 1247

De Flamingh J P G, Van der Merwe J V 1984 A serum biochemical profile of normal pregnancy. South African Medical Journal 65 : 552–555

Digre K B, Varner M W, Corbett J J 1984 Pseudotumor cerebri and pregnancy. Neurology 34 : 721–729

Donaldson J O 1978 Neurology of Pregnancy. Saunders, Philadelphia

Donaldson J O 1981 Stroke. Clinics in Obstetrics and Gynecology 24 : 825–835

Duff G B 1979 Preeclampsia and the patient with myasthenia gravis. Obstetrics and Gynecology 54 : 355–358

Dyck P J 1975 Inherited neuronal degeneration and atrophy affecting peripheral motor, sensory and autonomic neurons. In : Dyck P J, Thomas P K, Lambert E H (eds) Peripheral Neuropathy, vol 2. Saunders, Philadelphia, ch 41, pp 825–867

Eden R D, Gall S A 1983 Myasthenia gravis and pregnancy : a reappraisal of thymectomy. Obstetrics and Gynecology 62 : 328–333

Ellis C, Fidler J 1982 Drugs in pregnancy. Adverse reactions. British Journal of Hospital Medicine 28 : 575–584

Espir M L E, Hytten F E 1983 Pregnancy with epilepsy—the need for combined care. British Journal of Obstetrics and Gynaecology 90 : 1105–1106

Fehr P E 1982 Sagittal sinus thrombosis in early pregnancy. Obstetrics and Gynecology 59 : (6 suppl) 7S–9S

Fish S A, Morrison J C, Bucovaz E T, Wiser W L, Whybrew W D 1972 Cerebral spinal fluid studies in eclampsia. American Journal of Obstetrics and Gynecology 112 : 502–512

Flink E B 1978 Role of magnesium depletion in Wernicke-Korsakoff syndrome. New England Journal of Medicine 298 : 743–744

Froelich C J, Goodwin J S, Bankhurst A D, Williams R C 1980 Pregnancy, a temporary fetal graft of suppressor cells in autoimmune disease. American Journal of Medicine 69 : 329–331

Froescher W, Gugler R, Niesen M, Hoffman F 1984 Protein binding of valproic acid in maternal and umbilical cord serum. Epilepsia 25 : 244–249

Gaitz J P, Bamford C R 1982 Unusual computed tomographic scan in eclampsia. Archives of Neurology 39 : 66

Gandhi J, Ghosh S, Pillari V T 1978 Blindness and retinal changes with preeclamptic toxemia. New York State Journal of Medicine 78 : 1930–1932

Goebel H H, Zur P H-B 1976 Central pontine myelinolysis. In : Vinken P J, Bruyn G W (eds) Handbook of clinical neurology, vol 28 : The metabolic and deficiency diseases of the nervous system, part II. North Holland, Amsterdam, ch 11, pp 285–316

Goodman L A, Chang R J 1984 Pregnancy after bromocriptine-induced reduction of an extrasellar prolactin-secreting pituitary microadenoma. Obstetrics and Gynecology 63 (3 suppl) : 2S–7S

Graham J G 1982 Neurological complications of pregnancy and anaesthesia. Clinics in Obstetrics and Gynaecology 9 : 333–350

Hancock K W, Scott J S, Gibson R M, Lamb J T 1978 Pituitary tumours and pregnancy. British Medical Journal i : 1487–1488

Hibbard B M, Rosen M 1982 The management of eclampsia. Clinics in Obstetrics and Gynaecology 9 : 297–309

Hollingsworth M 1977 Drugs and pregnancy. Clinics in Obstetrics and Gynaecology 4 : 503–521

Holmes K K 1983 Syphilis. In : Petersdorf R G, Adams R D, Braunwald E, Isselbacher K J, Martin J B, Wilson J D (eds) Harrison's principles of internal medicine, 10th edn. McGraw-Hill, New York, ch 177, p 1041

Hopkins A 1977 Neurological disorders. Clinics in Obstetrics and Gynaecology 4 : 419–433

Ichikawa K, Kim R C, Givelber H, Collins G H 1980 Chorea gravidarum. Report of a fatal case with neuropathological observations. Archives of Neurology 37 : 429–432

Janz D 1982 Antiepileptic drugs and pregnancy : Altered utilisation patterns and teratogenesis. Epilepsia 23 (suppl 1) : S53–S63

Jewett J F 1973 Fatal intracranial edema from eclampsia. New England Journal of Medicine 289 : 976–977

Jones M W, Berry K 1981 Chronic relapsing polyneuritis associated with pregnancy. Annals of Neurology 9 : 413

Kassam S H, Hadi H A, Fadel H E, Sims W, Jay W M 1983 Benign intracranial hypertension in pregnancy : current diagnostic and therapeutic approach. Obstetrical and Gynaecological Survey 38 : 314–321

Keesey J, Lindstrom J, Cokeley H, Hermann C 1977 Anti-acetylcholine receptor antibody in neonatal myasthenia gravis. New England Journal of Medicine 296 : 55

Kelton J G, Hirsh J 1982 Venous thromboembolic disorders. In : Burrow G N, Ferris T F (eds) Medical complications during pregnancy, 2nd edn. Saunders, Philadelphia, ch 7, pp 169–186

Kirby J C, Jaindl J J 1984 Cerebral CT findings in toxemia of pregnancy. Radiology 151 : 114

Kline L B 1981 Retinopathy in toxemia of pregnancy. Southern Medical Journal 74 : 34–36

Koontz W L, Herbert W N P, Cefalo R C 1983 Pseudotumor cerebri in pregnancy. Obstetrics and Gynecology 62 : 324–327

Korn-Lubetzki I, Kahana E, Cooper G, Abramsky O 1984 Activity of multiple sclerosis during pregnancy and puerperium. Annals of Neurology 16 : 229–231

Kort H I, Cassel G A 1981 An appraisal of warfarin therapy during pregnancy. South African Medical Journal 60 : 578–579

Kriel R L, Cloyd J 1982 Clonazepam and pregnancy. Annals of Neurology 11 : 544

Kübler W 1981 Nutritional deficiencies in pregnancy. Biblioteca Nutritio et Dieta 30 : 17–29

Kusuyama Y, Tanaka S, Sakatsuji K, Nishihara T, Saito K, Ikeda K, Inui J, Iwahashi Y 1982 Central pontine myelinolysis. An Immunofluorescent study. Acta Pathologica Japonica 32 : 725–732

Lancet Editorial 1982 Valproate and malformations. Lancet 2 ; 1313

Lancet Editorial 1984 Lupus anticoagulant. Lancet 1 : 1157–1158

Laros R K, Alger L S 1979 Thromboembolism and pregnancy. Clinics in Obstetrics and Gynecology 22 : 871–888

Lavin P J M, Bone I, Lamb J T, Swinburne L M 1978 Intracranial venous thrombosis in the first trimester of pregnancy. Journal of Neurology, Neurosurgery and Psychiatry 41 : 726–729

Lavin P J M, Smith D, Kori S H, Ellenberger C 1983 Wernicke's encephalopathy : A predictable complication of hyperemesis gravidarum. Obstetrics and Gynecology 62 : (3 suppl) 13S–15S

Liebowitz H A, Hall P E 1984 Cortical blindness as a complication of eclampsia. Annals of Emergency Medicine 13 : 365–367

Lim V S, Katz A I, Lindheimer M D 1976 Acid base regulation in pregnancy. American Journal of Physiology 231 : 1764–1770

Lind T 1980 Clinical chemistry of pregnancy. Advances in Clinical Medicine 21 : 1–24

Lubbe W F, Walker E B 1983 Chorea gravidarum associated with circulating lupus anticoagulant : successful outcome of pregnancy with prednisone and aspirin therapy. Case report. British Journal of Obstetrics and Gynaecology 90 : 487–490

Lyle W H 1978 Penicillamine in pregnancy. Lancet 1 : 606–607

Magos A, Studd J 1985 Effects of the menstrual cycle on medical disorders. British Journal of Hospital Medicine 33 : 68–77

McEwan H P 1982 Drugs in pregnancy. Prescribing. British Journal of Hospital Medicine 28 : 559–565

Marchant D J 1978 Laboratory values and diagnostic tests. Clinics in Obstetrics and Gynecology 21 : 937–944

McGoogan L S 1942 Severe polyneuritis due to vitamin B deficiency in pregnancy. American Journal of Obstetrics and Gynecology 43 : 752–762

McNamee P T, McComb J M, O'Connor F A, Adgey A A J 1982 Complete recovery from late puerperal eclampsia with associated blindness. International Journal of Cardiology 1 : 327–328

Mjolnerod O K, Rasmussen K, Dommerud S A, Gjeruldsen S T 1971 Congenital connective tissue defect probably due to D-penicillamine treatment in pregnancy. Lancet 1 : 673–675

Moghissi K S 1981 Risks and benefits of nutritional supplements during pregnancy. Obstetrics and Gynecology 58 (5 suppl) : 68S–78S

Monteiro M L R, Hoyt W F, Imes R K 1984 Puerperal cerebral blindness. Transient bilateral occipital involvement from presumed cerebral venous thrombosis. Archives of Neurology 41 : 1300–1301

Montouris G D, Fenichel G M, McLain L W 1979 The pregnant epileptic : A review and recommendations. Archives of Neurology 36 : 601–603

Morrison J C, Whybrew D W, Wiser W L, Bucovaz E T, Fish S A 1972 Laboratory characteristics in toxemia. Obstetrics and Gynecology 39 : 866–872

Morton R S, Gollow M M 1978 Laboratory support in the management of syphilis. Medical Journal of Australia 1: 378–383

Moseley I In press. Imaging in neurological disease. Pitman, London

Naicker S N, Moodley J, van Middelkoop A, Cooper R C 1983 Serological diagnosis of syphilis in pregnancy. Experiences at King Edward VIII Hospital, Durban. South African Medical Journal 63: 536–537

Nausieda P A, Koller W C, Weiner W J, Klawans H L 1979 Chorea induced by oral contraceptives. Neurology 29: 1605–1609

Nel J T, Van Heyningen C F, Van Eeden S F, Labadarios D, Louw N S 1985 Thiamin deficiency gestational polyneuropathy and encephalopathy. South African Medical Journal 67: 600–603

Nelson K B, Ellenberg J H 1982 Maternal seizure disorder, outcome of pregnancy, and neurologic abnormalities in the children. Neurology 32: 1247–1254

Newsom-Davis J 1984 Myasthenia. In: Matthews W B, Glaser G H (eds) Recent advances in clinical neurology, No. 4. Churchill Livingstone, Edinburgh, ch 1, pp 1–18

Nightingale S, Bates D, Heath P D Barron S L 1982 Wernicke's encephalopathy in hyperemesis gravidarum. Postgraduate Medical Journal 58: 558–559

Nishimura R N, Koller R 1982 Isolated cortical blindness in pregnancy. Western Journal of Medicine 137: 335–337

Norenberg M D, Leslie K O, Robertson A S 1982 Association between rise in serum sodium and central pontine myelinolysis. Annals of Neurology 13: 232–242

Novak D J, Johnson K P 1973 Relapsing idiopathic polyneuritis during pregnancy. Immunological aspects and literature review. Archives of Neurology 28: 219–223

Novikov Y I, Palinka G K 1980 EEG changes in late toxemias of pregnancy. Human Physiology 6: 423–430

Olsson J E 1982 Comparison between induced platelet aggregation and circulating platelet aggregates as platelet function tests in patients with transient ischemic attacks. Acta Neurologica Scandinavica 65: 122–132

Palop R, Choed-Amphai E, Miller R 1979 Epidural anaesthesia for delivery complicated by benign intracranial hypertension. Anesthesiology 50: 159–160

Patterson J F 1979 Treatment of chorea gravidarum with haloperidol. Southern Medical Journal 72: 1220–1221

Philbert A, Dam M 1982 The epileptic mother and her child. Epilepsia 23: 85–99

Plauché W C 1979 Myasthenia gravis in pregnancy: An update. American Journal of Obstetrics and Gynecology 135: 691–697

Plauché W C 1983 Myasthenia gravis. Clinics in Obstetrics and Gynecology 26: 592–604

Pollock M, Nukada H, Kritchevsky M 1982 Exacerbation of Charcot-Marie-Tooth disease in pregnancy. Neurology 32: 1311–1314

Poser S, Poser W 1983 Multiple sclerosis and gestation. Neurology 33: 1422–1427

Poser S, Raun N E, Wikström J, Poser W 1979 Pregnancy, oral contraceptives and multiple sclerosis. Acta Neurologica Scandinavica 59: 108–118

Rail D L, Perkin G D 1981 Computerised tomographic appearances of hypertensive encephalopathy. Archives of Neurology 37: 310–311

Ramsay H 1984 Chorea gravidarum. Medical Journal of Australia 140: 631–632

Ramsay R E, Strauss R G, Wilder B J, Willmore L J 1978 Status epilepticus in pregnancy: Effect of phenytoin malabsorption on seizure control. Neurology 28: 85–89

Robert E, Löfkvist E, Mauguiere F 1984 Valproate and spina bifida. Lancet 2: 1392

Rocco C D, Iannelli A, Leone G, Moschini M, Valori V M 1981 Heparin-Urokinase treatment in aseptic dural sinus thrombosis. Archives of Neurology 38: 431–435

Savoiardo M, Bracchi M 1984 Neuroradiology of stroke. In: Callaghan N, Galvin R (eds) Recent research in neurology. Pitman, London, ch 11, pp 94–114

Schmidt D, Canger R, Avanzini G, Battino D, Cusi C, Beck-Mannagetta G, Koch S, Rating D, Janz D 1983 Change of seizure in pregnant epileptic women. Journal of Neurology, Neurosurgery and Psychiatry 46: 751–755

Shekleton P, Fidler J, Grimwade J 1980 A case of benign intracranial hypertension in pregnancy. British Journal of Obstetrics and Gynecology 87: 345–347

Snider D E, Layde P M, Johnson M W, Lyle M A 1980 Treatment of tuberculosis during pregnancy. American Review of Respiratory Disease 122: 65–79

So E L, Penry J K 1981 Epilepsy in adults. Annals of Neurology 9: 3–16

Solomon L, Abrams G, Dinner M, Berman L 1977 Neonatal abnormalities associated with

D-penicillamine treatment during pregnancy. New England Journal of Medicine 296 : 54–55

Srinivasan K 1983 Cerebral venous and arterial thrombosis in pregnancy and puerperium. A study of 135 patients. Angiology 34 : 731–746

Stafford C R, Fisher J F, Fadel H E, Espinel-Ingroff A V, Shadomy S, Hamby M 1983 Cryptococcal meningitis in pregnancy. Obstetrics and Gynecology 62 (3 suppl) : 35S–37S

Stevenson R E, Burton O M, Ferlauto G J, Taylor H A 1980 Hazards of oral anticoagulants during pregnancy. Journal of the American Medical Association 243 : 1549–1551

Thomas D, Byrne P D, Travers R L 1979 Systemic lupus erythematosus presenting as post partum chorea. Australian and New Zealand Journal of Medicine 9 : 568–570

Thompson P D, Gledhill R F, Quinn N P, Rossor M N, Stanley P, Coomes E N 1986 Neurological complications associated with parenteral therapy. Central pontine myelinolysis and Wernicke's encephalopathy. British Medical Journal 1 : 684–685.

Tooke J E, McNicol G P 1981 Thrombotic disorders associated with pregnancy and the pill. Clinical Haematology 10 : 613–630

Traviesa D C 1974 Magnesium deficiency : a possible cause of thiamine refractoriness in Wernicke-Korsakoff encephalopathy. Journal of Neurology, Neurosurgery and Psychiatry 37 : 959–962

Turkalj I, Braun P, Krupp P 1982 Surveillance of bromocriptine in pregnancy. Journal of the American Medical Association 247 : 1589–1591

Tuttelman R M, Gleicher N 1981 Central nervous system hemorrhage complicating pregnancy. Obstetrics and Gynecology 58 : 651–657

Victor M 1976 The Wernicke-Korsakoff syndrome. In : Vinken P J, Bruyn G W (eds) Handbook of clinical neurology, vol 28 : The metabolic and deficiency diseases of the nervous system, part II. North Holland, Amsterdam, ch 9, pp 243–270

Vir S C, Love A H G, Thompson W 1980 Thiamin status during pregnancy. International Journal for Vitamin and Nutrition Research 50 : 131–140

Warren T M, Datta S, Ostheimer G W 1982 Lumbar epidural anesthesia in a patient with multiple sclerosis. Anesthesia and Analgesia 61 : 1022–1023

Watanabe K, Tanaka K, Masuda J 1983 Wernicke's encephalopathy in early pregnancy complicated by disseminated intravascular coagulation. Virchows Archiv (A) 400 : 213–218

Whitfield L R, Lele A S, Levy G 1983 Effect of pregnancy on the relationship between concentration and anticoagulant action of heparin. Clinical Pharmacology and Therapeutics 34 : 23–28

Wood P, Murray A, Sinha B, Godley M, Goldsmith H J 1983 Wernicke's encephalopathy induced by hyperemesis gravidarum. Case reports. British Journal of Obstetrics and Gynaecology 90 : 583–586

Yiannikas C 1984 Chorea gravidarum. Medical Journal of Australia 140 : 631–632

Abdominal pain in pregnancy

It is a truism that virtually no pregnancy is completed without the occurrence of some degree of abdominal pain, not only during labour, but also in the antenatal period. The perception of pain by the pregnant woman may be heightened because of her concern that pain may signify some adverse event which will affect the outcome of her pregnancy. Conversely, some women will interpret significant pain as a consequence of pregnancy. The obstetrician therefore needs to make a number of important distinctions when assessing pain in pregnancy. Firstly he needs to distinguish the physiological from the pathological; secondly to decide whether the pain is pregnancy related, or incidental; and thirdly he needs to distinguish the trivial from the severe. These distinctions are made more difficult by the altered intra-abdominal anatomy and physiology of pregnancy, and the limitations which pregnancy imposes on investigation and interpretation of results. Such distinctions are not absolute; for example the physiological pain of labour may be regarded as pathological if it is premature or incoordinate. Degeneration of fibroids is not pregnancy-specific but is certainly more common in pregnancy, and oesophageal reflux is a trivial common occurrence, but it may occasionally lead to ulceration and haematemesis.

ANATOMY OF PAIN

It may be helpful to remember the innervation of the female pelvic organs in relation to pain perception. Pain from the body of the uterus is transmitted by sensory afferent fibres accompanying the sympathetic nerves to spinal segments T10 to L1 (Bonica, 1975) and the dermatomes corresponding to these spinal cord segments occupy the lower abdomen between the umbilicus and the symphysis pubis, a lateral area over the iliac crests, and posteriorly the area over the lower lumbar vertebrae and upper sacral spines.

Pain sensation from the cervix is transmitted to the same segments possibly with additional sensory fibres accompanying the parasympathetics to the 2nd, 3rd and 4th sacral segments (Cleland, 1933). Sensory afferent nerves from the ovary pass via the sympathetic nervous system to the 10th thoracic spinal segment. Since all these sensory nerves are common to other intra-abdominal organs, the site and nature of pain becomes particularly confusing. The perception of pain, and reaction to it, may vary considerably depending upon personality, cultural patterns, anxiety levels and other factors.

PREGNANCY RELATED PAIN

In order to form a structure to a discussion of pain in pregnancy it is helpful to consider first those conditions which, if not specific to pregnancy, are closely related to it. Although the division of pregnancy into three trimesters is somewhat artificial it may be helpful in this discussion.

First trimester

The commonest cause of pain in the first trimester is abortion. Although threatened abortion is characterised by painless bleeding there may be a dull suprapubic pain, but if this progresses to cramping colicky uterine pain, abortion is inevitable. If complete abortion occurs the pain subsides, but if the abortion is incomplete, some pain persists. Similarly if there is infection leading to so-called septic abortion, there is a persistence of pain. In missed abortion, pain does not usually occur until the uterus begins to expel the conceptus. Similarly hydatidiform mole only causes pain when expulsion of vesicles occurs. Physical signs of uterine size, and cervical dilatation, will be helpful in elucidating the type of abortion, and the addition of beta HCG assay and ultrasonic scan allows rapid diagnosis of the type of abortion.

Ectopic pregnancy is extremely important in the differential diagnosis of pain in the first trimester, as it is still a significant cause of maternal mortality and of much morbidity. The incidence in the United Kingdom is 1 in 200– 300 pregnancies, and there are suggestions that this is increasing; the incidence is considerably higher in some countries such as the West Indies. Classically pain precedes bleeding in ectopic pregnancy, but this is by no means universal. It should be suspected in any woman of childbearing age who has some or all of the following symptoms: amenorrhoea, lower abdominal pain, vaginal bleeding, shoulder-tip pain. It should be particularly considered if there is a past history of salpingitis, previous ectopic pregnancy, tubal surgery or IVF, or pregnancy in association with an IUCD or following sterilisation. The early use of laparoscopy has resulted in many ectopics being diagnosed before acute tubal rupture has occurred, so allowing conservative surgery rather than salpingectomy.

Although salpingitis and accidents to ovarian cysts are not specific to pregnancy, they are so important in the differential diagnosis of ectopic pregnancy that they must be considered here. Acute salpingitis is rarely seen, because the presence of a pregnancy in the uterus prevents ascending infection and if the disease is chronic infertility is likely to ensue. It is, however, possible for the pregnancy and gonococcocal infection to be acquired simultaneously, and post-abortal pelvic infection remains common.

Accidents to ovarian cysts occurring in early pregnancy include rupture, with or without haemorrhage, torsion, and haemorrhage into the cyst. The cyst may be a physiological corpus luteum, or a pathological neoplastic cyst. Pain from a haemorrhagic corpus luteum is usually unilateral but may become more generalised with rupture. There is minimal fever and tenderness is localised over the affected ovary. Conservative management is proper, but if a laparotomy has been performed the ovary should be repaired to obtain haemostasis. Torsion of an ovarian cyst, whether a corpus luteum or a pathological cyst, produces acute lower abdominal pain which may be unilateral or central. There is often vomiting and constitutional upset. Laparotomy and oophorectomy is required whatever the stage of pregnancy. If the corpus luteum is removed in early pregnancy, progesterone replacement will be required. Less severe episodes of pain may occur from repeated partial torsion which may resolve spontaneously. Another important cause of acute pain at the end of the first trimester of pregnancy is acute urinary retention, usually associated with a retroverted uterus at 12–14 weeks' gestation. The same problem may occur at an earlier stage of pregnancy if there is a uterine fibroid adding to the uterine enlargement. The patient becomes acutely uncomfortable and the bladder is palpable as an abdominal mass which may be confused with an ovarian cyst. Relief is quickly obtained by catheterisation and continuous drainage; within a few days the pregnant uterus will become an abdominal organ and the catheter can be removed.

Second trimester

Mid-trimester abortion is one of the commoner causes of pain at this stage of pregnancy, and the sequence of events as well as the aetiology are likely to be different from first trimester abortion.

Although every medical student knows that cervical incompetence classically causes relatively painless abortion, there is often some mild lower abdominal pain associated with an increased mucus discharge for several days prior to the miscarriage. Examination at this stage, and recognition of an effacing cervix, may allow the pregnancy to be saved by emergency insertion of a cervical circumsuture (Orr, 1973). More often, however, the classical sequence of membrane rupture followed by a rapid labour (with some painful contractions) will ensue. Mid-trimester abortion due to other causes follows a pattern similar to that of first trimester abortion. An important form of mid-trimester abortion to be aware of is that following amniocentesis. Sometimes there will be leakage of liquor soon after the amniocentesis, followed by painful contractions after a variable interval. On other occasions local amnionitis occurs, or retroplacental haemorrhage, and there may be pyrexia or pain preceding uterine contractions. Attempts to arrest threatened abortion in the mid-trimester with uterine relaxants are not conspicuously successful.

Variants of ectopic pregnancy which may occur in the mid-trimester are angular pregnancy, or rupture of a rudimentary horn. The patient presents with acute abdominal pain due to haemoperitoneum, with minimal vaginal bleeding. Damage to the uterus and haemorrhage may be so severe as to necessitate hysterectomy. Uterine fibroids are particularly liable to undergo necrobiosis (red degeneration) in the mid-trimester due to the rapid increase in size of both normal uterine muscle and the leiomyoma. The pain may be very severe, accompanied by vomiting. Palpation of an exquisitely tender firm mass in the uterus suggests the diagnosis, and ultrasound may help to confirm that the mass is a fibroid. Treatment is conservative with analgesics. If a laparotomy has been undertaken, the temptation to remove the fibroid must be resisted at all costs, excepting that a twisted pedunculated fibroid may be tied off and removed. Less severe pain may occur in milder cases of red degeneration.

Many women complain of pain in one or both iliac fossae between the 16th and 20th week of pregnancy; they often describe the pain as passing into the groin or down the thigh, and the pain improves on lying down. Such pain is attributed to stretching of nerve fibres in the round ligament. Certainly this is a period of pregnancy in which rapid elongation of the round ligaments occurs, but there is no firm proof as to the true cause of this pain. Provided all other causes of pain have been excluded, it may be reasonable to offer round ligament strain as an explanation to the pregnant woman for such pain.

Third trimester

It is in the third trimester that the diagnosis of abdominal pain becomes most difficult, because the pregnant uterus is in front of and masking the rest of the abdominal contents. Other intra-abdominal conditions may induce reflex uterine irritability, further confusing the issue.

Placental abruption is amongst the most important diagnoses to establish because of its grave consequences for the fetus. Although the physical symptoms and signs of abruption are well known (constant severe abdominal pain, and a tender, woody hard uterus, with or without some bleeding), there is often a delay in making the diagnosis, particularly in cases of concealed haemorrhage.

Case report

A 27-year-old gravida 2, booked for hospital delivery, developed abdominal pain and contractions at 39 weeks' gestation. Assuming this to be the onset of labour, she called the ambulance service. When they arrived they found her to be very distressed and, concluding that delivery must be imminent, declined to move her to hospital and sent for a midwife. When the midwife arrived she carried out a vaginal examination and found the cervix to be barely 2 cm dilated and, assuming her to be in early labour, advised an unhurried transfer to hospital. On arrival at hospital some 2 hours after the ambulance had arrived at her home, she was profoundly hypotensive with a tense tender uterus and an absent fetal heart. Delivery of a fresh stillbirth ensued, with a large retroplacental clot, and the patient required a transfusion of four units of blood.

A small abruption may be even more difficult to diagnose as the uterine pain and tenderness is localised. Ultrasound may reveal a retroplacental clot, and there may be some changes in FDP levels.

Another dramatic cause of pain in the third trimester is uterine rupture. Obstetricians and midwives are constantly looking for signs of rupture of a Caesarean scar in labour, but rupture of the uterus may occur in the late third trimester following a uterine perforation, hysterotomy, or myomectomy. There is likely to be a sudden onset of severe pain due to bleeding and leakage of liquor into the peritoneal cavity, and unless the diagnosis is made rapidly, and laparotomy carried out, fetal death will occur.

Fulminating pre-eclampsia is often associated with upper abdominal pain, thought to be due to oedema of the liver, and stretching of its capsule.

The third trimester is the time when most pregnant women will experience varying degrees of pressure symptoms which some will perceive as pain whilst those of a more stoical nature will describe them as 'discomfort'. Normal events causing pain at this stage include pain from vigorous fetal movements or engagement of the head, pain in the lower ribs associated with flaring of the ribs (particularly noticed in breech presentation), pain from distension of the abdominal wall, and Braxton Hicks contractions. The latter need to be differentiated from the onset of true labour. Although Braxton Hicks contractions are said to be painless, many women do in fact find them painful. They are, however, irregular in intensity and frequency, and cause no change in the cervix. Studies of uterine activity reveal that Braxton Hicks contractions are usually of 10–15 mmHg pressure, although they may reach 30 mmHg in the final week prior to labour. During labour, contractions increase from 25 mmHg in early labour to 50 mmHg or more as delivery approaches. Since the pain threshold is generally held to be 25 mmHg, it can be seen how difficult it may be to differentiate late strong Braxton Hicks contractions from early labour. False labour pains are similarly irregular, although they may mimic normal labour in starting in the back, radiating round to the front. False labour is of no great significance apart from the fact that it is a frequent cause of unnecessary admission to hospital, and anxiety to the mother. Vaginal examination, repeated after a few hours, is often the only satisfactory way to assess the significance of uterine contractions.

INCIDENTAL ABDOMINAL PAIN

Although a division between pregnancy-related and incidental causes of pain is helpful from a descriptive point of view, it must be realised that in the clinical problem it is just this distinction which is difficult to make. It is particularly important to make this distinction when a decision to perform a surgical operation is at stake. Incidental causes of abdominal pain have no respect for the trimesters of pregnancy, and although some are more common at one time or another, most can occur at any stage.

GASTROINTESTINAL CAUSES

Heartburn and hiatus hernia

Heartburn, a warm or burning sensation felt in the upper epigastrium and behind the sternum, sometimes with the regurgitation of a small amount of fluid into the mouth, is one of the commonest minor disturbances of pregnancy. It may be made worse by bending, lying flat or straining, and is accompanied by flatulence. Surveys have shown it to occur in 60–70 per cent of Caucasian pregnant women, but it may be less common in Negro races (Atlay et al, 1973). It is generally held to be due to the reflux of acid into the oesophagus as a result of hormone-induced relaxation of the lower oesophageal sphincter. There is some evidence that pyloric regurgitation of bile salts plays an important part in the symptom of heartburn, and certainly bile has been found in the oesophageal juices in women with heartburn (Gillison et al, 1971). There is reduced gastric acid secretion in pregnancy, at least in the first two trimesters, and a reduced response to histamine. The fact that dilute hydrochloric acid may relieve the symptoms of heartburn lends some support to the concept that it is regurgitation of bile which is responsible for the symptom.

Radiological studies which would not now be ethically justifiable have revealed that hiatus hernia is present in 7–22 per cent of pregnant women, the incidence increasing in later pregnancy (Sutherland et al, 1956). Gorbach and Reid (1956) found radiological evidence of hiatus hernia in 62 per cent of women with severe heartburn in the third trimester. Most of these hernias are small and regress after delivery but a minority will cause more serious problems such as vomiting and haematemesis. The treatment of heartburn, whether or not thought to be due to hiatus hernia, is with antacids and attention to posture. When vomiting is a problem the addition of metoclopramide may be justified.

Hernia through a congenital defect of the diaphragm is quite another matter and may result in herniation of large parts of the intestine into the chest. Severe pain, vomiting and shock may result, requiring urgent surgical treatment.

Constipation

Constipation is a frequent minor problem of pregnancy, often commencing early in the first trimester. It is principally due to the reduced peristalsis associated with progesterone, although reduced exercise and pressure of the uterus may contribute to this. If constipation is severe it may cause lower abdominal pain and pain in the left iliac fossa, sometimes of a colicky nature. Attention to diet by increasing fruit and bran will usually solve the problem, but a laxative, suppositories or even an enema may be required in more severe cases.

Peptic ulcer

Gastric and duodenal ulcer rarely occur for the first time in pregnancy, and patients with known ulcers usually improve considerably in pregnancy. This is presumably as a result of the reduced gastric acid secretion in the first two trimesters of pregnancy (Murray et al, 1957). After delivery there is a strong tendency to relapse (Clark, 1953). Although perforation or haematemesis is extremely rare, it can occur, particularly during or shortly after labour, and fatality may result. Perforation of a peptic ulcer results in acute generalised abdominal pain and shock, and needs to be distinguished from other shock-producing abdominal catastrophes. Plain abdominal X-ray may reveal the presence of gas under the diaphragm and early surgical treatment should be instituted after resuscitation.

Biliary disease

In view of the much-quoted aphorism that gallstones occur in the 'fair, fat, forty and fertile' it would be expected that biliary disease will occur in pregnancy. Biliary stasis and the raised cholesterol level in pregnancy may predispose to gallstone formation. Stauffer et al (1982) found an incidence of gallstones in 3·5 per cent of 338 pregnant women having routine ultrasound examinations. Only two of the patients had a history of biliary symptoms. Although 50 per cent of patients with gallstones are said to develop symptoms eventually, only a very small proportion of women with asymptomatic gallstones are likely to develop symptoms in pregnancy. Any of the complications of gallstones may occur in pregnancy (viz. cholecystitis, biliary colic, empyema or mucocoele of the gallbladder, or common bile duct obstruction). Management tends to be more conservative than in the non-pregnant, but cholecystectomy may be necessary in certain circumstances and appears to be a safe procedure in pregnancy (Hill et al, 1975).

Pancreatitis

Although pancreatitis is rare in pregnancy (1:4000 pregnancies), there is some evidence to suggest a causal relationship. The average age incidence in pregnancy is 27, compared with 50+ in the non-pregnant. Increase in blood lipids in early pregnancy, gallstones, and alcohol may all play a part in the aetiology. McKay et al (1980) found gallstones in 18 out of 20 patients with pancreatitis associated with pregnancy. Most patients with pancreatitis present with upper or central abdominal pain often radiating to the back, with vomiting and shock. Diagnosis depends upon the finding of a raised serum amylase, bearing in mind that amylase may be mildly raised in normal pregnancy (Kaiser et al, 1975). Treatment is as in the non-pregnant, with nasogastric aspiration and electrolyte replacement, with particular attention to glucose and calcium levels. Laparotomy should be avoided if at all possible. Wilkinson (1973) reported a mortality of 37 per cent in pancreatitis occurring in the third trimester of pregnancy, but with modern management a much lower mortality is to be expected, although there may be some fetal loss.

Acute appendicitis

The incidence of acute appendicitis in pregnancy is generally reported as 1:2500 pregnancies, and does not differ from that in a similar non-pregnant population. It has the reputation of carrying a high mortality, worsening with increasing gestation (Black, 1960) whilst Brant (1967) reported a mortality of 2 per cent in 256 cases. The symptoms and signs are the same as in the non-pregnant; that is central abdominal pain, later moving to the right iliac fossa, with variable gastro-intestinal upset, foetor, and fever. However, the upward displacement of the appendix may result in the pain being much higher so that cholecystitis may be suspected. Presence of the pregnant uterus in front of the appendix may mask tenderness and guarding, and reflex uterine contractions will frequently occur, confusing the diagnosis further. Displacement of abdominal organs by the uterus prevents the normal 'walling-off' of the inflamed appendix so that generalised peritonitis can ensue more readily.

The leucocytosis of pregnancy reduces the value of a white blood count, and if the diagnosis is seriously entertained it is better to carry out a laparotomy than delay unduly. The incision will need to be placed higher than usual, depending upon the site of maximal tenderness, and should allow generous access. Premature labour or abortion may ensue, especially if operation has been delayed. Coincidental Caesarean section is best avoided unless there are strong obstetric indications.

Acute intestinal obstruction

In healthy pregnant women, acute intestinal obstruction is rare. Most cases are due to bands or adhesions, external and internal hernias and volvulus, intussusception and neoplasms being other rarer causes. Ileostomy patients are particularly at risk of intestinal obstruction (Hudson, 1972). Presentation of intestinal obstruction would be with abdominal pain, nausea or vomiting, distension and constipation, all symptoms which may occur in normal pregnancy. However their simultaneous occurrence suggests intestinal obstruction; a plain X-ray will reveal a distended loop or loops of bowel with fluid levels, enabling the level of obstruction to be identified. Provided there are no signs of strangulation, conservative management of nasogastric aspiration and intravenous fluids should be tried for a few hours, but if clinical improvement does not occur, laparotomy should be carried out forthwith.

The rare condition of 'pregnancy ileus', in which there is gross distension of the large bowel and sometimes the ileum, is most likely to occur after delivery, especially Caesarean section. If unrecognised, perforation of the caecum may occur, and laparotomy may be required to prevent this (Harley, 1980).

Inflammatory bowel disease

Both ulcerative colitis and Crohn's disease may cause abdominal pain and diarrhoea, pain being a more marked feature of Crohn's disease except in the fulminating type of ulcerative colitis. It is beyond the scope of this chapter to give a full account of the influence of pregnancy on inflammatory bowel disease and the effects of the disease on pregnancy. Suffice it to say that Crohn's disease or ulcerative colitis may occur for the first time in pregnancy, albeit rarely; when it does, it tends to run a more serious course than pre-existing disease.

RENAL DISEASE AS A CAUSE OF ABDOMINAL PAIN

Pyelonephritis is by far the commonest and most important renal cause of abdominal pain in pregnancy, but renal calculi, pelvi-ureteric obstruction and hydronephrosis are other possible causes.

Pyelonephritis

It is well known that there is dilatation of the renal calyces, pelvis and ureter, starting quite early in pregnancy and continuing into the puerperium. This is attributed partly to the smooth muscle-relaxant effect of progesterone, and partly to mechanical compression of the ureter as it crosses the pelvic brim by the pregnant uterus. The stasis which occurs as a result of dilatation of the collecting system accounts for the predisposition of pregnant women to develop urinary infection, and the physiological dilatation makes interpretation of urinary tract obstruction more difficult. Pyelonephritis occurs in 1–2 per cent of pregnancies; 4–7 per cent of women have asymptomatic bacteriuria at the onset of pregnancy (Sweet, 1977) and approximately one-third of these will develop acute pyelonephritis during pregnancy. By treating asymptomatic carriers with antibiotics, the incidence of pyelonephritis may be reduced to 0·5 per cent (Harris and Gilstrap, 1981). Most cases of pyelonephritis occur in the second and third trimester. In the acute case the patient complains of severe pain in the lumbar region, sometimes radiating to the iliac fossa or vulva. More often the pain is on the right side, but may be on the left, or bilateral. The pain is usually accompanied by vomiting, tachycardia, and pyrexia, often with rigors. There may be marked tenderness of the loin and abdomen, and there is often reflex uterine irritability. The differential diagnosis includes appendicitis, torsion of an ovarian cyst, degeneration of a fibroid, abruption, and premature labour with infection. The diagnosis is confirmed by the finding of pus cells in a mid-stream specimen of urine, and culture of organisms in the laboratory. Energetic treatment with parenteral antibiotics, intravenous fluids and analgesia is required, because pyelonephritis is an infection with serious implications to both mother and fetus. Septicaemic shock may occur, and there may be permanent renal parenchymal damage. A severe attack may result in abortion or intra-uterine death, and less severe infection is associated with intra-uterine growth retardation and premature labour. Frequent follow-up urine cultures should be performed, and if there is a recurrent pyelonephritis or evidence of impaired renal function, intravenous pyelography should be carried out after delivery.

Renal calculi

Pregnancy does not predispose to the formation of renal stones, and the dilatation of the ureter may allow the passage of small ureteric calculi relatively painlessly. The incidence of calculi complicating pregnancy is estimated to be 1:1500 pregnancies (Lattonzi and Cook, 1980). A stone in the renal pelvis may cause some loin pain, but an acute clinical episode is likely to be due to the attempted passing of a ureteric calculus, giving rise to classical ureteric colic. Ultrasound may aid the diagnosis by showing unilateral dilatation of the collecting system, but a one-shot pyelogram is permissible if the diagnosis remains in doubt. Analgesia and a high fluid intake are given, and in more than half the cases the stone will pass. If obstruction persists, surgical intervention to remove the calculus may be necessary.

Pelvi-ureteric obstruction due to calculus, congenital obstruction or fibrosis may produce loin pain rarely.

MISCELLANEOUS CAUSES OF PAIN

Vascular accidents

Rectus sheath haematoma as a result of rupture of the inferior epigastric artery may occur in multiparous patients in late pregnancy, often associated with a bout of coughing. A severe pain with the development of a swelling in the lower abdominal wall occurs. Conservative treatment with analgesics is usually all that is required, but occasionally surgical evacuation of the haematoma and ligation of the artery is necessary.

Mesenteric thrombosis is an abdominal catastrophe unlikely to occur in pregnancy, but micro-infarction in sickle cell crisis is a not infrequent cause of abdominal pain in patients with sickle cell disease, and is a diagnosis not to be overlooked in patients of Negro origin.

A rupture of the spleen or a splenic aneurysm is a dramatic event which can occur in pregnancy, and may be confused with ectopic pregnancy, placental abruption or uterine rupture.

Malignant disease

Rarely, non-gynaecological malignancy may occur in pregnancy producing abdominal pain. Cases of carcinoma of the stomach, carcinoma of the rectum, Hodgkin's disease, and retroperitoneal rhabdosarcoma have all been seen in the writer's hospital in the past 5 years, presenting with abdominal pain. In all cases the presence of pregnancy delayed and obscured the diagnosis.

Porphyria

Acute porphyria presents with abdominal pain, psychiatric disturbance and autonomic effects. Pregnancy may precipitate an attack and so it may present for the first time during pregnancy. Any drug which may have initiated the attack should be stopped, and analgesics and anti-emetics prescribed.

CONCLUSION

Attempts should be made to reach a diagnosis in all cases of abdominal pain in pregnancy. Because of anatomical and physiological changes caused by the pregnancy, particular attention should be paid to detail of history and physical signs. The obstetrician should make use of those investigations which are available (see Tables 4.1–4.3), bearing in mind the limitations and constraints imposed by the pregnancy. Many of the conditions described should be managed in conjunction with specialist colleagues, and they

Table 4.1 Conditions where X-ray may be helpful

Suspected condition	Radiological investigation
1. Intestinal obstruction	Erect and supine plain film
2. Perforation of peptic ulcer	Erect abdominal plain film
3. Renal/ureteric calculi	Plain film and 'one-shot' IVP
4. Appendicitis	Plain abdominal film

Table 4.2   Conditions where ultrasound may be helpful

1. Gallbladder disease
2. Renal calculi
3. Ovarian cyst accident
4. Degenerating fibroids
5. Placental abruption
6. Rare intra-abdominal tumours

Table 4.3   Conditions where pathological tests may be helpful

Suspected condition	Test
1. Appendicitis	White blood count
2. Pyelonephritis	Urine microscopy and culture
3. Pancreatitis	Serum amylase
4. Biliary disease	Bilirubin and liver function tests
5. Sickle crisis	Hb and film
6. Porphyria	Urinary porphyrins
7. Placental abruption	Fibrinogen degradation products

should be reminded to consult with obstetric colleagues when pregnant patients present to them with abdominal pain. With prompt diagnosis and appropriate treatment, maternal morbidity can be reduced and the danger to fetal well-being minimised.

REFERENCES

Atlay R D, Gillison E W, Horton A L 1973 A fresh look at pregnancy heartburn. British Journal of Obstetrics and Gynaecology 80: 63–66
Black P 1960 Acute appendicitis in pregnancy. British Medical Journal 1: 1938
Bonica J J 1975 The nature of pain of parturition. Clinics in Obstetrics and Gynaecology 2: 499–516
Brant H A 1967 Appendicitis in pregnancy. Obstetrics and Gynaecology 29: 130
Clark D H 1953 Peptic ulcer in women. British Medical Journal 1: 1254–1257
Cleland J G P 1933 Paravertebral anaesthesia in obstetrics. Surgery, Gynaecology and Obstetrics 57: 51
Gillison E W, Nyhus L M, Duthie H L 1971 Bile reflux, gastric secretion and heartburn. British Journal of Surgery 58: 864
Gorbach A C, Reid D E 1956 Hiatus hernia in pregnancy. New England Journal of Medicine 255: 517–519
Harley J M G 1980 Caesarean section. Clinics in Obstetrics and Gynaecology 7: 529–557
Harris R E, Gilstrap L C 1981 Cystitis during pregnancy: a distinct clinical entity. Obstetrics and Gynaecology 57: 578–580
Hill L M, Johnson C E, Lee R A 1975 Cholecystectomy in pregnancy. Obstetrics and Gynaecology 46: 291–293
Hudson C N 1972 Ileostomy in pregnancy. Proceedings of the Royal Society of Medicine 65: 281–283
Kaiser R, Berk J E, Fridkinder L 1975 Serum amylase changes during pregnancy. American Journal of Obstetrics and Gynaecology 122: 283–286
Lattonzi D R, Cook W A 1980 Urinary calculi in pregnancy. Obstetrics and Gynaecology 56: 462–466
McKay A J, O'Neill J, Imrie C E 1980 Pancreatitis, pregnancy and gallstones. British Journal of Obstetrics and Gynaecology 87: 47–50

Murray F A, Erskine J P, Fielding J 1957 Gastric secretion in pregnancy. British Journal of Obstetrics and Gynaecology 64: 373–381

Orr C 1973 An aid to cervical cerclage. Australian and New Zealand Journal of Obstetrics and Gynaecology 13: 114

Stauffer R A, Adams A, Wygal J, Lavery J P 1982 Gallbladder disease in pregnancy. American Journal of Obstetrics and Gynaecology 144: 661–664

Sutherland C G, Atkinson J C, Brodgon B G 1956 Esophageal hiatus hernia in pregnancy. Obstetrics and Gynaecology 8: 261–264

Sweet R L 1977 Bacteriuria and pyelonephritis during pregnancy. Seminars in Perinatology 1: 25–40

Wilkinson E J 1973 Acute pancreatitis in pregnancy. Obstetrical and Gynaecological Survey 28: 281–303

Gestational diabetes

One can summarize the problem of gestational diabetes by noting that since 5 per cent of women are diabetic by the age of 50 years (Kriss & Futcher, 1948) there are 50 future diabetics in every 1000 antenatal patients. The perinatal mortality rate in the years before the emergence of clinical diabetes is approximately 10 per cent (see next section). Since perinatal mortality rates are of the order of 10 per 1000 births in developed countries, this simplistic calculation indicates that approximately 50 per cent of all perinatal deaths occur in women who will become diabetic. The challenge is to determine what proportion of these women are identifiable, and hence treatable, as gestational diabetics, by appropriate screening in pregnancy.

The main controversies in the subject of gestational diabetes are:

1. the criteria used for diagnosis,
2. the best method for screening the entire pregnant population,
3. the management of identified gestational diabetics.

This review examines these problems and also the effects of gestational diabetes on the fetus, and the subsequent long-term consequences for the mother and her child.

HISTORICAL PERSPECTIVE

Gilbert & Dunlop (1949) used the term *prediabetes* to refer to the time interval before the diagnosis of diabetes and, by retrospective analysis of the obstetric history in overt diabetics they found a fetal loss of 50 per cent for the 2-year interval preceding diagnosis. Subsequent writers confused the issue by using the term in a different sense. Jackson (1952) stated that prediabetes was a clinical diagnosis based on the previous obstetric history, whereas Lewis (1956) extended this definition and stated that in prediabetes the blood sugar levels were normal and that diagnosis rested upon evidence of overweight babies and high fetal loss, before there was any hyperglycaemia or an abnormal glucose tolerance curve.

Miller et al (1944) analyzed 252 prediabetic pregnancies occurring in women developing diabetes during the childbearing period. They found the maximum fetal loss rate of 35·4 per cent occurred during the 5 years immediately before the diagnosis of diabetes. This was considerably higher than the fetal loss rate of 23·6 per cent, which occurred in the 93 pregnancies among the same group of women, after the onset of diabetes. Mengert & Laughlin (1939) reported a fetal loss rate of 29·8 per cent in 84 pregnancies during the prediabetic period, whilst Jackson & Woolf (1958) found a stillbirth rate in prediabetic women of 29 per cent in the 5-year period directly preceding diabetes. Pedowitz & Shlevin (1957) found the fetal loss rate prior to and following clinical recognition of diabetes to be identical (20·5 per cent), and in the years immediately preceding the recognition of manifest diabetes the fetal loss rate rose rapidly, and sometimes exceeded that of known diabetics. Hagbard (1958) also found that the risk of perinatal death was almost as great during the time shortly before the diabetes was recognized as when it was clinically manifest. He calculated that the perinatal mortality for the deliveries 3–5 years before the onset of diabetes was 10·3 per cent in 68 pregnancies, and during the 2 years before the maternal diabetes was recognized it was 37·3 per cent in 52 pregnancies. Pomeranze et al (1959) examined the obstetric histories of 643 diabetic females and found that perinatal mortality was 12–16 per cent during the period 5–20 years before the clinical onset of diabetes, and 24–30 per cent during the 5 years preceding the clinical diagnosis.

The above studies provide ample retrospective evidence that, in the years prior to recognition of diabetes, the perinatal wastage is very high. For this reason the problem of prediabetes must be approached prospectively if treatment is to mitigate this high fetal wastage, and glucose tolerance testing must be available to permit identification of these patients.

PHYSIOLOGY

During pregnancy a number of factors act to alter the level of blood glucose. Hormones, such as human placental lactogen (Samaan et al, 1968), progesterone (Kalkhoff et al, 1970), prolactin (Landgraf et al, 1977) and cortisol (Rizza et al, 1982), have diabetogenic properties raising maternal blood glucose levels. These actions are counterbalanced by an increase in insulin concentrations reaching almost twice non-pregnant levels (Kuhl 1975). This rise is itself offset by increasing insulin resistance, the mechanism of which is not clearly understood (Kuhl et al, 1984). The vast majority of pregnant women (approximately 96 per cent) manage to maintain their blood glucose within normal limits, but around 2 per cent cannot do so, and become hyperglycaemic and a further 2 per cent hypoglycaemic (Abell & Beischer, 1975).

The consequence of this increasing resistance to insulin activity is that eventually, usually late in the second trimester of pregnancy, the capacity for insulin secretion is exceeded, glucose intolerance develops and the woman so destined becomes a gestational diabetic (Kuhl et al, 1984).

DEFINITION OF GESTATIONAL DIABETES

Considerable argument prevails with regard to the definition of gestational diabetes. The following definition has been adopted by the International Workshop Conference on Gestational Diabetes which was held under the joint sponsorship of four organisations concerned with the disease and its consequences—the Diabetic Pregnancy Study Group of the European Association for the Study of Diabetes, the American Diabetes Association, the American College of Obstetricians and Gynecologists, and the American Academy of Pediatrics.

They defined gestational diabetes mellitus as *carbohydrate intolerance of variable severity with onset or first recognition during the present pregnancy. The definition applies irrespective of whether or not insulin is used for treatment or the condition persists after pregnancy* (Freinkel & Josimovich, 1980). Previously used definitions stipulated that the glucose tolerance test must return to normal after delivery; if this did not occur the inference was that the condition predated pregnancy. This old definition was not helpful because the diagnosis must be made during pregnancy, and not after delivery, to allow proper management. The patient's prepregnancy glucose tolerance is irrelevant since the information will rarely be available, although one may find it easy to believe that the patient with diabetes mellitus at the postnatal visit may have had undiagnosed diabetes before the pregnancy.

Other terms such as *potential or latent diabetes*, as already explained, are best avoided, as a patient should be treated in terms of identified abnormal glucose tolerance, not clinical markers thought to be associated with an increased risk of development of the disease in later life. Two labels then remain: *diabetes mellitus* for women known to be diabetic before pregnancy and *gestational diabetes* for those diagnosed for the first time during pregnancy.

Diagnosis of gestational diabetes

The distribution curve of blood glucose levels in response to an oral glucose load is not bimodal, i.e. there is not a clear demarcation between normal and abnormal populations. The definition of abnormality must therefore be arbitrary (Hadden, 1975).

Some of the most widely used criteria chosen to define diabetes in both pregnant and non-pregnant subjects are summarized in Table 5.1.

The Expert Committee on Diabetes Mellitus of the World Health Organisation have introduced the subclassification of *impaired glucose tolerance* (Table 5.1) to denote those subjects who have an abnormal response to a glucose load but not yet of such magnitude to merit the label of diabetes. This committee specifically did not differentiate between the pregnant and non-pregnant subject (WHO, 1980); classification is based primarily on the fasting blood glucose, which ironically is significantly lowered in pregnancy

Table 5.1. Criteria used for classification of abnormal glucose tolerance

Criteria derived by	Oral glucose load (g)	Sample	Glucose tolerance test				Comment
			Fasting mmol/l	1-hour mmol/l	2-hour mmol/l	3-hour mmol/l	
O'Sullivan & Mahan	100	Venous plasma	5·8 (105)	10·6 (190)	9·2 (165)	8·1 (145)	Requires at least two samples to equal or exceed these levels
WHO	—	Venous plasma	⩾8·0 (144)				Diabetes
	75		6·0–8·0 (108) (144)	—	⩾11·0 (198)	—	Diabetes
			6·0–8·0 (108) (144)	—	⩾8·0–11·0 (144) (198)		Impaired glucose tolerance
Mercy Maternity Hospital	50	Capillary plasma	—	9·0 (162)	7·0 (126)	—	Must equal or exceed both values
British Diabetic Association	50	Venous plasma	6·7 (120)	10·0 (180)	6·7 (120)	—	Requires fasting or 2-hour value > 6·7 mmol/l and 1-hour > 10.0 mmol/l

Figures in parentheses denote equivalent values in mg/dl

(Victor, 1974). It is therefore not surprising that many authorities, including the NIH Diabetes Data Group and the groups whose definition of gestational diabetes was elaborated earlier in this section, strongly oppose this recommendation.

There are a number of important variables in the glucose tolerance test which need to be considered when attempting to compare one set of criteria with another. The actual amount of glucose ingested (50 g, 75 g, 100 g or 1·75 g per kg bodyweight) varies from one centre to another; European and British Commonwealth centres have tended to use a 50 g load in pregnancy mainly because it causes less vomiting, whereas North American centres tend to use 100 g. The WHO Committee has taken the middle ground of 75 g. Surprisingly a doubling of the glucose load from 50 to 100 g has a minimal effect on the peak blood glucose levels at 1 hour after ingestion; the difference is only apparent at the 2-hour sample, when levels are approximately 1 mmol/l higher (Castro et al, 1970).

The type and site of the blood sample taken is another important variable; whole blood glucose levels are about 14 per cent higher than serum and plasma levels as red cells bind this fraction of glucose (Lind et al, 1972). In the non-pregnant subject, capillary levels are 1 mmol/l higher than venous levels 2 hours after glucose ingestion, but do not differ significantly in the fasting state. Little information is available for pregnant women where the hyperdynamic cardiovascular state may lead to closer equilibration between the venous and capillary vascular beds.

In early studies the Somogyi-Nelson technique was used, which measures 5 mg/100 ml of non-glucose reducing substances. The specific glucose oxidase method is now the most widely used assay and consequently results are 5 per cent lower.

At the Mercy Maternity Hospital, Melbourne, it has been the policy to test all patients for glucose intolerance with a 50 g oral glucose tolerance test, the capillary plasma glucose levels being measured by the glucose oxidase method using a Beckman analyser. The criterion for diagnosis of gestational diabetes which we advocate was derived by analysis of the first 18 679 pregnancies tested and is *the combination of a 1-hour level of 9 mmol/l or more and a 2-hour level of 7 mmol/l or more*—this definition gave the most clinically significant values in terms of perinatal outcome (stillbirths, neonatal deaths, fetal growth retardation and congenital anomalies) (Table 5.2) and selected approximately 2·5 per cent of the population tested. The fasting and 3-hour levels did not prove to have useful predictive values.

When the results of glucose tolerance performed on 35 600 pregnancies investigated between 1971 and 1983 were analysed using the WHO criteria, 49 women were diabetic and 92 had impaired glucose tolerance (Table 5.3). This combined incidence of diabetes and impaired glucose tolerance is only 4/1000, which emphasises the unrealistic nature of the WHO Expert Committee's recommendation.

Two other methods of assessing glucose tolerance have been validated but are not widely used:

1. The *intravenous glucose tolerance test*, which measures the rate of disappearance of glucose denoted by the K value (Silverstone et al, 1961). O'Sullivan et al (1970) reported that the 90 per cent lower confidence limit of the K value was 1·34, but O'Sullivan and Hadden with their respective co-workers (Hadden et al, 1971) did not find that values below this figure predicted fetal mortality with significant accuracy.

Table 5.2 Pregnancy outcome according to glucose tolerance in 18 679 consecutive pregnancies

	Total study population (%)	Gestational diabetes[1] (%)	Gestational hypoglycaemia[2] (%)
Perinatal mortality	0·9	1·7	1·9
Major fetal malformations	2·6	2·6	3·2
Birthweight <10th percentile	10·0	8·7	15·8
Birthweight >90th percentile	10·0	13·4	6·3

[1] Gestational diabetes = 1-hour blood sugar value ⩾ 9 mmol/l + 2-hour ⩾ 7 mmol/l
[2] Gestational hypoglycaemia = fasting blood sugar value ⩽ 4 mmol/l + 3-hour ⩽ 3 mmol/l.

Table 5.3   Incidence of pregnancy complications according to severity of gestational diabetes in 35 629 consecutive pregnancies, Mercy Maternity Hospital, Melbourne

| Classification | Pregnancies | | Multiple births | Pre-eclampsia | APH[1] | Poly-hydramnios | Low oestriol excretion | Insulin therapy |
	No.	(%)	(%)	(%)	(%)	(%)	(%)	(%)
Current MMH	797	2·24	1·1	21·1†	3·5	1·0	16·9†	0·1
Original MMH[2]	212	0·60	2·4	21·7†	4·7	7·6*	17·9‡	2·4
WHO Impaired	92	0·26	2·2	30·4†	3·3	3·3	15·2	6·5
WHO Diabetic	49	0·14	4·1	26·5‡	6·1	6·1‡	20·4	42·9
Total	1150	3·23	1·6	22·2	3·8	2·6	17·1	3·0
Hospital incidence	40 982		1·4	10·6	3·8	0·8	10·6	

[1] Antepartum haemorrhage.
[2] Original MMH critera were 1-hour blood sugar value of 10 mmol/l or more *plus* 2-hour value of 7·8 mmol/l or more.
Incidence differing significantly from that classified by current MMH criteria: *$p<0.001$.
Incidence differing significantly from that of total hospital incidence: ‡$P<0.01$; †$p<0.001$.

2. The second method which utilises all the measured glucose values is the calculation of the *area under the blood glucose curve*. A refinement of this method measures only the incremental area, i.e. the area above the fasting level. These two methods suffer from requiring more complex computations and have not enjoyed wide usage.

Screening

The 'standard' indications for testing glucose tolerance in pregnancy have been:

1. family history in first-degree relatives,
2. previous delivery of large infants (birthweight > 4000 g),
3. poor obstetric history.
4. glycosuria during pregnancy.
5. obesity.

To these should be added polyhydramnios, early-onset pre-eclampsia or a macrosomic fetus in the current pregnancy.

Macafee and Beischer in 1974 reported the results of glucose tolerance testing in 1000 consecutive patients without regard to indications, and found that the only 'risk factor' with a significantly increased pick-up rate in comparison with the group as a whole, was maternal age over 30 years. O'Sullivan et al (1973b) had reported similar findings and noted that 44 per cent of their obstetric population had one or more 'risk' factors; interestingly in Macafee's series 44 per cent also had one or more of these factors. This association with age has now been examined and confirmed in a much larger series from the Mercy Maternity Hospital and the increasing incidence of gestational diabetes becomes highly statistically significant after the age of 30 years (Table 5.4). It should be noted that the importance of maternal age

Table 5.4 Incidence of gestational diabetes according to maternal age at diagnosis

Age in years	Total study population		Gestational diabetes (%)
	No.	(%)	
<20	1102	3·8	0·7
20–24	6714	23·1	1·9
25–29	12 690	43·6	3·0
30–34	6555	22·5	4·6
35–39	1683	5·8	7·6
>39	354	1·2	8·2
Total	29 098	100·0	3·3

as a marker for gestational diabetes has not been stressed in the literature until recently.

The prevalence of gestational diabetes is also significantly increased in twin pregnancy (5·6 per cent, Dwyer et al, 1982) and in women who develop early-onset pre-eclampsia (before 37 weeks gestation) (5·3 per cent, Long, 1983).

Fetal macrosomia is associated with maternal hyperglycaemia, the association being greater in overt diabetes (40 per cent, Beischer et al, 1968) than in gestational diabetes where 20 per cent of infants have a birthweight of 4000 g or more (Gabbe et al, 1977). The inference that mothers of macrosomic infants are likely to be gestational diabetics, however, does not follow. In a study of glucose tolerance in 137 pregnancies in which the infant weighed more than 4540 g (i.e. 99th percentile), only one mother (0·7 per cent) was a gestational diabetic (Oats et al, 1980); in other words in the community as a whole the majority of very large infants are not due to hyperglycaemia. It should be noted that when considering fetal macrosomia in gestational diabetics it is more correct to use weight for gestational age rather than absolute weight, since many of these patients are electively delivered before full term.

Maternal obesity, i.e. weight greater than 90 kg, is also considered to be a risk factor for developing gestational diabetes (Hadden et al, 1971). In an analysis of glucose tolerance tests performed in more than 18 000 pregnancies performed at the Mercy Maternity Hospital, we found that both extremes of maternal weight ($p < 0.001$) were associated with significantly increased incidences of gestational diabetes (Table 5.5).

Approximately 25 per cent of Australia's population are first-generation immigrants (Australian Bureau of Statistics, 1983) and analysis of our data shows that the incidence of gestational diabetes is increased by a factor of 2–3 in patients born in the Indian Subcontinent (8·2 per cent, $p < 0.05$), Italy (8·5 per cent, $p < 0.001$), China or Hong Kong (8·3 per cent, $p < 0.001$) and Malta (10·6 per cent, $p < 0.001$) in comparison with those born in Australia and New Zealand (3·0 per cent) (Table 5.6).

Table 5.5 Incidence of gestational diabetes according to maternal weight

Weight (kg)	Total study population No.	(%)	Gestational diabetes (%)
<55	790	4·3	5·7
55–59	1883	10·3	3·9
60–64	3425	18·6	3·2
65–69	4052	22·1	3·0
70–74	3279	17·9	2·4
75–79	2181	11·9	2·8
80–84	2155	6·3	3·5
85–89	723	3·9	4·1
>89	877	4·8	4·4
Total	18 365		3·3

The International Workshop Conference on Gestational Diabetes has recommended that *all* pregnant women should be screened between 24 and 28 weeks gestation for glucose intolerance unless testing earlier in the pregnancy, because of clinical indications, has already indicated gestational diabetes (Freinkel & Josimovich, 1980). Three methods of screening have been evaluated:

1. A 50 g oral glucose load is given to the pregnant women *without* regard to time of day or last meal. If the venous plasma glucose level measured 1 hour later is 7·8 mmol/l (140 mg/dl) or greater, a complete 3-hour glucose tolerance test is performed (Beard et al, 1980; O'Sullivan et al, 1973b).

Table 5.6 Incidence of gestational diabetes according to country of birth

Country of birth	Total no. tested	Gestational diabetes No.	(%)	
Australia, New Zealand	6538	197	3·0	
United Kingdom	572	13	2·3	
China, Singapore, Hong Kong, Philippines, Malaysia	458	38	8·3	†
Vietnam	352	15	4·3	
Greece	325	19	5·9	
Yugoslavia, Czechoslovakia, U.S.S.R., Poland	300	13	4·3	
Italy	295	25	8·5	†
Lebanon, Egypt, Jordan, U.A.E.	254	13	5·1	
Turkey	227	11	4·9	
Sri Lanka, Pakistan, Bangladesh, India	122	10	8·2	*
Malta	104	11	10·6	†
Others	602	28	4·7	
Total	10 149	393	3·9	

Incidence differing significantly from that of Australia and New Zealand born: *$p<0.05$; †$p<0.001$.

2. A plasma sample is taken on arrival at the antenatal clinic, irrespective of when the patient has last eaten. If this is within 2 hours the upper limit of normal is taken as 4·7 mmol/l (85 mg/dl), or if more than 2 hours from the last meal the upper limit is 4·1 mmol/l (74 mg/dl) Lind & McDougall, 1981). Again if these limits are exceeded, a complete glucose tolerance test is performed.
3. A 3-hour glucose tolerance test at 30 weeks on all patients. An additional advantage of measuring the fasting and 3-hour levels is that hypoglycaemia, which has significant associations with intrauterine growth retardation and perinatal mortality, is also identified (Abell & Beischer, 1975).

Glycosylated haemoglobin Hb.A$_{1c}$ has proved to be a useful indicator of average long-term blood glucose levels in diabetic and non-pregnant subjects (Gabbay et al, 1977), but is not an adequate screening test for gestational diabetes (Ross, 1984). This is not surprising since the hyperglycaemia that affects Hb.A$_{1c}$ needs to be long-standing, whereas the hyperglycaemia of gestational diabetes usually develops only after the first trimester (Jovanovic & Peterson, 1985).

Serum fructosamine concentrations are a measure of glycosylated protein and correlate closely with both fasting plasma glucose and glycosylated haemoglobin concentrations. Roberts et al (1983) reported that 85 per cent of women with gestational diabetes had serum fructosamine levels above the 95th percentile established for non-diabetic pregnant patients. The false-positive rate of 5 per cent is lower than the 13 per cent rate from the 50 g oral glucose screening test (O'Sullivan et al, 1973b) and therefore merits further evaluation. Interestingly, fructosamine levels are also higher in the cord blood of infants of mothers with gestational and established diabetes.

Another aspect of screening is to perform *amniotic fluid* and/or *cord blood insulin levels* on gestational diabetes since it has recently been reported that high levels are found when the fetus is macrosomic and in patients destined to develop overt diabetes (Weiss et al, 1984a,b).

MATERNAL MORBIDITY AND PERINATAL MORBIDITY AND MORTALITY

The main maternal hazards from gestational diabetes come from pre-eclampsia and polyhydramnios (Dandrow & O'Sullivan, 1966; Table 5.3), the incidences of which are 2–3 times higher than that of the total hospital population. Polyhydramnios is associated particularly with the more severe degrees of glucose intolerance (Table 5.3).

The fetus is at increased risk from *macrosomia* and conversely from poor *fetoplacental function* as indicated by subnormal oestriol excretion (Abell, 1983; Table 5.3). The increased incidence of *congenital malformations* in the offspring of women with pre-existing diabetes is well established (Pedersen et al, 1964) and a number of groups, including Fuhrmann et al (1983), report that this can be reduced by careful blood sugar control before conception and during organogenesis. The incidence of congenital malformations in infants born to mothers with gestational diabetes, however, is not increased (Dandrow & O'Sullivan, 1966; Beard & Hoet, 1982; Table 5.7) and since the vast majority of such women are normoglycaemic in early pregnancy, there seems little likelihood that any therapeutic measures would be applicable, presupposing that such women could be identified before pregnancy. Of course once identified, counselling is of value before any future pregnancies.

After birth the infant is at greater risk than those offspring of normoglycaemic mothers. *Hypoglycaemia*, although less common than in infants born to overt diabetics (who have a reported incidence of up to 77 per cent), occurs in 25 per cent (Haworth & Dilling, 1976). *Hypocalcaemia*, *hyperbilirubinaemia* and *polycythaemia* are also reported to occur more frequently in these infants (Coustan & Imarah, 1984) who therefore merit careful observation in the neonatal period.

Fetal macrosomia is due to an increase in body fat mass, fat cell weight and associated skinfold thickness. The mechanism that induces these changes is thought to be an insulin-induced enhancement of triglyceride synthesis and storage in the individual adipocytes (Enzi et al, 1980). Macrosomia carries increased risks of significant birth trauma (10 per cent, Gabbe et al, 1977) and exposes the mother to both vaginal and abdominal soft tissue injury.

Although most recent studies do not show any significant difference in perinatal mortality in pregnancies complicated by gestational diabetes when compared with normoglycaemic controls (Hadden, 1980), Pedersen (1984) emphasised that these were treated pregnancies. In an earlier study O'Sullivan et al (1973a) reported that the perinatal mortality was 6·4 per

Table 5.7 Pregnancy outcome according to severity of gestational diabetes in 35 629 consecutive pregnancies

Classification	No. of pregnancies	Stillbirth (%)	Neonatal death (%)	Major fetal malformation (%)	Birthweight > 90th percentile (%)	Birthweight < 10th percentile (%)
Current MMH	797	1·1	1·4	3·0	11·7	8·8
Original MMH	212	1·4	0·7	2·8	14·8	6·9
WHO Impaired	92	3·2	—	1·1	22·3†	3·2*
WHO Diabetic	49	—	5·9†	7·8*	37·3‡	9·8
Total	1150	1·3	1·0	3·0	14·2	8·1
Hospital incidence	40 982	1·3	1·4	3·3	10·0	10·0

Incidence differing significantly from that classified by current MMH criteria: *$p<0.05$; †$p<0.01$; ‡$p<0.001$.

cent amongst gestational diabetics compared with 1·5 per cent in a control group. In a subsequent study, treatment significantly reduced the perinatal wastage (O'Sullivan & Mahan, 1980). Abell et al (1976) reported similar results in a study from this institution, the perinatal mortality falling from 14·3 to 3·9 per cent ($p < 0·05$). The results in a series of 1150 pregnancies in 1016 patients with gestational diabetes treated at the Mercy Maternity Hospital are shown in Table 5.7. As might be expected the incidence of macrosomia, the use of insulin and the perinatal mortality rate are greater in those patients classified with the far more restrictive WHO criteria that diagnosed diabetes and impaired glucose tolerance in only 4/1000 patients. Since diagnosis of gestational diabetes is usually only made between 30 and 32 weeks gestation, comparison of perinatal mortality rates with those of the total hospital population can be misleading since one of the main causes of perinatal wastage, prematurity, has been largely eliminated by the time of diagnosis.

Management

The objectives of diagnosis of gestational diabetes are:

1. to avoid the increased risk of intrauterine death in late pregnancy by fetal monitoring and by induction of labour at 38–40 weeks' gestation when indicated;
2. to minimise the risk of complications of overt diabetes in the patient herself by proper follow-up.

Once a woman is identified as being a gestational diabetic, attention needs to be directed to her blood glucose levels. *Dietary manipulation* is usually all that is needed to maintain the fasting blood glucose below 6 mmol/l (105 mg/dl) and the 2-hour postprandial level below 7 mmol/l (120 mg/dl). Brunzell et al (1971) reported that a high-carbohydrate diet resulted in lower fasting insulin and plasma glucose levels and improved glucose tolerance. Nolan (1984) also reported improved glucose tolerance in gestational diabetics using a low-fat, high-fibre, high-unrefined carbohydrate diet.

In the short time available to the clinician following diagnosis, weight reduction in the obese gestational diabetic is unlikely to significantly improve blood glucose control. If the fasting blood glucose levels cannot be maintained below 6 mmol/l and the 2-hour postprandial below 7 mmol/l, then *insulin therapy* is indicated (Freinkel & Josimovich, 1980) and requires the same tight control, using personal blood glucose analysers where possible, that overt diabetes demands. However there is much individual variation on the part of the physician in the use of insulin in gestational diabetes—e.g. at the King George V Hospital, Sydney the figure is 55 per cent (Plehwe et al, 1984) whereas at the Mercy Maternity Hospital, Melbourne it is 3 per cent (Table 5.3).

The place of low-dose insulin therapy for prevention of macrosomia is more controversial. Coustan & Imarah (1984) reported an incidence of macrosomia of 7 per cent in women given insulin compared with 18 per cent in the untreated group; operative deliveries (16·3 per cent versus 28·5 per cent) and birth trauma (4·8 versus 20·4 per cent) were also significantly reduced. Moreover the incidence of birthweight below the 10th percentile was not increased. The possible influence of treatment on the incidence of fetal macrosomia will depend upon the period of gestation at which gestational diabetes is diagnosed, and is an important reason why screening should be done by 30 weeks gestation.

The importance of careful observation of maternal blood pressure, early detection of proteinuria and polyhydramnios is self-evident.

Fetal monitoring

Fetal monitoring using biochemical means (oestriol, human placental lactogen) kick charts, and antenatal cardiotocography is indicated in these high-risk pregnancies. Ultrasound surveillance should detect most major congenital malformations that would alter management and abnormal growth patterns resulting in either macrosomia or intrauterine growth retardation.

Providing close surveillance of fetoplacental well-being is maintained, labour need not be induced before full term (Gabbe et al, 1977). If induction of labour is performed electively before full term because of gestational diabetes, fetal pulmonary maturity should be ascertained by estimation of amniotic fluid L/S ratio—one of the advantages of allowing diabetic pregnancies to proceed to full term, when tests of fetoplacental function are normal, is that many patients come into spontaneous labour and the need for amniocentesis is avoided. Electronic fetal heart rate monitoring during labour and anticipation of dystocia due to fetal macrosomia are also important considerations.

LONG-TERM IMPLICATIONS OF GESTATIONAL DIABETES

From the mother's viewpoint the major advantage is that once identified long-term follow-up offers the possibility of early diagnosis or prevention of overt diabetes. O'Sullivan's study of women diagnosed as having gestational diabetes in Boston, now comprises 615 women with 328 negative controls followed for up to 28 years—he has reported that 50 per cent of the gestational diabetics and 7 per cent of the negative controls have developed diabetes, 50 per cent of these being decompensated diabetics requiring specific therapy. Using cumulative life table analysis 73 per cent of the gestational diabetics and 11·2 per cent of the controls followed for 24 years or more have developed diabetes. Furthermore gestational diabetics, as a group, had a greater frequency of hypertension, hyperlipidaemia, proteinuria, abnormal electrocardiograms and a higher mortality rate (O'Sullivan, 1984). The criteria used for diagnosis of diabetes in this follow-up study are a variant on those of the USPHS and requires that after a 100 g glucose load three or more plasma values, or the fasting and 3-hour values, should equal or exceed fasting 6·6 mmol/l, 1 hour 10·3 mmol/l, 2 hour 7·4 mmol/l, and 3 hour 6·6 mmol. Again it is important to recognise when comparing one study with another that these standards differ from the WHO criteria.

Grant et al (1986) have performed follow-up glucose tolerance testing of women diagnosed as having gestational diabetes at the Mercy Maternity Hospital, Melbourne (Table 5.8). Since it has been the policy to test the entire antenatal population for glucose intolerance, this study will enable the prevalence of emerging diabetes to be determined in an unselected group, which is not the case in any other reported series. As of November 1985, 447 women had been retested at intervals ranging from 1 to 13 years from the index pregnancy in which gestational diabetes was diagnosed. Using the WHO criteria for classification of diabetes mellitus 49 (11.0 per cent) are now *diabetic* and 35 (7·8 per cent) have *impaired glucose tolerance*; of the 50 women who have been retested 9 or more years after the index pregnancy eight (16 per cent) are diabetic and six (12 per cent) have impaired glucose tolerance. In this study factors that had a predictive value in selecting those who would develop diabetes were:

1. recurrance in a subsequent pregnancy;
2. a first family history of diabetes;
3. weight greater than 70 kg;
4. an abnormal postnatal glucose tolerance test (Table 5.8).

The benefit to the mother may be inferred from the study of Stowers (1984) who treated women who had an abnormal intravenous glucose tolerance test

Table 5.8 Incidence of abnormal glucose tolerance at follow-up according to results of the postnatal glucose tolerance test

Postnatal glucose tolerance test	No.	Normal		Follow-up glucose tolerance test			
				Impaired glucose tolerance		Diabetes	
		No.	(%)	No.	(%)	No.	(%)
Normal	40	31	78	1	3	8	20
Abnormal per Mercy Maternity criteria	13	5	38	3	23	5	38
Impaired glucose tolerance	5	0	0	2	40	3	60
Diabetes	5	0	0	0	0	5	100
Total	63	36	57	6	10	21	33

at 6 weeks postpartum with chlorpropamide. Only 1·3 per cent per annum of this group developed overt diabetes compared with 2·2 per cent of a control group. Sartor et al (1980) have demonstrated that dietary treatment of patients with impaired glucose tolerance reduced the emergence of overt diabetes by more than 50 per cent. This does mean that there is the opportunity to reduce the otherwise inevitable emergence of diabetes with all its consequent medical problems. We, however, are somewhat puzzled by this report because in our experience of follow-up studies, dietary management of gestational diabetics is unlikely to be possible in a controlled study, as women know that they are at risk and many of the obese patients are likely to take the obvious remedy, and we consider that it would be unethical to dissuade them from so doing.

One other aspect of the Boston study of interest for the prevention of the eventual emergence of overt diabetes is the observation that the subgroup of gestational diabetics treated during with insulin pregnancy, who gave birth to macrosomic infants or had a family history of diabetes, had a significantly lower incidence of decompensated diabetes 16 years later (O'Sullivan & Mahan, 1980). This implies that insulin therapy may not only reduce the incidence of macrosomia but also have long-term preventative benefits for the mother.

Gestational diabetes may have long-term implications for the infant since in overt diabetics a number of studies have demonstrated that the incidence of juvenile diabetes in the offspring is 20 times higher than that in a control population (Farquhar, 1969). It is suggested that the fetal pancreas is affected both morphologically and functionally by maternal diabetes, and that the stimulation of the beta cells is responsible for the increase in childhood obesity (Pettitt et al, 1983).

Van Assche and others have demonstrated both pancreatic islet hypertrophy and beta cell hyperplasia in fetuses of gestational diabetics, and that this can be prevented by careful control of maternal blood sugar levels; they postulate that careful maternal metabolic control prevents fetal beta cell exhaustion and perhaps later progression to diabetes (Van Assche, 1984). The answer to this and many other of the problems associated with gestational diabetes referred to above will only come from long-term follow-up studies.

Despite the confusion of terminology and of diagnostic criteria, gestational diabetes remains an important medical disorder of pregnancy. It places the mother and fetus at risk during the pregnancy and has serious implications for their long-term well-being.

ACKNOWLEDGEMENTS

The collation of data on the incidence of gestational diabetes by race, age and weight was done by Miss A. Beischer and Dr J. Gordon, and the pregnancy data by Ms J. Drake. These studies were supported by the Mercy Maternity Hospital Research Foundation.

REFERENCES

Abell D A 1983 Diabetes and gestational diabetes. In: Beischer N A, Abell D A (eds) Third clinical report, Mercy Maternity Hospital Melbourne, for the Years 1978–80. Ramsay Ware, Melbourne, pp 17–19

Abell D A, Beischer N A 1975 Evaluation of the 3-hour oral glucose tolerance test in detection of significant hyperglycemia and hypoglycemia in pregnancy. Diabetes 24: 874–880

Abell D A, Beischer N A, Wood C 1976 Routine testing for gestational diabetes, pregnancy hypoglycaemia and fetal growth retardation and results of treatment. Journal of Perinatal Medicine 4: 197–212

Australian Bureau of Statistics. Births Australia 1983, Canberra

Beard R W, Hoet J J 1982 Is gestational diabetes a clinical entity? Diabetologia 23: 307–312

Beard R W, Gillmer M D G, Oakley N W, Gunn P J 1980 Screening for gestational diabetes. Diabetes Care 3: 468–471

Beischer N A, Holsman M, Kitchen W H 1968 Relation of various forms of anemia to placental weight. American Journal of Obstetrics and Gynecology 101: 801–809

Brunzell J D, Lerner R L, Hazzard W R, Porte D Jr, Bierman E L 1971 Improved glucose tolerance with high carbohydrate feeding in mild diabetes. New England Journal of Medicine 284: 521–524

Castro A, Scott J P, Grettie D P, MacFarlane D, Bailey R E 1970 Plasma insulin and glucose responses of healthy subjects to varying glucose loads during three hour oral glucose tolerance tests. Diabetes 19: 842–851

Coustan D R, Imarah J 1984 Prophylactic insulin treatment of gestational diabetes reduces the incidence of macrosomia, operative delivery and birth trauma. American Journal of Obstetrics and Gynecology 150: 836–842

Dandrow R V, O'Sullivan J B 1966 Obstetric hazards of gestational diabetes. American Journal of Obstetrics and Gynecology 96: 1144–1147

Dwyer P L, Oats J N, Walstab J E, Beischer N A 1982 Glucose tolerance in twin pregnancy. Australian and New Zealand Journal of Obstetrics and Gynaecology 22: 131–134

Enzi G, Inelmen E M, Caretta F, Villani F, Zanardo V, De Biasi F 1980 Development of adipose tissue in newborns of gestational-diabetic and insulin-dependent diabetic mothers. Diabetes 29: 100–104

Farquhar J W 1969 Prognosis for babies born to diabetic mothers in Edinburgh. Archives of Diseases in Childhood 44: 36–40

Freinkel N, Josimovich J 1980 Summary and recommendations of American Diabetic Association Workshop conference on gestational diabetes. Diabetes Care 3: 499–501

Fuhrmann K, Reiher H, Semmler K, Fischer F, Fischer M, Glockner E 1983 Prevention of congenital malformations in infants of insulin dependent diabetic mothers. Diabetes Care 6: 219–223

Gabbay K H, Hasty K, Breslaw J L, Ellison R C, Bunn H F, Gallop P M 1977 Glycosylated hemoglobins and long-term glucose control in diabetes mellitus. Journal of Clinical Endocrinology and Metabolism 44: 859–864

Gabbe S C, Mestman J H, Freeman R K, Anderson G V, Lowensohn R I 1977 Management and outcome of class A diabetes mellitus. American Journal of Obstetrics and Gynecology 127: 465–469

Gilbert J A L, Dunlop D M 1949 Diabetic fertility, maternal mortality and foetal loss rate. British Medical Journal 1: 48–51

Grant P T, Oats J N, Beischer N A 1986 The long-term follow-up of women with gestational diabetes. Australian and New Zealand Journal of Obstetrics and Gynaecology 26: 17–22

Hadden D R 1975 Glucose tolerance tests in pregnancy. In: Sutherland H W, Stowers J M (eds) Carbohydrate metabolism in pregnancy and the newborn. Churchill Livingstone, Edinburgh, pp 19–40

Hadden D R 1980 Screening for abnormalities of carbohydrate metabolism in pregnancy 1966–77. The Belfast experience. Diabetes Care 3: 440–446

Hadden D R, Harley J M G, Kajtar T J, Montgomery D A D 1971 A prospective study of three tests of glucose tolerance in pregnant women selected for potential diabetes with reference to the fetal outcome. Diabetologia 7: 87–93

Hagbard L 1958 The prediabetic period from an obstetric point of view. Acta Obstetrica Gynecologica Scandinavica 37: 497–518

Haworth J C, Dilling L A 1976 Relationships between maternal glucose intolerance and neonatal blood glucose. Journal of Pediatrics 89: 810–813

Jackson W P U 1952 Studies in prediabetes. British Medical Journal 2: 690–696

Jackson W P U, Woolf N 1958 Maternal prediabetes as a cause of the unexplained stillbirth. Diabetes 7: 446–448

Jovanovic L, Peterson C M 1985 Screening for gestational diabetes optimum timing and criteria for retesting. Diabetes 34 Suppl 2: 21–23

Kalkhoff R K, Jacobson M, Lemper D 1970 Progesterone, pregnancy and the augmented plasma insulin response. Journal of Clinical Endocrinology 31: 24–28

Kriss J P, Futcher P H 1948 The relation between infant birth weight and subsequent development of maternal diabetes mellitus. Journal of Clinical Endocrinology 8: 380–389

Kuhl C 1975 Glucose metabolism during and after pregnancy in normal and gestational diabetic women. Influence of normal pregnancy on serum glucose and insulin concentration during basal fasting conditions and after a challenge with glucose. Acta Endocrinologica 79: 709–719

Kuhl C, Hornnes P J, Andersen O 1984 Aetiological factors in gestational diabetes. In: Sutherland H W, Stowers J M (eds) Carbohydrate metabolism in pregnancy and the newborn. Churchill Livingstone, Edinburgh, pp 12–22

Landgraf R, Landgraf-Leurs M M C, Weissman A, Horl R, Van Werder K, Scriba P C 1977 Prolactin: a diabetogenic hormone. Diabetologia 13: 99–104

Lewis T L T 1956 Pregnancy and Diabetes. In: Lewis T L T (ed) Progress in clinical obstetrics and gynaecology. Churchill, London, pp 98–115

Lind T, McDougall A N 1981 Antenatal screening for diabetes mellitus by random blood glucose sampling. British Journal of Obstetrics and Gynaecology 88: 346–357

Lind T, Van C de Groot H A, Brown G and Cheyne G A 1972 Observations on blood glucose and insulin determinations. British Medical Journal 3: 320–323

Long P A 1983 Preeclampsia. In: Beischer N A, Abell D A (eds) Third clinical report, Mercy Maternity Hospital Melbourne, for the Years 1978–80. Ramsay Ware, Melbourne pp 17–19

Macafee C A J, Beischer N A 1974 The relative value of the standard indications for performing a glucose tolerance test in pregnancy. Medical Journal of Australia 1: 911–914

Mengert W F, Laughlin K A 1939 Thirty-three pregnancies in diabetic women. Surgery, Gynecology and Obstetrics 69: 615–617

Miller H C, Hurwitz D, Kuder K 1944 Fetal and neonatal mortality in pregnancies complicated by diabetes mellitus. Journal of the American Medical Association 124: 271–275

National Diabetes Data Group 1979 Classification and diagnosis of diabetes mellitus and other categories of glucose intolerance. Diabetes 8: 1039–1057

Nolan C J 1984 Improved glucose tolerance in gestational diabetic women on a low fat high unrefined carbohydrate diet. Australian and New Zealand Journal of Obstetrics and Gynaecology 24: 174–177

Oats J N, Abell D A, Beischer N A, Broomhall G R 1980 Maternal glucose tolerance during pregnancy with excessive size infants. Obstetrics and Gynecology 55: 184–186

O'Sullivan J B 1984 Subsequent morbidity among gestational diabetic women. In: Sutherland H W, Stowers J M (eds) Carbohydrate metabolism in pregnancy and the newborn. Churchill Livingstone, Edinburgh, pp 174–180

O'Sullivan J B, Mahan C M 1980 Insulin treatment and high risk groups. Diabetes Care 3: 482–485

O'Sullivan J B, Snyder P J, Sporer A C, Dandrow R V, Charles D 1970 Intravenous glucose tolerance test and its modification by pregnancy. Journal of Clinical Endocrinology and Metabolism 31: 33–37

O'Sullivan J B, Charles D, Mahan C M, Dandrow R V 1973a Gestational diabetes and perinatal mortality rate. American Journal of Obstetrics and Gynecology 116: 901–904

O'Sullivan J B, Mahan C M, Charles D, Dandrow R V 1973b Screening criteria for high risk gestational diabetic patients. American Journal of Obstetrics and Gynecology 116: 895–900

Pedersen L M 1984 Perinatal mortality in gestational diabetes. In: Sutherland H W, Stowers J

M (eds) Carbohydrate metabolism in pregnancy and the newborn. Churchill Livingstone, Edinburgh, pp 196–197

Pedersen L M, Tygstrup I, Pedersen J 1964 Congenital malformations in newborn infants of diabetic women. Lancet 1 : 1124–1126

Pedowitz P, Shlevin E L 1957 Perinatal mortality in the unsuspected diabetic. Obstetrics and Gynecology 9 : 524–532

Pettitt D J, Baird H R, Aleck K A, Bennett P H, Knowler W C 1983 Excessive obesity in offspring of Pima women with diabetes during pregnancy. New England Journal of Medicine 308 : 242–245

Plehwe W E, Shearman R P, Turtle J R 1984 Management of pregnancy complicated by diabetes : experience with 232 patients in a four year period. Australian and New Zealand Journal of Obstetrics and Gynaecology 24 : 167–173

Pomeranze J, Stone M L, King E J 1959 The obstetric importance of obesity and 'benign' glycosuria in prediagnosis diabetes. Obstetrics and Gynecology 13 : 181–184

Rizza R A, Mandarino L J, Gerich J E 1982 Cortisol-induced insulin resistance in man : impaired suppression of glucose production and stimulation of glucose utilization due to a postreceptor defect of insulin action. Journal of Clinical Endocrinology and Metabolism 54 : 131–138

Roberts A B, Baker J R, Court D J, James A G, Henley P, Ronayne I D 1983 Fructosamine in diabetic pregnancy. Lancet 998–1000

Ross I S 1984 Glycosylated haemoglobin in the detection of gestational diabetes in an unselected population. In : Sutherland H W, Stowers J M (eds) Carbohydrate metabolism in pregnancy and the newborn. Churchill Livingstone, Edinburgh, pp 206–208

Samaan N, Yen S C C, Gonzalez D, Pearson O H 1968 Metabolic effect of placental lactogen (HPL) in man. Journal of Clinical Endocrinology and Metabolism 28 : 485–491

Sartor G, Schersten B, Carlstrom S, Melander A, Norden A, Persson G 1980 Ten year follow up of subjects with impaired glucose tolerance. Diabetes 29 : 41–49

Silverstone F A, Solomons E, Rubricius J 1961 The rapid intravenous glucose tolerance test in pregnancy. Journal of Clinical Investigation 40 : 2180–2189

Stowers J M 1984 Follow-up of gestational diabetic women treated thereafter. In : Sutherland H W, Stowes J M (eds) Carbohydrate metabolism in pregnancy and the newborn. Churchill Livingstone, Edinburgh, pp. 181–183

Van Assche 1984 Fetal islets in gestational diabetes. In : Sutherland H W, Stowers J M, Carbohydrate metabolism in pregnancy and the newborn. Churchill Livingstone, Edinburgh, pp. 184–186

Victor A 1974 Normal blood sugar variation during pregnancy. Acta Obstetrica Gynecologica Scandinavica 53 : 37–40

Weiss P A M, Hofmann H, Purstner P, Winter R, Lichtenegger W 1984a Fetal insulin balance : gestational diabetes and postpartal screening. Obstetrics and Gynecology 64 : 65–68

Weiss P A M, Purstner P, Winter R, Lichtenegger W 1984b Insulin levels in amniotic fluid of normal and abnormal pregnancies. Obstetrics and Gynecology 63 : 371–375

WHO 1980 World Health Organization Expert Committee on Diabetes Mellitus 1980, WHO. Technical Report Series No 646, Geneva

Triplet pregnancy

Guttmacher (1953) agreed with previous opinions that the Hellin–Zeleny hypothesis ('if $1/N$ is the proportion of twin births to all births in a large population during any period, then the proportion of triplet births during the same period is very near to $1/N^2$') (Hellin, 1895; Zeleny, 1921) is more of a mathematical approximation than a mathematical law. Guttmacher believed that there was one consistent error in the statistics of plural gestations for which no exact or even approximate correction could be made. Vital statistics record only viable births, not total pregnancies, so the unknown abortion rate, which is higher with multiple pregnancies, prevents the hypothesis holding true.

There are other aspects affecting the incidence of triplet pregnancy besides the *abortion rate aspect*. Guttmacher reviewed the incidence of triplets in the U.S.A. from 1928 to 1949 and reported a *racial* aspect in that the highest incidence is amongst Negro races, the lowest amongst Mongoloid people, with Caucasians occupying an intermediate position. Guttmacher also considered *national aspects* and listed 10 nations, from highest to lowest frequency (Italy, Netherlands, Germany, Hungary, U.S.A., France, Bulgaria, Australia, Argentina, Japan).

If the most recent national rates are considered for twins (Brown & Daw, 1980) and if the Hellin–Zeleny hypothesis is applied, a theoretical triplet rate can be deduced and then compared with actual reported rates (Table 6.1). For most countries there appears to be a fair correlation with the Hellin–Zeleny hypothesis.

There is also a *time sequence variation* with the incidence of triplets, though other factors may influence this, as reported below. In England and Wales the incidence has varied as follows: 1:9650 (1945–49); 1:8275 (1955–59); 1:10 657 (1965–69); 1:8445 (1975–79) (Macdonald-Davies, 1983).

James (1980), of the Galton Laboratory, University College, London, found good evidence of a *seasonal variation* with twin and triplet births (higher in December than June). Seasonal variations reported from both Canada and Japan were also considered by James, who hypothesised that the variation may be related to seasonal food consumption variations rather than coital rate, spontaneous abortion rate or probability of fertilisation.

Table 6.1   The racial incidence of twin pregnancy compared to singleton pregnancy; the theoretical incidence of triplets using the Hellin–Zeleny hypothesis; actual incidence of triplets

	National incidence, twins		Theoretical incidence, triplets	Actual incidence, triplets
Nigeria	1:25		1:625	1:425
Scotland	1:86		1:7396	1:8880
Manchester	1:90		1:8100	1:8034
England	1:81	1945–9	1:6561	1:9650
		1955–9		1:8275
	1:92	1965–9	1:8464	1:10 657
	1:104	1975–9	2:10 816	1:8445
U.S.A.	1:97		1:9409	1:9428
Japan	1:160		1:25 600	

One factor, besides being a factor in its own right, also influences the time sequence; this is *artificial induction of ovulation* in use since the late 1960s. In two recent series from Israel the incidence of triplets was 1:1696 and 1:3412 (Ron-el et al, 1981; Holcberg et al, 1982) with one-third of each series of triplets resulting from the use of artificial induction of ovulation. The chances of multiple pregnancy after the use of clomiphene have been reported as seven per 100 for twins, five per 1000 for triplets and three per 1000 for quadruplets. The use of different agents for artificial induction of ovulation may influence the ratio of triplets:twins. This may explain the variation in triplets:twins in the England and Wales series of Macdonald-Davies (1983): 1:102 (1955–59); 1:114 (1965–69); 1:81 (1975–79).

The use of artificial induction of ovulation may simulate the higher serum-follicle-stimulating hormone (FSH) levels seen in Nigerian women, who are recognised as having the highest incidence of twin pregnancy (Sogbanmu, 1981).

Efforts to reduce the risk of multiple pregnancy when inducing ovulation may fail, as for example using pulsatile administration of gonadotrophin releasing hormone (GhRH) if the GhRH overcomes the normal inhibition of hypophyseal follicle stimulating hormone release by oestradiol (Bogchelman et al, 1982).

In vitro fertilisation (IVF) and embryo transfer now coming into vogue proposes the reimplantation of several fertilised ova into the uterine cavity (Kerin et al, 1983), obviously resulting in a high incidence of multiple pregnancy (35 per cent in Kerin et al's 1983 series); so high that Kerin et al proposed a restriction of the number of embryos transferred to limit multiple pregnancy to twins. The use of IVF may account for the already recorded increasing incidence of triplets (Syrop & Varner, 1985).

Triplet pregnancy has occurred in various sites in the female genital tract from unilateral tubal triplet pregnancy (Forbes & Natale, 1968) to triplets in a double uterus, with two infants in one horn and another in the other horn (Varma, 1980). In another similar case there was a 72-day interval between delivery of infants A and B (A by the vaginal route, B by Caesarean section) and infant C, by Caesarean section (Maschiach et al, 1981). A triplet pregnancy has been reported with abortion of one fetus at 16 weeks, then insertion of a cervical cerclage and tocolysis with delivery of the other twins 131 days later, at 35 weeks gestation, by Caesarean section (Banchi, 1984).

One mother tolerated a triplet birth following a successful mitral valve operation (Holland, 1955).

Extreme rarities have been reported amongst the infants of triplet pregnancy; for example, all three with pyloric stenosis (Gillespie et al, 1982); all three with hypodontia (Möller et al, 1981); two of the three triplets with endocardial fibroelastosis (EFE) (Seibold et al, 1980); a craniothoracopagus associated with a normally developed infant in uniovular triplets (Hioki et al, 1982)—one of triplets being an acardiac, acephalic monster (Kirkland, 1982), now reported in 11 cases.

Although multiple pregnancy is associated with anencephalus only a few cases have been reported with triplets (Greenberg et al, 1981), even so monozygous anencephalic triplets have been reported (Scott & Paterson, 1966). Hausknecht et al, (1980) reported a technique for amniocentesis for prenatal diagnosis in triplet gestation. The incidence of triplet births rises with *maternal age* in a comparable way to the incidence of twins (Fig. 6.1)

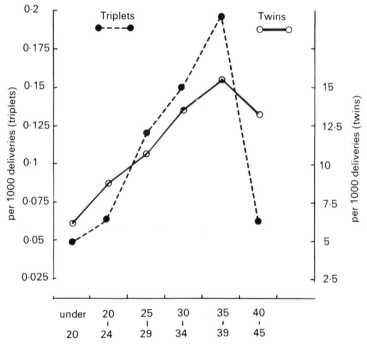

Fig. 6.1   Incidence of triplets (and twins) England and Wales, 1971–75, in relation to maternal age. (Reproduced with kind permission of the Editor, *British Journal of Clinical Practice*.)

(Brown & Daw, 1980). Parity has been considered an important factor influencing pregnancy duration with triplets, with multiparous patients having a pregnancy lasting 2 weeks longer than nulliparous patients. Nulliparous patients may benefit more than multiparous patients from prolonged bed rest, beta-mimetics and gestagens (Ron-el et al, 1981).

Placentation and zygosity

Corney (1975) recorded how triplets may originate from three zygotes (TZ), less commonly from two (DZ), and rarely from one (MZ). In the commonest form (TZ) three ova are fertilised by three sperms, whilst the other two varieties involve the division of a single zygote as in monozygotic twinning (Fig. 6.2). In the case of DZ triplets the combination is a pair of MZ twins and an individual embryo, meaning that the principles of both dizygotic and monozygotic twinning are operating in the same pregnancy.

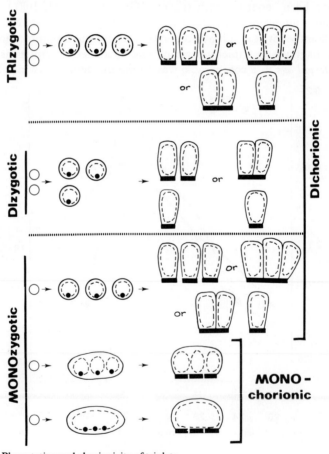

Fig. 6.2 Placentation and chorionicity of triplets.

As with twin births monochorionic placentation is the least common. The usual factors, such as race, will affect triplets so that the highest number of chorionic membranes (trichorionic) are much commoner in Nigeria than amongst Caucasians (Corney, 1975).

Monoamniotic triplet pregnancy, the rarest type, has been reported (Sinykin, 1958) and his paper reviews the aetiological theories.

In appearance the human triplet placenta is usually a single structure weighing over 1500 g on occasions. Its appearance is as a single organ when viewed from the maternal aspect because of fusion during growth even if originating from two or three zygotes. When viewed from the fetal aspect the various components may be divided according to zygosity (Fig. 6.3) very accurately by recording the number of membranes (Bernischke, 1961). Various investigations can be undertaken to check the zygosity; these were recorded by Ganda et al (1977) whilst investigating monozygotic triplets with discordance for diabetes mellitus.

The clinical accuracy of recording zygosity can be checked roughly using Weinberg's method (Daw, 1974). Weinberg's method of statistically sorting one-egg twins (monozygotic) from two-egg twins (dizygotic) consists of subtracting from the total number of like-sexed the total number of unlike-sexed, the remainder being the number of one-egg pairs. This is based on the premise that in any large population sample there are the same number of two-egg male–male plus two-egg female–female pairs as there are male–female plus female–male pairs: the two latter by necessity being dizygotic. The ratio is 1:3 theoretically for twins. When applied to triplets the ratio is 1:5, remembering that the 5 will include di- and tri-zygotic (James, 1980).

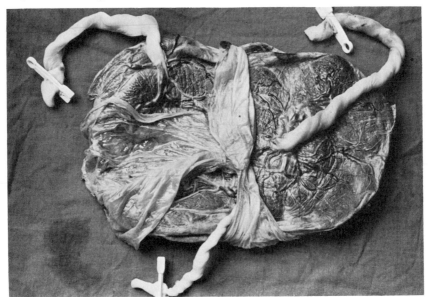

Fig. 6.3   Human dizygotic placenta: fetal aspect.

Placental function tests and triplet pregnancy

Many studies have been undertaken to evaluate antenatal screening procedures where it was hoped high values would suggest multiple pregnancy (or a single large infant) and low values a small-for-dates infant. Most conclude that inexpensive epidemiological and clinical data readily available in the clinic are of more value.

Figure 6.4 shows levels of human placental lactogen (HPL) serially taken from three cases in a series of 14 triplet pregnancies (Daw, 1978). The levels consistently remain above the +2 standard deviation values for both singleton and twin pregnancy. With only three cases significance cannot be applied, but high levels of HPL should encourage the exclusion of multiple pregnancy. Spellacy et al (1978) also found consistently high values of HPL in a single case of triplet pregnancy.

Placental protein 5 has been found to consistently have elevated levels in *twin* pregnancy but is also raised in pre-eclampsia, diabetes and intra-uterine growth retardation (Obiekwe and Chard, 1981).

Antepartum diagnosis

Unfortunately the diagnosis of triplet pregnancy is often only made during delivery. This can occur even when ultrasonic screening or X rays has been used, and a misdiagnosis of only twins made. However in special groups of

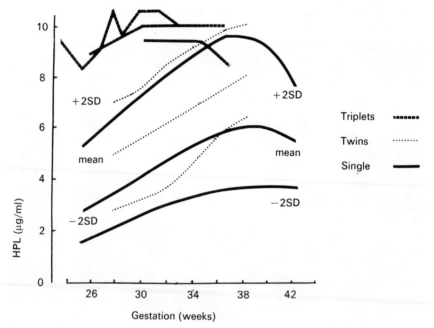

Fig. 6.4   Human placental lactogen values in triplet pregnancy, compared with twin and singleton values.

patients early diagnosis may be made and subsequent treatment may help survival as maturity is so important (Holcberg et al, 1982). If multiple pregnancy is suspected, repeated, serial investigations are indicated until the *exact* number of infants is determined. Itzkowic (1979) suggested that whenever multiple pregnancy is diagnosed an X-ray of the abdomen should be performed before 33 weeks to exclude triplets.

Most authorities would recommend hospitalisation, as soon as the diagnosis is made, with prolonged bed rest. Prophylactic cervical cerclage or beta-mimetic therapy is more debatable and must be on the individual clinician's decision.

Antepartum problems

The main problems that arise with triplet pregnancy are anaemia in the mother (? due to the excessive demands of three infants), pregnancy-induced hypertension (? related to placental size and function), threatened abortion and antepartum haemorrhage (? related to extra-large placenta overlapping the lower segment), and premature labour (? related to overdistension of the uterus). Various prophylactic measures have been attempted to overcome premature labour problems, such as cervical cerclage (as soon as the diagnosis is made), and beta-adrenergic mimetic agents; however, bed rest and particularly hospitalisation still appear to carry the best results.

Growth rates

If the birthweight of individual triplets is plotted against the completed weeks of gestation and compared with the centiles for singleton pregnancy a poor growth record is seen (Fig. 6.5). This poor growth record has been

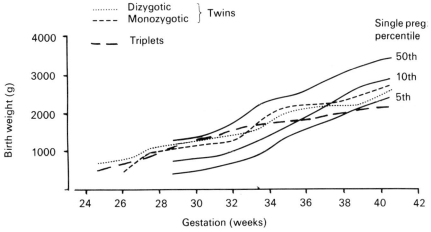

Fig. 6.5 Birthweight of triplets against completed weeks of gestation. (The singleton pregnancy birthweight centiles are those given by Walker (see Daw, 1978).)

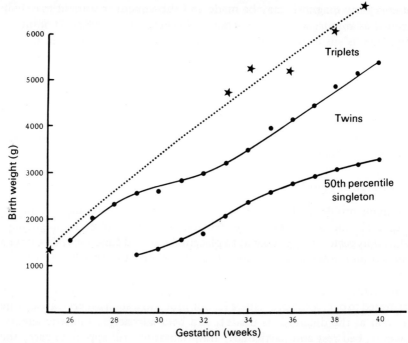

Fig. 6.6   Combined weight of triplet set against completed weeks of pregnancy.

noted in all the reported series of triplet pregnancy and is in accordance with the 'uterine crowding' theory of McKeown and Record (Daw, 1978) but is completely masked if the combined weights of the triplets are considered (Fig. 6.6). However, the poor growth rate for triplet pregnancy does not increase the incidence of *fetus papyraceus*, which is a rare condition with the intra-uterine death and subsequent retention of one or more fetuses (Daw, 1983). There is evidence that cord complications are the predisposing cause and consumptive coagulopathy may follow fetal death *in utero*.

Birthweight

As will be reported later, *maturity* rather than *birthweight* is the determinant for fetal survival in triplet pregnancy. Itzkowic (1979) reported the first-born infant to be the heaviest, but this has not been substantiated in other series, though there is evidence that the lung maturity of the first triplet may determine the onset of labour.

Sex of infants

The sex ratio (proportion of male births) in triplet pregnancy has been analysed in some detail. The sex ratio is lower in triplets than in twins or the general population. There is a variation between countries, from 0·480 (England and Wales), 0·471 (France), 0·487 (Italy), 0·498 (USA—Whites), 0·502 (USA—Negro) to 0·515 (Japan). Imaizumi (1982) thought that in Japan the male triplets were selectively spontaneously aborted compared with twins and the general population.

Fetal presentation and birth order

The fetal presentation at delivery is vertex/vertex/breech; vertex/vertex/ vertex; vertex/breech/breech; or vertex/breech/vertex, according to the various published reports, though all reports agree that the first triplet is most likely to present by the vertex. The first triplet presenting by the breech may therefore be an indication for Caesarean section delivery (Daw & Brown, 1982). The presentation of the second and third infants prior to labour does not need to influence the mode of delivery except in so far as spontaneous breech delivery has carried the greatest mortality rate in some series, particularly for the second and third (Daw, 1978).

The indications for Caesarean section delivery have been given as: malpresentation of the first fetus regardless of the gestational age, prolonged premature rupture of the membranes, dysfunctional labour, and all the other medical or obstetric complications, as with singletons (Ron-el et al, 1981).

Elective Caesarean section has been proposed for all triplet deliveries for optimum management of neonatal problems. On this principle a high Caesarean section rate can produce a lower perinatal mortality (Michlewitz et al, 1981; Ron-el et al, 1981; Loucopoulos et al, 1982).

Time interval between deliveries

Kurtz et al (1958) reported that if the time interval between deliveries was less than 5 minutes the perinatal mortality was half that for an interval over 5 minutes (for both first–second and second–third intervals). They felt that this was a direct result of progressive fetal anoxia due to changes in uteroplacental haemodynamics. Subsequent reports have not mentioned the time interval between deliveries, but the theory of Kurtz et al is sound, and an essential component of Caesarean section delivery, which has been advocated as an aid to reduction of perinatal mortality.

Duration of pregnancy at delivery

The main complication of triplet pregnancy has already been stated to be premature delivery with increasing mortality and morbidity. Up to 80 per cent of triplets will be delivered before the 37th week of pregnancy, and maturity rather than birth weight is the determinant of fetal survival. Any procedure to prolong the pregnancy will improve the survival rates, as is reflected in special groups such as those with induced ovulation, early diagnosis of triplet pregnancy and subsequent hospitalisation (Holcberg et al, 1982; Loucopoulos et al, 1982).

There is evidence that the onset of labour in multiple pregnancy may be determined by the fetus with the most mature lungs who also, it appears, is commonly the presenting fetus and firstborn (Wilkinson et al, 1982).

Perinatal mortality

The stillbirth rate for triplets is four times that of singleton births (Daw & Brown, 1982) (see Fig. 6.7) and the perinatal mortality rate five times that of singleton pregnancy (Macdonald-Davies, 1983). In the large series of 354 sets of triplets reported by Macdonald-Davies it appears that both the stillbirth and perinatal mortality rates are higher for monozygous infants (by applying Weinberg's method to determine the zygosity). Male triplets have a higher mortality rate whether dizygotic or monozygotic (Brown & Daw, 1980).

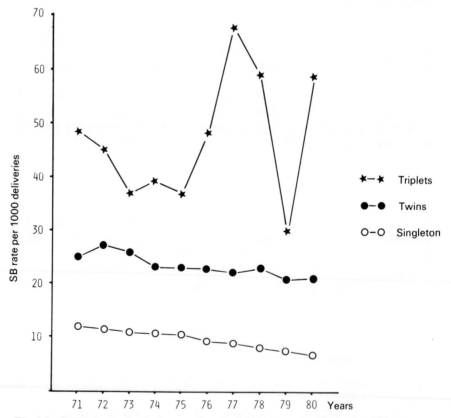

Fig. 6.7   Stillbirth rates for singleton, twin and triplet pregnancies, England and Wales 1971–80. (Reproduced from *Maternal and Child Health* 1980; 7:447, by permission of Barker Publications Ltd.)

Both Daw (1978) and Itzkowic (1979) noted that the second and third infants had an increased perinatal loss compared with the first (a ratio in the order of 1:2:3), probably related to breech delivery of the second and third infants.

Stillbirth is least likely to occur where there is a mixture of the sexes (i.e. some dizygosity). This is related to the higher mortality rate of monozygous infants (see above) and the belief that 'antigenic dissimilarity . . . enhances fetal growth' and also 'immunological differences would be greater . . . for male fetuses . . . than female' (Daw, 1978).

The highest mortality rates among second and subsequent infants in multiple pregnancies may in part be due to delayed pulmonary maturation because of uterine position (Wilkinson et al, 1982).

Postpartum problems

The main postpartum complication of triplet pregnancy is haemorrhage, whether the delivery was by the vaginal or abdominal route, and such atony of the uterus may occur that hysterectomy is necessitated (Ron-el et al, 1981; Holcberg et al, 1982). Secondary (late) postpartum haemorrhage may be just as severe.

Conclusions

1. Early diagnosis of triplet pregnancy is essential if any attempt is to be made to increase the survival rates of triplets.
2. Prolonged bed rest, preferably in hospital, with other preventative measures, may avoid premature labour.
3. Maturity, rather than weight, of the infants is a better guide to survival.
4. Malpresentation of the first fetus regardless of the gestational age is an indication for delivery by Caesarian section. Some would argue that liberal use of Caesarean section improves the survival rate.
5. The second and third infants have a higher perinatal loss.
6. Monozygous infants have a higher perinatal loss.
7. Male infants have a higher perinatal loss, whether mono- or dizygotic.
8. Postpartum haemmorhage due to atony of the uterus remains a serious complication.

REFERENCES

Banchi M T 1984 Triplet pregnancy with second trimester abortion and delivery of twins at 35 weeks' gestation. Obstetrics and Gynecology 64: 728–729
Bernischke K 1961 Accurate recording of twin placentation. Obstetrics and Gynecology 18: 334–347
Bogchelman D, Lappohn R E, Janssens J 1982 Triplet pregnancy after pulsatile administration of gonadotrophin releasing hormone. Lancet ii: 45–46

Brown G, Daw E 1980 Some aspects of triplet pregnancies in England and Wales 1971–1975. British Journal of Clinical Practice 34: 134–135

Corney G 1975 Placentation. In: MacGillivray I, Nylander P P S, Corney G (eds) Human multiple reproduction. Saunders, London, pp 72–76

Daw E 1974 Twin pregnancy—the effects of recent socio-ecological factors. Health Bulletin XXXII: 1–4

Daw E 1978 Triplet pregnancy. British Journal of Obstetrics and Gynaecology 85: 505–509

Daw E 1983 Fetus papyraceus—11 cases. Postgraduate Medical Journal 59: 598–600

Daw E, Brown G 1982 Triplet and twin stillbirth rates—a cause for concern. Maternal and Child Health 7: 447–450

Daw E, Walker J 1975 Biological aspects of twin pregnancy in Dundee. British Journal of Obstetrics and Gynaecology 82: 29–34

Forbes D A, Natale A 1968 Unilateral tubal triplet pregnancy. Obstetrics and Gynecology 31: 360–362

Ganda O P, Soeldner J S, Gleason R E, Smith T M, Kilo C, Williamson J R 1977 Monozygotic triplets with discordance for diabetes mellitus and diabetic microangiopathy. Diabetes 26: 469–479

Gillespie J C, Peterson G H, Lehocky R, Shearer L 1982 Occurrence of pyloric stenosis in triplets. American Journal of Diseases of Children. 136: 746–747

Greenberg M, Krim E Y, Mastrota V F, Rosenfeld D L, Goldman M, Fenton A N 1981 Discordant anencephalus in a pergonal-induced triplet pregnancy. Journal of Reproductive Medicine 26: 593–594

Guttmacher A E 1953 The incidence of multiple births in man and some of the other unipara. Obstetrics and Gynecology 2: 22–35

Hausknecht R U, Yem M C, Godmilow L 1980 Prenatal genetic diagnosis in a triplet gestation. Obstetrics and Gynecology 58: 382–385

Hellin D 1895 Die Ursache der Multiparität der Uniparen Tiere überhaupt und der Zwillingschwanderschaft beim Menschen. Seitz and Schauer, Munich

Hioki T, Tominaga Y, Maeda K, Matsui K 1982 A craniothoracopagus associated with a normally developed newborn infant in uniovular triplets. Asia Oceania Journal of Obstetrics and Gynaecology 8: 29–35

Holcberg C, Biale Y, Lewenthal H, Insler V 1982 Outcome of pregnancy in 31 triplet gestations. Obstetrics and Gynecology 59: 472–476

Holland R M 1955 Triplet birth following mitral commissurotomy. Obstetrics and Gynecology 5: 107–108

Imaizumi Y 1982 Sex ratio of triplet births in Japan. Human Heredity 32: 114–120

Itzkowic D 1979 A survey of 59 triplet pregnancies. British Journal of Obstetrics and Gynaecology 86: 23–28

James W H 1980 Seasonality in twin and triplet births. Annals of Human Biology 7: 163–175

Kerin J F, Quinn P J, Kirby C, Seamark R F, Warnes G M, Jeffrey R, Matthews C D, Cox L W 1983 Incidence of multiple pregnancy after in-vitro fertilisation and embryo transfer. Lancet ii: 537–540

Kirkland J A 1982 An acardiac, acephalic monster in a triplet pregnancy. Australian and New Zealand Journal of Obstetrics and Gynecology 22: 168–171

Kurtz G R, Davis L L, Loftus J B 1958 Factors influencing the survival of triplets. Obstetrics and Gynecology 12: 504–508

Loucopoulos A, Jewelewicz R, Vande Wiele R L 1982 Multiple gestations. Acta Geneticae Medicae et Gemellologiae 31: 263–266

Macdonald-Davies I 1983 Mortality in multiple births. Medical Statistics Division, Office of Population Censuses and Surveys

Maschiach S, Ben-Rafael Z, Dor J, Serr D M 1981 Triplet pregnancy in uterus didelphys with delivery interval of 72 days. Obstetrics and Gynecology 58: 519–521

McKendrick M W, Fitzgerald M G 1978 Diabetes in identical triplets. British Medical Journal i: 482

Michlewitz H, Kennedy J, Kawada C, Kennison R 1981 Triplet pregnancies. Journal of Reproductive Medicine 26: 243–246

Möller P, Berg K, Ruud A F, Kvien T K 1981 Variable expression of familial hypodontia in monozygotic triplets. Scandinavian Journal of Dental Research 89: 16–18

Obiekwe B C, Chard T 1981 Circulating levels in twin pregnancy. European Journal of Obstetrics, Gynaecology and Reproductive Biology 12: 135–141

Ron-el R, Caspi E, Schreyer P, Weinraub Z, Arieli S, Goldberg M D 1981 Triplet and quadruplet pregnancies and management. Obstetrics and Gynecology 57: 458–463

Scott J M, Paterson L 1966 Monozygous anencephalic triplets—a case report. Journal of Obstetrics and Gynaecology of the British Commonwealth 77: 147–151

Seibold H, Mohr W, Lehmann W D, Lang D, Spanel R, Schwarz J 1980 Fibroelastosis of the right ventricle in two brothers of triplets. Pathology, Research and Practice 170: 402–409

Sinykin M B 1958 Monoamniotic triplet pregnancy with triple survival. Obstetrics and Gynecology 12: 78–82

Sogbanmu M O 1981 Triplet pregnancy in Nigeria. International Journal of Gynaecology and Obstetrics 19: 301–304

Spellacy W N, Buhi W C, Birk S A 1978 HPL levels in multiple pregnancy. Obstetrics and Gynecology 52: 210–212

Syrop C H, Varner M W 1985 Triplet gestation: maternal and neonatal implications. Acta Geneticae Medicae et Gemellologiae 34: 81–88

Varma T R 1980 Double uterus with twin pregnancy in the left and singleton in the right horns: a case report. Journal of Obstetrics and Gynaecology 1: 36–37

Wilkinson A R, Jenkins P A, Baum J D 1982 Uterine position and fetal lung maturity in triplet and quadruplet pregnancy. Lancet ii: 663

Zeleny C L 1921 The relative numbers of twins and triplets. Science 53: 262

Uterine contractions and the fetus

The powers of labour are generated by uterine contractions and are responsible for the progress of labour. Adequate labour progress and delivery are entirely dependent on effective contractions. The passenger within the amniotic cavity has to tolerate variations in oxygen supply during contractions without becoming compromised. The capacity of the fetoplacental unit to tolerate such stress will determine whether fetal distress occurs.

Contractions have been studied for many years but it was the introduction of oxytocic drugs such as oxytocin, ergometrine and prostaglandins that stimulated interest in the uterine and fetal response to such agents. The contribution of dystocia to rising Caesarean section rates in the USA has recently prompted the National Institutes of Health to recommend examination of the diagnostic criteria of dystocia and research to clarify the factors which affect the progress of labour (Caesarean childbirth: NIH consensus statement).

This chapter reviews the field of research on uterine activity measurements, equipment used and the spectrum of activity in spontaneous normal labour. Based on these findings an approach to oxytocin titration to optimise length of induced labour without compromising the fetus is discussed. The theory of cervical and pelvic tissue resistance according to parity and cervical score is explored. A rational approach to augmenting labour in high-risk situations with the help of a uterine catheter and uterine activity measurements is elaborated.

Historical background

Although external tocography is more widely used in clinical practice than internal tocography the latter method preceded the former historically. Schatz (1872) was the first investigator to insert a probe into the human uterus to measure intrauterine pressure. Schaffer (1898) subsequently devised an instrument which was applied to the abdomen overlying the distended abdomen by means of straps, and estimated the force exerted by the contracting uterus.

Sir Henry Dale (1906) had recorded the action of pituitary gland extract on uterine tissue in animal experiments, and Blair Bell (1909) recommended its use but considered it dangerous prior to delivery of the fetus. Hofbauer in 1911 was the first to suggest its use in established labour (Hofbauer & Hoerner, 1927) and Blair Bell also recommended this later (Blair Bell 1925). The structure of oxytocin itself was not discovered until 1953 (Du Vigneaud et al, 1953) leading to its synthesis in 1954 (Du Vigneaud et al, 1954).

Embrey (1940) used external techniques to assess the effects of various pharmacological agents. His comments are as relevant today as in 1940, when he stated that there can be no doubt that efficiency of the expulsive forces is indirectly responsible for many of the disasters of midwifery. Delay consequent on poor contractions increases the incidence of interference to expedite delivery which, in turn, especially if universally applied, may be a cause of lacerations, haemorrhage and sepsis. Many of the complications of labour become increasingly dangerous and difficult to manage in the presence of inefficient uterine contractions. Reynolds et al (1948), also using external techniques but having a multi-channel device, introduced the concept of fundal dominance of contractions spreading inferiorly on the uterus. Smyth (1957) described the guard ring tocodynamometer, claiming accurate measurement of contractions, and Bell (1981) further developed this technique for use in the antenatal patient with intact membranes to predict preterm labour.

Although external tocography or a hand placed on the abdomen will provide an indication of the frequency and duration of contractions they provide no information about intra-uterine pressure. Bourne and Burn (1927), working in Queen Charlotte's Hospital, inserted a fluid-filled bag mounted on the end of a catheter through the cervix. The bag was placed in an extra-amniotic position under general anaesthesia: rupture of the membranes was considered undesirable because of the risks of infection and the bad reputation of 'dry' labour. Williams and Stallworthy (1952) used an intra-amniotic technique with the amniotic sac itself acting as a balloon (Fig. 7.1). The catheter was passed through the vagina and cervix, anaesthesia not being considered necessary. Alvarez and Caldeyro (1950) had already reported the insertion of a fluid-filled catheter through the anterior abdominal wall (Fig. 7.2), performing multiple insertions at different stages of pregnancy. Their unit in Uruguay performed very important work but an abdominal insertion of a catheter would today be considered hazardous and unethical, as it was by Williams and Stallworthy. Turnbull (1957) conducted extensive studies using a transcervical intra-amniotic approach, and this method has been most popular subsequently. More recent work has seen the evolution of materials and methods as described in the following paragraphs.

Intra-uterine catheters

Disposable, fluid-filled, plastic catheters connected to a transducer dome (Fig. 7.3) have been used for much of the work on uterine activity. They are

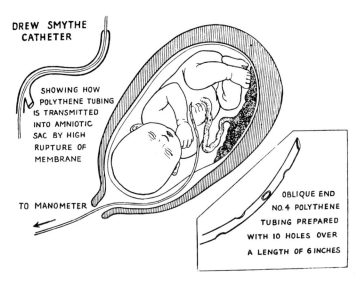

Fig. 7.1   Transcervical intra-amniotic technique of Williams & Stallworthy (1952).

awkward to set up, demanding maintenance of the column of fluid during insertion. Odendaal et al (1976) showed that pressure-recording using such devices may be unreliable due to blockage by vernix, blood clot or fetal parts. The signal may be attenuated by the presence of air bubbles, and zeroing of

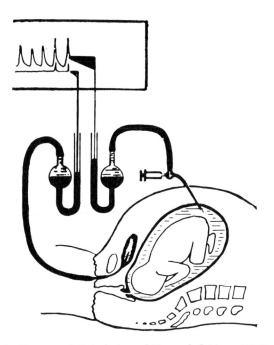

Fig. 7.2   Abdominal intra-amniotic technique of Alvarez & Caldeyro (1950).

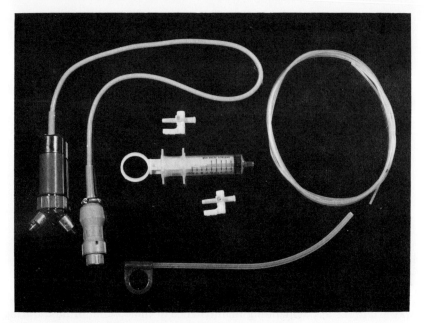

Fig. 7.3   Plastic fluid-filled cather kit, transducer dome and cable.

the system is difficult. This is because the transducer dome must be placed at a level with respect to the mother's abdomen where the catheter tip is thought to be. Reports have appeared of fetal, cord or placental damage associated with such a system (Tutera & Newman, 1975; Nuttall, 1978; Trudinger & Pryse Davies, 1979).

Steer et al (1978) introduced the transducer-tipped catheter (Figs 7.4a, b Sonicaid—Gaeltec Ltd), which is easy to insert, not associated with fetal damage, capable of producing good-quality recordings, but expensive. When not in use it is stored in a plastic tube filled with activated glutaraldehyde attached to the fetal monitor. They found no demonstrable morbidity especially due to infection associated with its use. The expense of such a device is offset by greater reliability of recording, and reusability. Each catheter may be used for more than 100 patients if handled with care. A fibre optic pressure transducer has recently been introduced (Svenningsen et al, 1984) which might prove to be more robust but has yet to be fully tested clinically.

QUANTIFICATION OF UTERINE ACTIVITY

The terminology used to describe a tocographic tracing is shown in Fig. 7.5. Active pressure, duration and contraction interval (related to frequency) are easy to quantify but coordination is more difficult. The average active pressure, average duration and average frequency of contractions have been

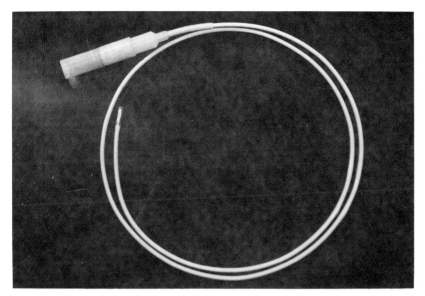

Fig. 7.4a   Sonicaid Gaeltec catheter.

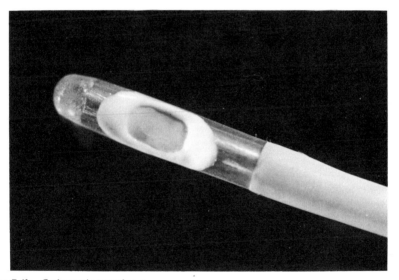

Fig. 7.4b   Catheter tip transducer.

used to quantify activity; however all may change over a period of time and serial observations are cumbersome. Bourne and Burn (1927) suggested that the area under the tocographic curve represented uterine work being affected by all three variables; this concept has subsequently been used as an integral part of several methods of quantification.

The Montevideo unit was introduced by Caldeyro-Bracia et al in 1957.

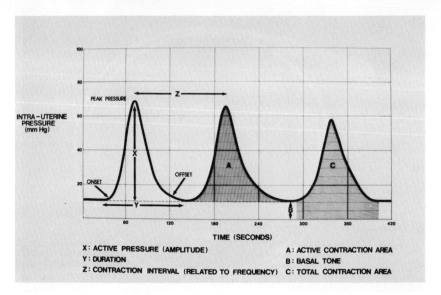

Fig. 7.5   Terminology of uterine contractions.

Figure 7.6 shows how Montevideo units are calculated. Average duration is multiplied by average frequency over a period of 10 minutes. Two problems are apparent. The measurement does not include contraction duration, and Montevideo units are difficult to quantify on-line whilst labour is in progress. El Sahwi et al (1967) devised the Alexandria unit to solve the first problem by including a multiplication factor of the mean contraction duration in minutes. DeHart et al (1977) subsequently devised electronic methods to quantify Montevideo units on line.

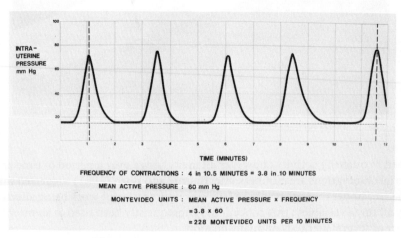

Fig. 7.6   Calculation of Montevideo units.

Hon and Paul (1973) described the on-line quantitation of total contraction area. They proposed that 1 uterine activity unit (UAU) be defined as 1 torr-minute. This means that it is equivalent to a rectangle 1 mm high which lasts for 1 minute. Torr-minutes are much less cumbersome than Torr-seconds.

Harbert (1982) compared quantification using Montevideo units, Alexandria units, UAU and average pressures, finding similarities evidenced by statistically significant linear correlation coefficients.

Analysis of records suggested that the area under basal pressure contributed a large amount to the total area, whilst this component might not represent useful activity as far as the dynamic process of labour was concerned. Steer (1977) therefore proposed using the active contraction area derived by an electronic subtraction technique on-line. This was termed the uterine activity integral (UAI) and was processed in Système International (SI) units. The SI unit of pressure is the kiloPascal, being equivalent to 7·5 millimetres of mercury. A pressure of 1 kiloPascal for a duration of 1 second is 1 kiloPascal second (kPas). This has to be measured over a period of 15 minutes although UAUs had been measured over 10-minute intervals. A period of 15 minutes was chosen because this coincides with the length of time taken to establish a stable response to short-term changes in oxytocin infusion rate. Sequential values are therefore obtained at 15-minute intervals throughout labour using a Sonicaid FM3R or FM6 fetal monitor. Steer et al (1984) measured contraction frequency, active pressure, Montevideo units and active contraction area in the same subjects finding that active contraction area correlated better than any of the other measures with the rate of cervical dilatation in the active phase of labour. The relationship between 1 UAU and 1 kPas is a purely arithmetical one, as shown in Figure 7.7.

Care should be exercised in the interpretation of UAI values when

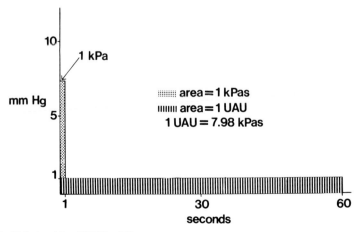

Fig. 7.7   Relationship of UAU to kPa.

inspection of the trace reveals excessive frequency or incoordination, because both of these may lead to high UAI values in a suboptimal labour.

PHYSIOLOGY OF UTERINE ACTIVITY

Although uterine contractions have been studied in some detail the endocrinological events of parturition present a complex picture which has been recently reviewed by Fuchs and Fuchs (1984).

Neurological control of uterine activity does not appear to be important. This observation is supported by the findings of Sjoberg (1967), showing tha myometrial cells have a sparse innervation further reduced during pregnancy, and by the observation of normal labour and delivery in paraplegic patients (Mulla, 1957). The contractile function of the uterus is largely humoral or myogenic.

There is no anatomical pacemaker governing the pattern of uterine contractions. The contraction usually arises in the uterine fundus and spreads from cell to cell through a syncytium. This may explain why patterns of incoordination have a tendency to recur throughout one individual labour (Gibb et al, 1984a). Effer et al (1969) proposed an index of uterine arrhythmia demonstrating that there appears to be an intrinsic pattern of uterine contractile rhythm each patient assumes once labour is established. Schulman and Romney (1970) confirmed these observations, emphasising the variability of uterine contractions. Gap junction formation appears to be a key to synchronisation of uterine activity (Garfield & Hayashi, 1981). This is oestrogen-dependent and these junctions provide low-resistance pathways for the conduction of electrical activity from cell to cell. Electromyographic recordings made in women during labour indicate increasing synchronisation with advancing labour (Wolfs & Van Leeuwen, 1979).

Uterine contractions are asymmetrical with the increase of pressure being more rapid than the decrease. Harbert (1982) documented the cardiovascular changes associated with uterine contractions in Rhesus monkeys. The pulse rate rises, as do the systolic and diastolic blood pressures, with increasing intra-amniotic pressure. Vena caval pressure also increases but rather later than uterine artery blood flow, which begins to decrease within seconds after a detectable rise in intra-amniotic pressure. Minimal flow usually occurs during the ascending phase of a uterine contraction and stabilises until after the peak intensity is reached. Flow then returns to the precontraction level or slightly above. Myometrial venous channels appear to be emptied of blood during contractions. The observation that arterial inflow ceases before intra-amniotic pressure rises above arterial pressure suggests that mechanisms other than relative pressures govern blood flow. These may involve a sphincteric-like action of the myometrium on the vessels. The intervillous space acting as a reservoir is likely to play an important role in fetal oxygenation during the periods of reduced blood flow. Bleker et al (1975) showed expansion of this space measured by ultrasond during contractions in normal patients. Borell et al (1964), using arteriographic techniques, also demonstrated the trapping of intervillous blood during a contraction but found no correlation between slowing of arterial blood flow and intra-amniotic pressure. These considerations may be important when considering the concept of fetoplacental reserve.

CLINICAL STUDIES

Different types of patients might be expected to exhibit different uterine activity profiles. Parity, age, race, fetal weight, maternal height, multiple pregnancy, fetal presentation and position could all be expected to play a role. Patients in abnormal labour, augmented labour and induced labour might behave differently. Events occurring in labour—such as the administration of drugs, epidural anaesthesia, retention of urine, rupture of the membranes and changes of posture—could affect uterine contractions.

The understanding of labour was much advanced by the introduction of the graphic analysis of labour by Friedman (1954). This enabled different types of labour progress to be identified. Philpott and Castle (1972) developed this concept using alert lines and action lines to facilitate labour management in rural Africa. Studd (1973) introduced this to the United Kingdom and evolved a nomogram of labour progress based on a study of 15 000 labours. O'Driscoll et al (1969) had introduced basic partograms and an expected labour progress line of 1 cm/h in their historic study of the active management of labour. O'Driscoll's approach results in oxytocin augmentation in about 50 per cent of primigravidae, whilst that of Studd results in an equivalent figure of 25 per cent.

Any study of labour must involve the analysis of labour progress and recognition of types of abnormal progress: prolonged latent phase, primary dysfunctional labour and secondary arrest (Cardozo et al, 1982).

In view of all these variable factors it is important to specify the existing conditions in a particular patient before interpreting uterine activity values.

Normal levels of uterine activity previously reported in the literature have been in Montevideo units or uterine activity units. Most of these reports have not documented cervical dilatation–specific values, and many of them have not taken all variables into account. Comparison is therefore difficult.

Spontaneous labour

There have been three recent reports using comparable methods: Cowan et al (1982), Steer et al (1984) and Gibb et al (1984a). Cowan et al (1982) studied African patients of rather short stature with 30 per cent being delivered instrumentally. They found a slow rise of uterine activity during the first stage of labour in nulliparous patients with an overall median of 1824 k/Pas/15 min during relatively short labours: median duration 2·65 h. Steer et al (1984), in a small group of mixed parity including two patients delivered by Caesarean section, found a steady rise in uterine activity with a mean activity value of 1099 kPas/15 min. Gibb et al (1984a), studying Singaporean patients of Chinese origin adhering to strict criteria of normality, found a slow rise in activity during the first stage of labour with a peak in the late first stage prior to unassisted delivery (Fig. 7.8). Their overall median value was 1440 kPas/15 min, falling midway between those of the other two studies.

All of these studies have shown wide ranges of activity; however it is important to establish a normal range if such values are to be used to guide the management of abnormal labour. The differing findings may in part be explained by differing patient characteristics and differing interpretation of the concept of normal labour progress. Use of a nomogram proposed by Studd (1973), and allowing progress to deviate up to 2 h to the right of the nomogram before augmentation is instituted, would include the slower as well as the faster normal labours: such a method was adopted by Gibb et al (1984a).

It is striking that these three studies were performed in different countries and possible racial variation should be considered. The incidence of diseases may vary on a racial basis but human physiology is universal. Any effect of race on labour may be expected to be due to the physical characteristics of different racial groups rather than intrinsic differences in uterine function. It is probably valid to extrapolate normal values from one race to another but this requires further study.

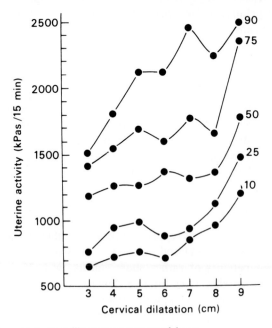

Fig. 7.8   Uterine activity in nulliparous spontaneous labour.

The effect of parity

Arulkumaran et al (1984a) performed a study in multiparous Singaporean women of Chinese origin adhering to the same criteria of normality as the previously reported nulliparous group. Cervical dilatation-specific uterine activity values are shown in Figure 7.9. Once again there was a wide range, but a steady rise of activity was seen in the first stage of labour with a steeper rise towards the end. The overall median value was 1130 kPas/15 min and Figure 7.10 shows a comparison of median values. The median values at 3, 4, 5, and 6 cm dilatation were significantly lower in the multiparous group, permitting the conclusion that the parous uterus requires to expend significantly less effort to effect normal vaginal delivery than its nulliparous counterpart. This supports the findings of Huey et al (1976) and Turnbull (1957), but contradicts those of Steer et al (1984) who studied only 21 patients of mixed parity.

The clinical impression of many experienced obstetricians and midwives that parous patients tend to labour more easily appears to have some substance.

Induced labour

Labour should be induced so as to mimic the physiological process of

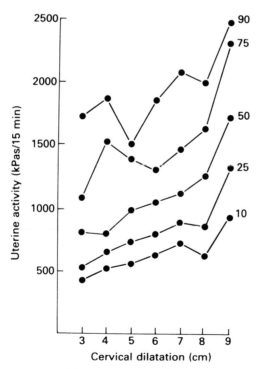

Fig. 7.9   Uterine activity in multiparous spontaneous labour.

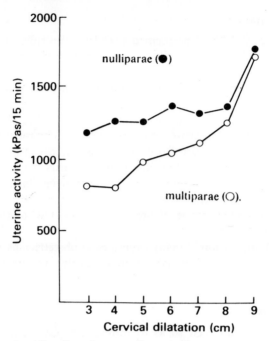

Fig. 7.10   Comparison of median values according to parity.

spontaneous labour. The aim should be to generate uterine activity similar to that found in spontaneous labour.

Oxytocin is usually infused at a starting dose of 2 milliunits/min. There are several incremental dosage schedules; doubling the dose at regular intervals by titrating against uterine contractions (Turnbull & Anderson, 1968), regular constant increases in arithmetic form (Woolfson et al, 1976) or a combination of both. Based on the observation of pulsatile release of oxytocin during human labour (Gibbens et al, 1972), Pavlou et al (1978) compared continuous and pulsed oxytocin infusion in the induction of labour. The induction–delivery and induction-full dilatation intervals were similar but the total dose of oxytocin required was significantly lower in the pulsed group. Toaff et al (1978) studied induction of labour by pharmacological (2·6 mU/min to 422·4 mU/min) and physiological (2·6 mU/min to 13·2 mU/min) doses of intravenous oxytocin. Pharmacological doses gave better results in terms of induction–delivery intervals, incidence of failed inductions and puerperal morbidity. The incidence of hypertonus was similar in both groups and unrelated to oxytocin doses. The principle was to titrate oxytocin to generate a prescribed level of uterine activity to achieve successful induction of labour. Beazley et al (1975) found that induced labour, once established, could be maintained with a lower dose of oxytocin than initially required.

Krapohl et al (1965) developed equipment which electronically monitored and controlled labour. The system automatically changed the infusion rate in response to the nature of the uterine contractions. It was too complex, not allowing for the essential variability of normal contraction patterns which makes a closed-loop system difficult to operate. Francis et al (1970) developed an automatic infusion system (Cardiff pump) of the open-loop type not being directly dependent on input from contraction assessment. It ensured efficient administration of oxytocin, doubling the dose every 12·5 min, but the operator had to select the appropriate maximum dose based on contractions assessed manually or by intra-uterine catheter. This is comparable to an intravenous infusion regulated by a peristaltic infusion pump but with automatic preset increments of dose rate. Such a system requires careful supervision to avoid hyperstimulation.

Carter and Steer (1980) described a closed-loop automatic infusion system (AIS) entirely dependent on uterine activity assessment using an intra-uterine catheter (Fig. 7.11a). The loop mechanism is shown diagrammatically in Figure 7.11b. This system functions according to a present programme, aiming for UAI values in the range of 700–1500 kPas/15 min.

Gibb et al (1984b) studied the outcome of labour in patients induced using such a system compared to that in a control group induced using a peristaltic infusion pump (IVAC) infusing oxytocin in a semi-arithmetic dose schedule to attain uterine activity values similar to those in their previous studies of spontaneous labour. 121 patients were classified according to parity and cervical score. They were nulliparous or multiparous, the modified cervical score being good ($\geqslant 6/10$) or poor ($\leqslant 5/10$) and patient characteristics being similar in all groups. They were allocated to AIS or peristaltic infusion pump system. Labour was significantly longer in those induced by AIS, particularly in nulliparae and patients with poor cervical scores. In nulliparae with poor cervical scores the AIS proved inadequate to effect vaginal delivery in about half the cases. There were no significant differences in neonatal outcome as measured by umbilical vein pH.

Uterine activity during such labours was studied according to phase of labour rather than cervical dilatation because of great variation in length of labour. Irrespective of parity there appeared to be an initial incremental phase when activity increased to a plateau followed by a terminal rise prior to the second stage (Figs 7.12 and 7.13). The plateau phase and terminal rise were divided into four equal parts. The feature of a plateau phase confirms the findings of Steer et al (1975) but its level appeared to be dependent on mode of oxytocin infusion. Those patients having oxytocin infused by peristaltic infusion pump had a higher plateau level and delivered earlier without undue stress to the fetus as measured by umbilical vein pH. It is the programme incorporated in the AIS pump that is inadequate, and not the system itself. Another programme based on aiming for uterine activity values previously observed in spontaneous labour (Gibb et al, 1984a; Arulkumaran et al, 1984a), and on which the control of the peristaltic infusion system were based, might lead to improved results.

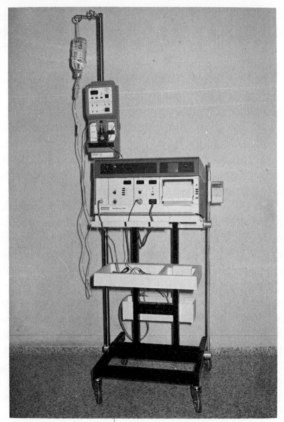

Fig. 7.11a   Automatic infusion system.

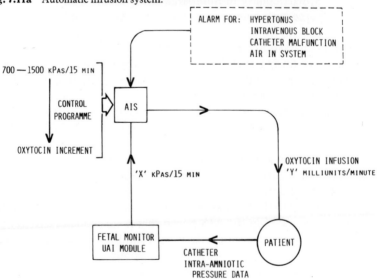

Fig. 7.11b   Diagrammatic representation of AIS closed loop.

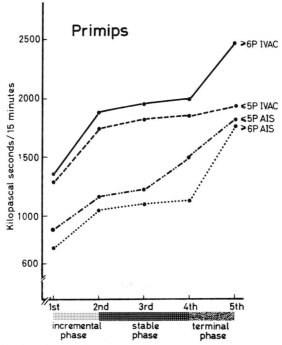

Fig. 7.12 Profile of uterine activity during induced labour in Prirnips according to mode of oxytocin infusion: peristaltic infusion pump (IVAC) or automatic infusion system (AIS).

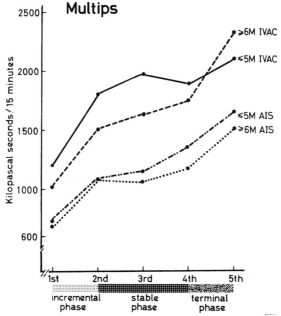

Fig. 7.13 Profile of uterine activity during induced labour in multips according to mode of oxytocin infusion: peristalic infusion pump (IVAC) or automatic infusion system (AIS).

AIS does present other problems of sensitivity of alarm settings and expense of the equipment. Whilst theoretically attractive the current climate of obstetric opinion against undue intervention and unnecessary technology makes its acceptance difficult in clinical practice.

Total uterine activity—cervical and pelvic tissue resistance

Rossavik (1978) proposed that a certain total uterine activity in labour was needed to overcome cervical and pelvic tissue resistance. He calculated the uterine work as the product of active pressure in kiloPascals and the duration of contractions in seconds, and called it the total uterine impulse. He showed a positive correlation between total uterine impulse (and hence resistance) between 5 and 10 cm cervical dilatation and the frequency of operative vaginal deliveries especially in nulliparae.

Arulkumaran et al (1984b) used such a concept but calculated cumulative UAI values throughout the induced labours reported by Gibb et al (1984b). This was termed the total uterine activity (TUA). Table 7.1 shows the total uterine activity in induced labour according to parity, cervical score and mode of oxytocin infusion. There were no significant differences in TUA required to induce labour with respect to mode of infusion. The AIS generated the same amount of uterine activity as the peristaltic infusion system within each parity and cervical score group at the expense of a longer duration of labour.

Nulliparae with a poor cervical score required the greatest amount of uterine activity 60 000 kPas (Fig. 7.14), whilst nulliparae with good score and multiparae with a poor score required 30 000 kPas and multiparae with a good score required the least, being about 15 000 kPas. These differences were all statistically significant. Cases requiring Caesarean section were excluded from the analysis. These values are entirely consistent with the theory that the uterus has to generate enough activity to overcome the cervical and pelvic tissue resistance presented to it. In induced labour, if the TUA exceeds the value expected for the relevant parity and cervical score, the possibility of cephalopelvic disproportion, malposition or failed induction of labour should be considered. In situations of borderline fetoplacental

Table 7.1 Total uterine activity in induced labour according to parity, score and mode of oxytocin infusion

Parity	Cervical score	Total uterine activity (kPas)	
		IVAC	AIS
Nulliparae	$\leqslant 5$	56 878	61 685
	$\leqslant 6$	27 065	35 619
Multiparae	$\leqslant 5$	27 633	35 155
	$\leqslant 6$	15 632	14 488

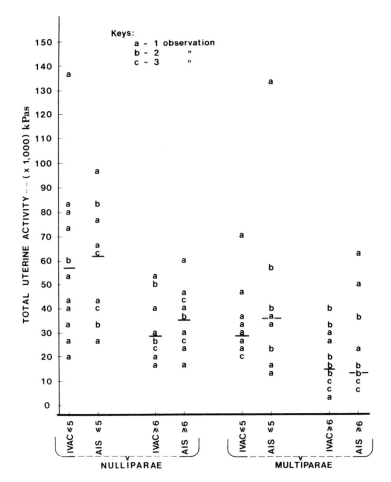

Fig. 7.14 Comparison of total uterine activity according to parity score and mode of oxytocin infusion.

function it may be possible to effect delivery with lower uterine activity values over a longer period of time.

Further work is required to elaborate the prognostic value of cumulative uterine activity in difficult labours.

CLINICAL APPLICATIONS

Intra-uterine pressure measurements are not useful when cervimetric labour progress is normal, and such patients do not require catheters. When oxytocin is being used for induction or augmentation, especially if labour is prolonged, they contribute to management. Oxytocin infusion can be regulated to optimise contractions and to complete an adequate trial of labour in reasonable time. The duration of abnormal labour is directly related to deteriorating fetal and maternal condition. A decision for Caesarean section may be made at the appropriate time. Concern has been expressed about the dangers of oxytocin-induced labours to fetuses (Liston & Campbell, 1974). Ghosh & Hudson (1972) reported a relationship between oxytocin and neonatal hyperbilirubinaemia. McKenna & Shaw (1979) documented hyponatraemic fits in oxytocin-augmented labours. Iatrogenic fetal hypoxia due to poorly controlled oxytocin infusions was described by Kubli & Ruttgers (1961). Careful control of oxytocin infusion by a peristaltic infusion pump is essential, preferably based on accurate assessment of uterine contractions. Uterine activity measurement provides the necessary information to limit the dose and duration of oxytocin infusion, thereby minimising such undesirable effects.

The relationship between fetal distress and uterine contractions is a complex one. Steer (1977) specified that fetal distress was likely to occur at levels above 1500 kPas/15 min but Gibb et al (1984a) found no evidence of this in spontaneous labours. In induced labours there could be some degree of placental compromise which may have been the indication for induction. Uterine activity could unmask this but it seems unlikely that activity in excess of 1500 kPas/15 min *per se* precipitates fetal distress. An important factor must be fetoplacental reserve, and we have seen growth-retarded fetuses distressed by a very small amount of activity. Conversely well-grown, uncompromised fetuses can tolerate activity values in excess of 2500 kPas/15 min in spontaneous labour. It is desirable to assess activity in labours where the fetus is already known to be compromised, especially if oxytocin is to be used.

The management of labour in patients who have had a previous Caesarean section is a dilemma when progress is slow. We have used activity measurements to permit augmentation of such labours with good result. The characteristics of uterine activity associated with a scar rupture are unknown but it seems reasonable to augment activity at least to the appropriate 50th centile level when there is no reason to doubt scar integrity. Augmentation of labour when the presentation of the fetus is breech remains controversial. It has been suggested that abnormal labour progress in such cases is a manifestation of fetopelvic disproportion and augmentation is contraindicated (Duignan, 1982). If a breech presentation has been thoroughly assessed prior to labour then fetopelvic disproportion should have been excluded. As inefficient uterine action is a potent cause of poor labour progress in a cephalic presentation, so it is likely to be so in a breech. We therefore insert intra-uterine catheters in such cases and carefully augment labour, with a good result. Grand multiparity is another condition where augmentation of labour may be hazardous. Again it appears that measurement of activity allows such a decision to be made more rationally and the oxytocin dose to be controlled carefully. Our experience in this field has been encouraging. Uterine activity measurements in these clinical situations require further study but should prove valuable.

CONCLUSION

Intra-uterine catheters and uterine activity assessment have a role to play in the control of the inexorable rise of Caesarean section rates due to dystocia. Time spent in abnormal labour may be reduced with consequent improvement in fetal and maternal condition at delivery. The contribution of inefficient uterine action to poor progress of labour can be objectively assessed, permitting rational clinical management. The technique is simple and safe. All hospitals should be able to offer such a facility to the minority of patients who would benefit from it.

REFERENCES

Alvarez H, Caldeyro R 1950 Contractility of human uterus recorded by new methods. Surgery, Gynecology and Obstetrics 91 : 1–13

Arulkumaran S, Gibb D M F, Lun K C, Heng S H, Ratnam S S 1984 The effect of parity on uterine activity in labour. British Journal of Obstetrics and Gynaecology 91 : 843–848

Arulkumaran S, Gibb D M F, Ratnam S S, Heng S H, Lun K C 1985 Cervical and pelvic tissue resistance or total uterine activity in induced labour. British Journal of Obstetrics and Gynaecology 92 : 693–697

Beazley J M, Banovic I, Feld M S 1975 Maintenance of labour. British Medical Journal 2 : 248–250

Bell R 1981 Measurement of spontaneous uterine activity in the antenatal patient. American Journal of Obstetrics and Gynecology 140 : 713–715

Blair Bell W 1909 The pituitary body. British Medical Journal ii : 1609–1613

Blair Bell W 1925 Infundibulin. British Medical Journal ii : 1027–1031

Bleker O P, Kloosterman G J, Mieras D J, Oosting J, Salle H J A 1975 Intervillous space during uterine contractions in human subjects. An ultrasonic study. American Journal of Obstetrics and Gynecology 123 : 697–699

Borell U, Fernstrom I, Ohlson L and Wiqvist N (1964) Effect of uterine contractions on the human uteroplacental blood circulation. American Journal of Obstetrics and Gynaecology 89(7) : 881–890

Bourne A, Burn J H 1927 The dosage and action of Pituitary Extract of the Ergot Alkaloids on the uterus in labour, with a note on the action of adrenaline. Journal of Obstetrics and Gynaecology of the British Empire 34 : 249–272

Caesarean childbirth : Summary of a National Institute of Health Consensus Statement (1981). British Medical Journal 282 : 1600–1604

Caldeyro Barcia R, Sica-Blanco Y, Poseiro J J, Gonzalez-Panizza U, Mendez Bauer C, Feilitz C, Alvarez H, Pose S V and Hendricks C H (1957) A quantitative study of the action of synthetic oxytocin on the human uterus. Journal of Pharmacology and Experimental Therapeutus 121 : 18–31

Cardozo L D, Gibb D M F, Studd J W W, Vasant R V, Cooper D J 1982 Predictive value of cervimetric labour patterns in primigravidae. British Journal of Obstetrics and Gynecology 89 : 292–295

Carter M C and Steer P J (1980) An automatic infusion system for the measurement and control of uterine activity. Medical Instrumentation 14(3) : 169–173

Cowan D B, Van Middelkoop A and Philpott R H (1982) Intrauterine pressure studies in African nulliparae : normal labour progress. British Journal of Obstetrics and Gynaecology 89 : 364–369

Dale H H 1906 On some physiological actions of Ergot. Journal of Physiology 34: 163–205

DeHart W R, Laros R K, Witting W C, Work B A 1977 System for computing Montevideo units for monitoring progress of labour. IEEE Transactions on Biomedical Engineering 24: 94–101

Duignan N M 1982 The management of breech presentation. In: Studd J (ed.) Progress in obstetrics and gynaecology, vol 2. Churchill Livingstone, London, pp 73–84

Du Vigneaud V, Ressler C, Trippett S 1953 The sequence of amino acids in oxytocin with a proposal for the structure of oxytocin. Journal of Biological Chemistry 205: 949

Du Vigneaud V, Ressler C, Swan J M, Roberts C W, Katsoyannis P G 1954 The synthesis of oxytocin. Journal of the American Chemical Society 76: 345

Effer S B, Bertola R P, Vrettos A, Caldeyro-Barcia R 1969 Quantitative study of the regularity of uterine contractile rhythm in labor. American Journal of Obstetrics and Gynecology 105: 909–915

El-Sahwi S, Gaafar A A and Toppozada H K (1967) A new unit for evaluation of uterine activity. American Journal of Obstetrics and Gynecology 98: 900–903

Embrey M P (1940) External hysterography. A graphic study of the human parturient uterus and the effect of various therapeutic agents on it. Journal of Obstetrics and Gynecology of the British Empire 371–390

Francis J G, Turnbull A C and Thomas F F (1970) Automatic oxytocin infusion equipment for induction of labour. Journal of Obstetrics and Gynaecology of the British Commonwealth 77: 594–602

Friedman E A (1954) The graphic analyses of labour. American Journal of Obstetrics and Gynecology 68: 1568–1575

Fuchs A R, Fuchs F 1984 Endocrinology of human parturition: a review. British Journal of Obstetrics and Gynecology 91: 948–967

Garfield R E, Hayashi R H 1981 Appearance of gap junctions in the myometrium of women during labour. American Journal of Obstetrics and Gynecology 140: 254–260

Ghosh A, Hudson F P 1972 Oxytocin and neonatal hyperbilirubnaemia. Lancet ii: 823

Gibb D M F, Arulkumaran S, Lun K C, Ratnam S S 1984a Characteristics of uterine activity in nulliparous labour. British Journal of Obstetrics and Gynecology 91: 220–227

Gibb D M F, Arulkumaran S and Ratnam S S (1985) A comparative study of methods of oxytocin administration for induction of labour. British Journal of Obstetrics and Gynaecology 92: 688–692

Gibbens D, Boyd N R H, Chard T 1972 Spurt release of oxytocin during human labour. Journal of Endocrinology 53: 54–55

Harbert G M 1982 Uterine contractions. Clinics in Obstetrics and Gynaecology 25(1): 177–187

Hofbauer J, Hoerner J K 1927 The nasal application of pituitary extract for the induction of labour. American Journal of Obstetrics and Gynecology 2: 137–148

Hon E H, Paul R H 1973 Quantitation of uterine activity. Obstetrics and Gynecology 42: 368–370

Huey J R, Al Hadjiev A, Paul R H 1976 Uterine activity in the multiparous patient. American Journal of Obstetrics and Gynecology 126: 682–686

Krapohl A J, Devries J H, Evans T N 1965 Electronic control of induction of labour. Obstetrics and Gynecology 25: 334–339

Kubli F, Ruttgers H 1971 Iatrogenic fetal hypoxia. In: Gevers R H, Ruys J H (eds) Physiology and pathology in the perinatal period. Leiden University Press, pp 57–75

Liston W A, Campbell A J 1974 Dangers of oxytocin-induced labour to fetuses. British Medical Journal 3: 606–607

McKenna P, Shaw R W 1979 Hyponatraemic fits in oxytocin-augmented labours. International Journal of Obstetrics and Gynaecology 17: 150–252

Mulla N 1957 Vaginal delivery in a paraplegic patient. American Journal of Obstetrics and Gynecology 73: 1346–1348

Nuttall I D 1978 Perforation of a placental fetal vessel by an intrauterine pressure catheter. British Journal of Obstetrics and Gynaecology 85: 573–574

Odendaal H J, Neves Dos Santos L M, Henry M J, Crawford J W 1976 Experiments in the measurement of intrauterine pressure. British Journal of Obstetrics and Gynaecology 83: 96–100

O'Driscoll K, Jackson R H A, Gallagher J T 1969 Prevention of prolonged labour. British Medical Journal 2: 477–480

Pavlou C, Barker G H, Roberts A, Chamberlain G V P 1978 Pulsed oxytocin infusion in the induction of labour. British Journal of Obstetrics and Gynaecology 85 : 96–100

Philpott R H, Castle W M 1972 Cervicographs in the management of labour in primigravidae. Journal of Obstetrics and Gynaecology of the British Commonwealth 79 : 592–598

Reynolds S R M, Hellman L M, Bruns P 1948 Patterns of uterine contractility in women during pregnancy. Obstetrical and Gynaecological Survey, 629–646

Rossavik I K 1978 Relation between total uterine impulse, method of delivery and one-minute apgar score. British Journal of Obstetrics and Gynaecology 85 : 847–851

Schaffer O 1898 Quoted in Embrey (1940).

Schatz F 1872 Arch Gynakol iii : 58–144. Quoted in Bourne & Burn (1972).

Schulman H, Romney S L (1970) Variability of uterine contractions in normal human parturition. Obstetrics and Gynecology 36 : 215–221

Sjoberg N-O (1967) The adrenergic transmitter of the female reproductive tract : distribution and functional changes. Acta Physiologica Scandinavica (Suppl) 305 :5

Smyth C N 1957 The guard ring tocodynamometer. Absolute measurement of intra-amniotic pressure by a new instrument. Journal of Obstetrics and Gynaecology of the British Empire 64 : 59–66

Steer P J 1977 The measurement and control of uterine contractions. In : The current status of fetal heart rate monitoring and ultrasound in obstetrics. RCOG London, pp 48–68

Steer P J, Little D J, Lewis W L, Kelly M C M E, Beard R W 1975 Uterine activity in induced labour. British Journal of Obstetrics and Gynaecology 82 : 433–441

Steer P J, Carter M C, Gordon A J, Beard R W 1978 The use of cathetertip pressure transducers for the measurement of intrauterine pressure in labour. British Journal of Obstetrics and Gynaecology 85 : 561–566

Steer P J, Carter M C, Beard R W 1984 Normal levels of active contraction area in spontaneous labour. British Journal of Obstetrics and Gynaecology 91 : 211–219

Studd J W W 1973 Partograms and nomograms of cervical dilatation in primigravid labour. British Medical Journal 4 : 451–455

Svenningsen L, Jensen O, Dodgson M S 1984 A fibre-optic pressure transducer for intrauterine monitoring (unpublished)

Toaff M E, Hezrone J, Toaff R 1978 Induction of labour by pharmacological and physiological doses of intravenous oxytocin. British Journal of Obstetrics and Gynaecology 85 : 101–108

Trudinger B J and Pryse Davies J (1979) Fetal hazards of the intrauterine pressure catheter : five case reports. British Journal of Obstetrics and Gynaecology 85 : 567–572

Turnbull A C 1957 Uterine contractions in normal and abnormal labour. Journal of Obstetrics and Gynaecology of the British Empire 64 : 321–332

Turnbull A C, Anderson A B M (1968) Induction of labour. Journal of Obstetrics and Gynaecology of the British Commonwealth 75 : 32–41

Tutera G, Newman R L 1975 Fetal monitoring : its effect on perinatal mortality and Caesarean section rates and its complications. American Journal of Obstetrics and Gynaecology 122 : 750–754

Williams E A, Stallworthy J A 1952 A simple method of internal tocography. Lancet i : 330–332

Wolfs G M J A, Van Leeuwen M 1979 Electromyographic observations on the human uterus during labour. Acta Obstetrica Gynaecologica Scandinavica (Suppl) 90 : 1–61

Woolfson J, Steer P J, Bashford C C, Randall N J 1976 The measurement of uterine activity in induced labour. British Journal of Obstetrics and Gynaecology 83 : 934–937

Fetal blood gases and pH: current application

The human fetus has not been an easy subject for investigation, given the impropriety of invading its domain without good reason. Clearly, an ideal opportunity for obtaining physiological information with minimal fetal harm is during labour. Landmark investigators took advantage of this time to unravel some of the physiological mysteries of the fetus. Fetal blood gas physiology was one of the first areas investigated. Erich Saling, a pioneering researcher in fetal blood gas physiology in the early 1960s, first described a useful technique for fetal scalp blood sampling to help recognize fetal distress (Saling, 1963). When electronic fetal monitoring (EFM) became widespread, the combination of abnormal fetal heart-rate (FHR) patterns and fetal scalp blood sampling to assess acid-base changes during labour were used to determine optimal labour management.

Over the next decade EFM and fetal blood-gas monitoring each developed supporters who tended to favour either EFM alone or EFM in combination with fetal scalp blood sampling. The ease with which EFM could be done, in contrast to the relative difficulty in obtaining a sample of fetal blood, led to a decline in the use of fetal scalp blood sampling. The introduction of a workable classification of the FHR patterns added further support to EFM alone (Hon & Quilligan, 1967). In countries where the technique of fetal scalp blood sampling has received greater support, acceptance has still not been universal. In the United Kingdom, for example, only 40 per cent of the major obstetric units use it as an adjunct to EFM (Gillmer & Combe, 1979). The evidence in support of doing fetal blood-gas assessment to diagnose fetal distress is abundant (Tejani et al, 1976; Zanini et al, 1979) and its impact on lowering the Casarean delivery rate is clear (Zalar & Quilligan, 1978). These facts alone suggest that it is time to take a second look at fetal acid–base monitoring. Its successful re-emergence will depend to some degree on clinicians having an understanding of the relevant physiology.

FETAL ACID–BASE PHYSIOLOGY

The human fetus is entirely dependent on an adequate uterine blood flow and a well-oxygenated mother to satisfy its own oxygen needs. Unless the mother is suffering from severe anaemia or a major respiratory impediment, maternal oxygenation will almost certainly be adequate. Maintenance of an optimal uterine blood flow, however, is subject to many factors, including acute and chronic changes in the maternal blood pressure (Bonica & Figge, 1969) and maternal diseases, of which diabetes mellitus, chronic renal disease, and various cardiac disorders comprise only a few.

The normal uterine blood flow at term is approximately 110 ml/kg per minute, based on the weight of the uterus and its contents (Blechner et al, 1974). The partial pressure of oxygen (Po_2) in the spiral artery is approximately 100 torr (14 kPa) but because of the haemodynamics of the uteroplacental circulation this is not the tension of oxygen to which the fetal blood ultimately equilibrates. The anatomical arrangement of the uteroplacental interface deserves further examination, if the physiology of gas exchange is to be understood more clearly.

The fetal umbilical artery transports the most highly desaturated blood to the placenta. The artery subdivides into 60–100 branches and each supplies a portion of the placenta or a lobule. The end arteries then subdivide into complex capillary networks covered by trophoblast, which are called villi, and which project into the intervillous space. The lobule actually consists of multiple villi arranged in the shape of a hemisphere. The fetal end artery enters at the pole of the hemisphere and divides into multiple capillary loops within each villus. The hemispherically arranged villi cover a single spiral artery which spurts highly oxygen-saturated maternal blood against them. The blood circulates against the villi exchanging gases and metabolites, finally exiting as desaturated blood, coursing towards the uterine veins. In this arrangement the least saturated fetal blood first meets the most saturated maternal blood. A rapid exchange of gases occurs since the pressure gradient between the gases is high due to the large difference in tensions between the two blood flows. The highly oxygenated maternal blood soon gives up its oxygen (O_2) and the partial pressure Po_2 falls quickly. At the same time, under the influence of the pressure gradients, the fetal blood is exchanging carbon dioxide (CO_2) for O_2. The high pressure gradient for O_2 lasts for approximately 1 second and the drive to exchange gases weakens considerably as the maternal Po_2 falls and the fetal Po_2 increases (Power et al, 1971). The blood entering the fetal villi closer to the equator of the hemisphere will exchange with maternal blood which is now moderately desaturated, resulting in a much poorer gas exchange. In reality the flow of each circulation is not so ideal. The maternal blood swirling through the intervillous space will not always desaturate as progressively as the model predicts, resulting in oxygen tension gradients at variance with the predicted value. Nevertheless, the basic concept of the maternal blood becoming progressively desaturated of oxygen, as the fetal blood becomes more saturated, holds true.

Once the fetal–maternal gas exchange has occurred, the fetal blood returns through the umbilical vein to the inferior vena cava where slight admixture occurs with the desaturated blood returning from the lower limbs, and from the superior vena cava. The blood which is least admixed with desaturated fetal blood enters the coronary sinuses and the carotid arteries via the foramen ovale. Through this arrangement, the vital structures (the liver, heart, and brain) receive the most highly oxygenated blood (Fig. 8.1). The non-vital organs receive less well-oxygenated blood due to the characteristics of the laminated blood flow, which directs the most desaturated blood through the right ventricle, the pulmonary artery, and via the ductus arteriosus, to the aorta. During hypoxaemic episodes blood flow to the vital organs is protected because arterial vasoconstriction occurs in the lower extremities (Boddy, 1976).

THE FETAL BLOOD-GASES

P_{O_2}

Since the final equilibration of the fetal blood-gases with the mother's blood occurs as the maternal blood becomes 'venous', the oxygen level of the

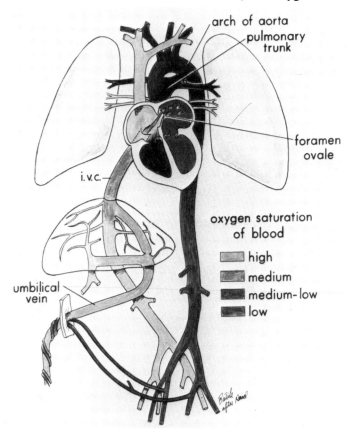

Fig. 8.1. The fetal circulation.

villous (umbilical venous) blood can only approximate the maternal venous values. Because of the separation of the two circulations, the fetal blood is prevented from achieving Po_2 values as high as the maternal venous Po_2 (Rankin et al, 1971). This limits the fetal Po_2 to maximum values of 35–40 torr (5–5·4 kPa), which represents an oxygen saturation of about 50–55 per cent (Pearson, 1976).

Using the transcutaneous technique for fetal oxygen measurements we demonstrated fetal $tcPo_2$ values in the range of 14–33 torr (2–4·7 kPa) in the early part of labour, providing the FHR pattern was normal (Willcourt et al, 1981). While oxygen values in this range appear low by neonatal standards, clearly they are sufficient to maintain fetal growth. The mean fetal O_2 consumption has been estimated at approximately 6·0 ml/kg per minute (Longo et al, 1971). Provided that the fetal cardiac output remains at an optimal rate to ensure a normal flow of blood through the placental villi, there will be enough oxygen being transported for fetal consumption. Umbilical flow rates have been calculated at 200 ml/min (Makowski et al, 1968) which would supply the average fetus at term with oxygen at the rate of 8 ml/kg per minute (at 60 per cent oxygen saturation). This does not leave a great margin of reserve. Using the transcutaneous technique we, and other workers, have shown that decreases in the fetal $tcPo_2$ can be brought about by factors such as a slight decrease in the maternal blood pressure or by uterine hyperactivity (Huch et al, 1977; Willcourt et al, 1981, 1982). These changes in the uteroplacental circulation can affect the exchange of oxygen in the placenta and, hence, the fetal $tcPo_2$ (Fig. 8.2). Other factors, such as supine hypotension, pre-eclampsia and other hypertensive states, may produce more subtle alterations in oxygenation, but of a longer duration (Lumley et al, 1969). While these changes are not desirable, a number of

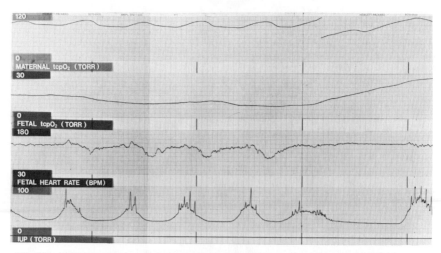

Fig. 8.2.   This late deceleration pattern occurred in the presence of increasing uterine activity following the onset of an epidural block.

factors exist which buffer the fetus from the adverse effects of decreased oxygenation.

GAS TRANSPORT AND BUFFERS AND FETAL HAEMOGLOBIN

Why the fetus is usually happy

One of the factors enabling the fetus to adapt to its apparent intra-uterine oxygen deprivation, lies in the special character of fetal haemoglobin. The fetal red cell contains lower amounts of 2,3-diphosphoglycerate (2,3-DPG) than adult red cells. Because the affinity of haemoglobin for oxygen is inversely proportional to the quantity of 2,3-DPG present in the cell, the fetal haemoglobin is able to pick up more oxygen in a less well-oxygenated environment than adult haemoglobin. The affinity for oxygen increases as the O_2 saturation of the fetal falls below 50 per cent. This is clearly an advantage to the fetus since it can never avail itself of the Po_2 of 150 torr (20 kPa) to which the mother is usually exposed. Therefore, for any given Po_2, the fetal haemoglobin is more highly saturated than the maternal haemoglobin. Indeed, the fetus is capable of transporting approximately 22 ml of oxygen per 100 ml of blood compared to 15 ml per 100 ml of maternal blood at full O_2 saturation. Given the oxygen tensions to which the fetus must equilibrate, the actual volume of oxygen transported in the fetal umbilical vein is still an impressive 13 ml per 100 ml of blood—ergo the fetus is happy.

Factors affecting blood-gas equilibrium

The Bohr effect

During normal metabolism the pH falls as a result of an accumulation of hydrogen ion (H^+), and this causes saturated haemoglobin to release oxygen. This applies to both fetal and maternal haemoglobin. The fetal blood returning through the umbilical arteries is low in O_2 concentration and high in H^+ ions. As the H^+ ions are transferred to the maternal blood, the fetal pH rises and the maternal pH falls. The increase in H^+ ion in the maternal blood accelerates the off-loading of oxygen to the fetal blood, at the maternal–fetal interface (the Bohr effect). At the same time the fetal blood increases its affinity for oxygen as its pH rises (Fig. 8.3). The complementary effect of the fetal to maternal passage of H^+ ion on the efficient transfer of oxygen to the fetus is called the 'double Bohr effect'. The fetus is thus able to avail itself of a reasonable supply of oxygen under the usual intra-uterine conditions.

The decline in the oxygenation of the fetal blood as it circulates through the peripheral tissues should, in theory, hinder further release of the remaining oxygen molecules because of the affinity of fetal haemoglobin for oxygen at low oxygen tensions. This effect is partially offset by the declining

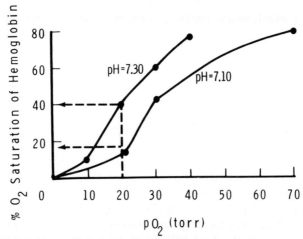

Fig. 8.3. The Bohr effect. There is a marked difference in the values for the pO_2 when the blood samples are of a different pH for a given oxygen saturation.

pH in the actively metabolising tissues, allowing more oxygen to be released than would occur under less acidotic conditions. This effect is probably protective during episodes of acidosis. As the pH falls, the liberation of the oxygen molecules decreases the oxygen saturation of the haemoglobin but maintains the tissue Po_2. Therefore, acidosis raises the Po_2 for a given haemoglobin saturation. This effect must be taken into account when evaluating a scalp blood gas Po_2, or a transcutaneous Po_2 ($tcPo_2$) tracing, since the amount of oxygen actually being transported in the fetal blood may be dangerously low while the Po_2 is in the normal range (Fig. 8.3).

CO_2

The amount of carbon dioxide (CO_2) in the fetal blood is a reflection of its accumulation through tissue metabolism balanced against its placental clearance. A large accumulation of CO_2 indicates that fetal to maternal clearance is impaired. Profound uteroplacental insufficiency and cord compression will lead to a marked retention in fetal CO_2. The CO_2 in fetal blood is present as carbaminohaemoglobin, carbonic acid (H_2CO_3) or as a gas in solution. In normal labour the plasma Pco_2 lies between 37 and 46 torr (Jacobson & Rooth, 1971). Almost one-third of the CO_2 is transported as carbaminohaemoglobin. In the erythrocyte the major portion of CO_2 is present as H_2CO_3 which dissociates into bicarbonate (HCO_3^-) and H^+. The HCO_3^- passes out of the cell in exchange for chloride (Cl^-) ions, permitting more CO_2 to enter the cell and continue the cycle. The H^+ ion is buffered by haemoglobin causing little, if any, change in pH within the cell (see below).

During placental exchange with maternal blood the fetal CO_2 passes to the maternal compartment quite rapidly. More CO_2 is liberated from the fetal erythrocytes to compensate for that lost by diffusion from the fetal

plasma. The HCO_3^- in the fetal erythrocytes combines with H^+ ion forming more CO_2. This drops the intracellular HCO_3^- level rapidly, causing plasma HCO_3^- to enter the cells which combines with H^+ ion and releases more CO_2.

The Haldane effect

The release of CO_2 is also dependent on the availability of oxygen, which encourages its release from the haemoglobin molecule. More CO_2 can be taken up by haemoglobin for a given P_{CO_2}, when oxygen is being released. This is called the 'Haldane effect'. The CO_2 content of fetal plasma depends on how readily CO_2 can diffuse across the placental membrane and how much HCO_3^- is present in the erythrocyte, to be converted to CO_2 and water. As H^+ ion reacts with HCO_3^- to form CO_2 in the erythrocyte, the intracellular pH rises, i.e. H^+ is being used up. More H^+ ion will then pass from the plasma into the red blood cells to be buffered (Power et al, 1971). The rising intracellular CO_2 will cause an increase in carbaminohaemoglobin and HCO_3^-, while the H^+ ion formed at this time is buffered by the haemoglobin. As the carbaminohaemoglobin concentration rises, less H^+ ion can be buffered, causing a fall in both the intracellular and plasma pH. The increased carbaminohaemoglobin content also reduces the ability of the red cells to transport oxygen. The type of fetal distress in which these changes are exaggerated is called an asphyxial or respiratory acidosis. Typically, in severe cases, the fetal P_{O_2} is less than 15 torr (2 kPa) and the P_{CO_2} is greater than 60 torr (8·3 kPa). The pH will decline rapidly under these conditions. From the above it can be seen that the hydrogen ion concentration is dependent on the buffering capacity of the system, which in turn is dependent on the concentration of CO_2, O_2, and HCO_3^- present.

pH and lactic acid

Since H^+ ion accumulation is a result of decreased fetal oxygenation it would seem useful to measure the blood pH to determine the degree of hypoxaemia. It should be noted that H^+ ion accumulation is not a cause of 'fetal distress'. It is only during severe acidosis that the H^+ ion concentration will disrupt cellular metabolism and compound the effects of the existing state of diminished oxygenation (Pearson, 1976). Not only is H^+ ion accumulation a result of CO_2 retention, but it also results from the production of metabolic by-products and intermediaries, such as lactic and pyruvic acids. Lactic acid is produced in greater amounts if insufficient oxygen is present to permit normal aerobic glycolysis (equations 8.1 and 8.2).

$$Glucose + O_2 \text{ (hypoxaemia)} = lactate + H^+ \qquad (8.1)$$
anaerobic glycolysis

$$Glucose + O_2 \text{ (normoxaemia)} = CO_2 + H_2O \qquad (8.2)$$
aerobic glycolysis

The H^+ ion produced is buffered by the mechanisms described previously. While a reduced oxygen environment may result in a partial increase in anaerobic glycolysis, CO_2 exchange may still occur normally. Vital organs will maintain relatively normal perfusion through redistribution of the fetal blood flow (Cohn et al, 1974). However, accumulation of lactic acid will occur in suboptimally perfused tissues leading to a generalised acidosis. This mechanism probably exists in some cases of intra-uterine growth retardation (IUGR) and pre-eclampsia (Wood, 1978). In our own unpublished observations of fetuses with IUGR during labour, we have observed very little aberration in the Po_2 and Pco_2 values, while fetal pH and lactic acid have been only slightly, but not statistically abnormal. The acidosis in this instance is referred to as a metabolic acidosis. A mixed type of acidosis will occur if acute fetal distress is superimposed. In addition, a mixed acidosis will also occur if an acute fetal distress continues without relief.

Interpretation of pH; pH qu 40

The pH value is influenced by both CO_2 and lactic acid, and since each of these components may imply a different aetiology, the pH qu 40 can help to determine the underlying pathology. The pH qu 40 is the pH measurement made after the sample of blood has been equilibrated (hence the 'qu') to a Pco_2 of 40 torr (5·4 kPa). Carbon dioxide in excess of a Pco_2 of 40 torr (5·4 kPa) will be 'washed out' of the blood sample. A change in pH after equilibration would indicate that the CO_2 content of the blood contributed to the pH value. Little alteration in the pH after equilibration implies that the main component of the pH value is from lactic acid, and not CO_2. The literature is replete with tables of values for fetal blood gas parameters. One should derive standard values for one's own institution since it is clear that the selection of patients, the techniques, and the technicians introduce variables that negate the utility of a universal standard table. For institutions unable to produce their own table the following figures may be useful. It is generally agreed that a pH of 7·25 or less on a fetal scalp blood sample indicates some degree of fetal hypoxemia. Values of 7·20 and less have been used to recommend immediate delivery (Wood, 1978). Unless many samples have been taken to provide a trend, such an approach does not take into account the possibility that the fetus has recovered from a previous insult and is not in immediate jeopardy.

Since false-positive or false-negative results can occur in up to 10 per cent of samples (Beard, 1970), attempts are being made to improve the reliability of fetal scalp blood analysis. Smith and colleagues (1979) made whole-blood lactate estimations on maternal and fetal blood samples obtained either at Caesarean delivery or in labour. The lactate levels bore a strong correlation with neonatal outcome, being markedly elevated in depressed babies. To insure that fetal lactate values are not influenced by maternal levels, the difference between maternal and fetal levels can be determined. Evaluations of the maternal-minus-fetal values did not identify more precisely the difference between the normal and the hypoxaemic fetuses (Smith et al, 1979; Lawrence et al, 1982). It is important to realise that lactic acid does not readily cross the placenta, and may remain in the fetal compartment for some hours after its initial accumulation (Shelley, 1973), making it difficult to identify fetal recovery. Conversely, a fetal scalp blood sample obtained in the recovery phase might demonstrate normal pH and gas tensions with an elevated lactic acid concentration as the only remaining evidence of prior hypoxaemia.

It has been reported that lactic acid accumulation can lead to brain oedema and cerebral necrosis (Myers, 1979). This may be one of the mechanisms involved in the pathogenesis of cerebral palsy. Recently it has been shown that rapidly infusing 10 per cent dextrose solutions to mothers during labour to treat ketonuria can elevate both maternal and fetal lactic acid levels (Lawrence et al, 1982). A fall in fetal pH occurred as the fetal plasma glucose concentrations reached 150 mg/dl (8·3 mmol/l), primarily through an increase in fetal lactate. This has practical implications, since it is customary to increase the rate of intravenous infusion during episodes of fetal distress. If a glucose solution is used, fetal lactate levels may be further increased during prolonged hypoxaemia, worsening the acid–base state of the fetus. It is now a policy in our institution to use non-dextrose solutions in the mainline, supplementing the mother with intermittent 5 per cent dextrose infusions as shown by the presence of ketonuria, but only if further hydration fails to decrease the presence of ketones.

Another cause of fetal hyperglycaemia comes from the use of B-sympathomimetic agents (Epstein et al, 1973). Might this have an effect on the fetal acid–base state during long-term labour inhibition? We use non-dextrose solutions for the treatment of preterm labour, and have found that the maternal glucose and lactic acid levels return to normal within 48–72 h of tocolytic treatment. In patients who are maintained on B-sympathomimetics for longer than 3 days, we have noted that the maternal and fetal glucose and lactate levels, at delivery, are not significantly different from those patients not receiving tocolytic therapy.

The extreme acidaemia noted in deteriorating fetuses of diabetic mothers may occur through a similar mechanism. If uteroplacental insufficiency exists and produces a suboptimal rate of aerobic glycolysis, excessive lactic acid accumulation will occur. Additional acute hypoxaemic episodes in the presence of fetal hyperglycaemia may elevate the lactic acid levels further, resulting in a profound lactic acidosis.

Hypoxanthine

Recently a metabolite of ATP has been investigated, which shows some promise as another marker of fetal hypoxaemia (Saugstad & Gluck, 1982).

This substance is called hypoxanthine (Fig. 8.4). Hypoxanthine accumulates during periods of fetal hypoxaemia and may be assayed in cord blood after delivery (Swanstrom & Bratteby, 1982). Currently, 0·6 ml of blood are required for the analysis, which is too large a quantity for scalp blood analysis. It has been shown that the concentration of hypoxanthine in cord blood at delivery is able to define, at least as well as lactate does, the presence of recent hypoxaemia. What is urgently required is a marker of longer-standing hypoxaemia. Harkness et al (1983), have shown that, in women judged to be high-risk, the levels of hypoxanthine in the amniotic fluid were elevated compared to normal low-risk patients. Hypoxanthine was found to be as good a marker of fetal hypoxaemia as was lactate, which is currently the standard by which tests of fetal acid–base status should be compared. Since hypoxanthine is eliminated rapidly once the hypoxaemic insult is over, it may be far more useful than pH or lactic acid in determining the rate of fetal recovery after an hypoxic insult, since the latter are cleared more slowly from the fetal circulation.

Hypoxanthine may be elevated in babies with IUGR even when the other blood-gas parameters are normal (Thiringer, 1983). In the study reported by Thiringer, there were two babies with acceptable Apgar scores who later

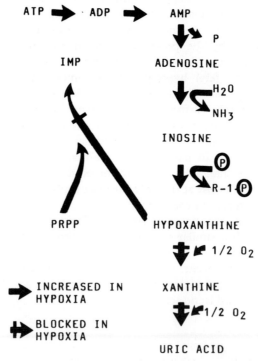

Fig. 8.4. Hypoxanthine is produced in greater quantities when there is impaired oxygenation. This substance can be measured, and may provide evidence for past hypoxia.

developed neurological signs despite blood-gas values which were abnormal except for elevated hypoxanthine.

Therefore if hypoxanthine proves to be a practical marker for discovering antepartum hypoxic insults, and in the identification of newborns at risk for cerebral dysfunction, it may eventually become part of routine perinatal assessment.

The assumption that the brain-damaged child is the result of obstetric negligence, is proving to be fallacious in the majority of instances, yet the practising obstetrician is falling prey to a greedy legal profession and a gullible public. Tests which disclose prior hypoxic insults will be the basis of a good defence, and it is clear that there is an urgent need to evaluate these tests to help re-establish some order in the obstetric medico-legal chaos that has mushroomed in the United States in recent years.

THE TECHNIQUES AND TECHNOLOGIES OF BLOOD-GAS ASSESSMENT

Intermittent scalp blood sampling

The most universal means of assessing the blood-gas and acid–base status of the fetus is to obtain a scalp blood sample. After the technique was first described, improvements were made in order to reduce the incidence of artifactual changes in the collected samples. A recent review of the technique has been presented by Willcourt & Queenan (1981), in which the major sources of errors in collecting fetal scalp blood, and how to minimise them, are described. A brief review of the technique is presented.

Since blood-gas and acid–base interactions are dynamic, a single scalp blood sample will provide only limited information about the degree to which the system has been assaulted, and no information about the direction the trend is taking. Therefore, frequently repeated samples must be obtained to demonstrate the trends. Portable pH analysers are now available which require samples of only 15 µl of blood and which provide reliable results within seconds (Stewart et al, 1983). This is in contrast to the standard analysers which need at least 50 µl of blood and, depending on the distance from the labour and delivery area, the results may not be available for 5–10 minutes. Despite the positive features of the portable analysers, the discontinuous nature of this form of blood-gas assessment has generated a search for continuous blood-gas and acid–base monitoring.

Transcutaneous Po_2

The Clark electrode, used for measuring oxygen tensions in standard blood-gas devices, has been modified to allow measurements of Po_2 to be made on the surface of the skin (Clark, 1956). The technique involves applying the electrode to the skin using glue to secure it firmly. The electrode contains a heating element which raises the skin temperature by user selection to 42–45°C. Oxygen is liberated from the underlying capillaries as the temperature is raised. The O_2 molecules pass from the skin through the electrode membrane and, by an electrochemical reaction, produce an electrical current proportional to the oxygen tension.

The results of transcutaneous oxygen (tcP_{O_2}) measurements made during labour on the scalp of the human fetus were reported by Huch and colleagues (Huch et al, 1977). The technique is based on the assumption that the P_{O_2} on the skin will reflect reliably the central P_{O_2}, and that the peripheral circulation will remain relatively intact during episodes of fetal hypoxaemia. Under normal circumstances the fetal scalp receives the most highly oxygenated blood, as does the fetal brain; however, it is not clear whether the integrity of the scalp circulation is maintained during fetal distress.

To validate the technique in the fetus, intermittent scalp blood samples have been compared to the tcP_{O_2} values, and in general there has been good agreement (Huch et al, 1977; Fall et al, 1979). The static P_{O_2} and P_{CO_2} values obtained by intermittent sampling are not clinically useful since they vary widely from minute to minute (Fig. 8.2) but can be used to verify transcutaneous blood-gas values, provided they are collected meticulously (Willcourt & Queenan, 1981). The range of the tcP_{O_2} values during normal labours with normal FHR tracings, was found to be in the range of 15–25 torr (2–3·7 kPa), which agrees fairly well with the values obtained by intermittent scalp blood sampling (Saling, 1966; Kunzel & Wulf, 1976). The continuous and non-invasive nature of the method is attractive, but it is prone to errors which have limited its widespread acceptance in obstetrics. Excessive compression of the electrode by the pelvic tissues, for example, may lower the value (Huch et al, 1977; O'Connor et al, 1979), while acidosis, through the Bohr effect, may raise the value. Nevertheless, it has proved a useful research tool in the investigation of factors that affect fetal oxygenation in labour (Huch et al, 1977; Willcourt et al, 1981, 1982).

Our studies on the fetal tcP_{O_2} electrode with abnormal fetal heart rate patterns have underscored the need for a more specific means of identifying the 'stressed' from the 'distressed' fetus than is provided for in conventional FHR monitoring (Willcourt et al, 1981). These studies demonstrated a close relationship between certain FHR patterns and changes in fetal oxygenation. Some of these findings are presented.

Variable decelerations precede a fall in the fetal tcP_{O_2} with some correlation between the magnitude of the deceleration and the decrease in the fetal tcP_{O_2}. The occlusion of the umbilical arteries and vein, separately or together, will reduce the rate of blood flow through the placenta. A baroreceptor response causes a sudden drop in the heart rate (Lee & Hon, 1963). As a result of the decreased blood flow there will be a decrease in the delivery of oxygen molecules to the skin and with the added effect of impaired gas exchange in the placenta, the tcP_{O_2} will decline.

A late deceleration pattern is associated with a decline in the fetal tcP_{O_2}

and does not occur at a specified level of fetal oxygenation (Fig. 8.2). It has been stated that the late deceleration pattern begins when the fetal Po_2 falls below some absolute value (James et al, 1972). It is more probable that it is the decline in the fetal $tcPo_2$ which, in part, generates the late deceleration pattern (Willcourt et al, 1981, Itskovitz et al, 1982). The decline in the fetal $tcPo_2$ may be either so large that recovery to normal values cannot occur, or the frequency of uterine contraction prevailing during this period may reduce and maintain the Po_2 to low levels. Once the fetus has become 'stressed' and acidotic, the late deceleration pattern may be produced through a direct myocardial response to hypoxaemia. Blood samples taken at this time will exhibit low Po_2 values, and this association has presumably led to the concept of a 'critical' level Po_2 needed to generate this heart-rate pattern.

The relationship between the late deceleration pattern and Apgar scores has been evaluated. In one study 63 per cent of newborns had an Apgar score of 6 at 1 minute, despite a late deceleration pattern existing before delivery (Tejani et al, 1976). Similar results have been found in other studies (Low et al, 1973). These findings suggest that further investigation of an abnormal FHR pattern is required, if true fetal distress, as a distinction from stress, is to be recognised clearly.

Lack of variability of the fetal heart rate has been used to identify periods of fetal hypoxaemia. Yet it is only when a late deceleration pattern occurs, in addition, that decreased FHR variability signifies hypoxaemia (Paul et al, 1975). Despite this knowledge many clinicians have come to view decreased FHR variability alone as an ominous sign of fetal compromise. Indeed, recent studies have shown decreased FHR variability occurs frequently as the $tcPo_2$ rises (Willcourt et al, 1981; Kurz et al, 1981). This supports the findings of Zalar & Quilligan (1978) who, using scalp pH assessment of FHR patterns, found that decreased variability alone was rarely a sign of fetal compromise. It is clear that decreased variability may occur at extremes of fetal well-being and, as a result, its significance needs to be viewed in light of other FHR changes that may be present, and by use of scalp blood analysis. Increased variability with an acute decrease in oxygen tension has been reported using continuous $tcPo_2$ measurements (Gauwerky et al, 1981; Willcourt et al, 1981) as well as from direct arterial catheterisation (Ikenoue et al, 1981).

Transcutaneous Pco_2

There have been some recent developments in the area of Pco_2 monitoring in the fetus by the transcutaneous technique (Lysikeiwicz et al, 1981). The technique is so new that the reliability of the electrodes has yet to be determined. The physical appearance of the electrode is similar to the $tcPo_2$ electrodes and uses the principle of liberation of gas from the skin capillaries. Some electrodes require heating, in a manner similar to the $tcPo_2$ electrodes, while others do not (Severinghaus, 1981). Attachment of the electrode is the same as for the tcPo_2 electrode. An early observation shows that a rising tcPco_2 occurs during hypoxaemic episodes but a direct relationship between the tcPco_2 and the FHR pattern has yet to be elucidated. However, it may be a better means of monitoring the fetus in labour since an accumulation of CO_2 is more readily interpretable and hence carries more significance than a marginally decreased Po_2. Further research is needed before a commitment can be made to either fetal transcutaneous technique for the management of obstetric patients. Their use in a research setting may provide greater insights into the significance of the FHR patterns, making FHR monitoring a more precise method than it is now.

Continuous scalp pH monitoring

Since it has been shown that fetal pH measurement is a useful adjunct to FHR monitoring, a considerable effort has been applied to the design of a continuous pH electrode, similar in concept to that embodied in the transcutaneous Po_2 and Pco_2 electrodes. The major difference from the clinician's point of view is that the pH electrode needs to be imbedded in the fetal scalp rather than attached superficially with glue, as in the other methods (Stamm et al, 1976). A large spiral screw is used to secure the glass electrode into the fetal scalp after making a cruciate incision in the skin (Fig. 8.5). The glass tip is held in the incision below the skin surface, while the spiral screw serves not only to keep the electrode attached, but also to conduct the fetal electrocardiogram. The electrode functions reliably in approximately 60 per cent of applications (Sturbois et al, 1977; Flynn &

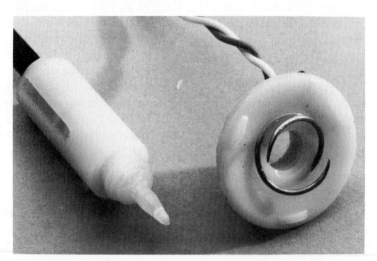

Fig. 8.5. The larger pH electrode must be embedded in the fetal scalp, which makes this a more traumatic means of monitoring than either by fetal EKG or by intermittent scalp blood sampling. (Reproduced by kind permission of Kontron SA, France)

Kelly, 1978) but is prone to splintering in the fetal scalp, either on insertion or during the period of monitoring. Small particles of glass may become embedded in the scalp, and may not be retrievable. Scalp lacerations requiring sutures have occurred (Janecek & Bossart, 1978).

When the electrode appeared to be working reliably the correlations between the values obtained and a fetal scalp blood sample were statistically significant at the $P=0.001$ level. Fetal pH values showed a decline during heart rate decelerations, with a return to normal levels in 30 min. Compared to tcPo_2 and tcPco_2 changes the fetal pH alterations are less acute. The more rapid fluctuation in the tcPo_2 and tcPco_2 values can be correlated to the FHR changes more readily, while the continuous tissue pH defines the directions in which the fetal acid–base state is going. In view of the difficulty in attaching the electrode, its invasive nature and the fragility of the glass electrode, the method has not gained wide acceptance.

It is clear that continuous acid–base assessment is possible with the techniques just described. However, all current methods present problems of reliability and difficulty of application to the fetal scalp, and neither method alone can be expected to provide a precise representation of the acid–base status.

Lactic acid pH and hypoxanthine estimation

It has been shown that lactic acid measurements are superior to other blood-gas and acid–base parameters in assessing the extent of tissue hypoxia (Weil & Afifi, 1970). Lactic acid can now be measured readily with an instrument suitable for placement in the labour and delivery area (Soutter et al, 1978). Lactic acid levels can be determined on samples of 150 µl of fetal blood obtained by the scalp sampling technique. Previously, lactic acid values could only be obtained on larger samples, rendering the concept useless for fetal assessment. Also, it took, on average 30–40 min to obtain the results. In a report by Smith et al (1979), 34 babies had scalp blood samples taken during labour which were analysed by the new technique. Lactic acid values were obtained within 5 min. The correlation between fetal outcome and lactic acid levels was striking, although lactic acid was no better a predictor of fetal compromise than pH (Smith et al, 1983). Recognising that it may take many hours for the fetal lactic acid levels to return to the former values after recovery from a hypoxaemic insult, there appears to be a place for pH and hypoxanthine measurements, which will show an earlier return to normal.

PRACTICAL APPLICATIONS

The following cases illustrate how blood gas and acid base values could have been used to assess the fetus in labour.

In *Case A* the mother, who was a G_1P_0, was admitted in labour at term.

The antenatal course had been uneventful. Premature rupture of the membranes occurred, predating the onset of uterine contractions by 16 h. During labour, which proceeded rapidly once it established, the maternal temperature rose to 101°F (37·9°C). Intermittent variable decelerations occurred, which disappeared at the end of the first stage of labour, though the FHR continued to show decreased short-term variability and a baseline of 190 bpm (Fig. 8.6a). An attempt at a forceps delivery was abandoned when the FHR dropped to 45 bpm on inserting the first blade. A female infant with Apgar scores of 4 at 1 min and 8 at 5 min was delivered by Caesarean delivery. The umbilical venous blood-gases showed a pH of 7·05, Po_2 of 11 torr (1·4 kPa), a Pco_2 of 53 torr (7·3 kPa) and a lactic acid level of 12·2 mmol/l (N 1–4 mmol/l). The FHR pattern was not considered serious enough to warrant scalp blood analysis. Certainly, the Apgar scores did not reflect the extent of the metabolic acidosis. Yet would not the fetus have benefited from an earlier delivery? A comprehensive blood gas assessment may have spared this baby from the hazards of prolonged hypoxaemia and lacticacidemia.

In *Case B* a variable deceleration pattern occurred in a term fetus, without antecedent high-risk factors. Fetal HR variability was judged to be normal. In the second stage of labour a series of profound variable decelerations occurred which led to a decision to perform a Caesarean delivery (Fig. 8.6b). Meconium was noted at the time of making the uterine incision, and

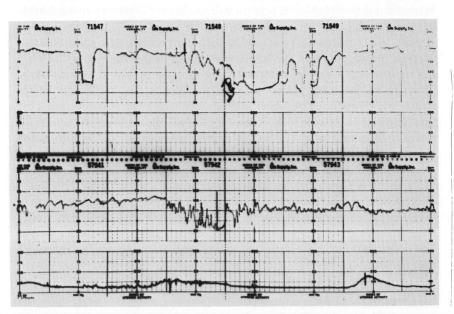

Fig. 8.6(a)   The smoother tracing in Figure 8.6(a) is more suggestive of acidosis than the tracing in Figure 8.6b. The Apgar scores for the baby in 8.6b were worse than for the baby in 8.6a because of the extensive suctioning to remove meconium in the baby in 8.6b. The blood gases proved more reliable in correlating the fetal heart rate tracing than the Apgar scores.

suctioning of the oropharynx was performed as soon as the head was delivered. Apgar scores were 1 at 1 min and 3 at 5 min. The cord venous blood-gas values were: pH 7·36, Po_2 of 31 torr (4 kPa), Pco_2 of 42 torr (6·3 kPa) and a lactic acid level of 4·9 mmol/l.

In this case the Apgar scores did not reflect the intra-uterine blood-gas environment, but rather the effects of suctioning the airways to clear meconium. Had scalp blood sampling been performed, the second stage may not have been interrupted by Caesarean delivery. The low Apgar scores were initially attributed to intrapartum asphyxia. This would have been the second error of assessment made in this delivery. It has been our recommendation to collect fetal cord blood at delivery in all cases where fetal hypoxaemia is suspected. This confirms the diagnosis of fetal distress and provides a baseline for the paediatrician. It also ensures that when a baby is assigned low Apgar scores, it is for the right reason.

SUMMARY

Fetal heart rate monitoring remains the mainstay of intrapartum fetal assessments. Subtle changes of the FHR, such as mild late decelerations, or diminished FHR variability, will not be perceived by the nurse or physician using non-electronic means, no matter how zealously sought. Intermittent blood sampling for pH is usually reliable enough to permit clinical judgments to be made, notwithstanding the fact that errors may occur due to technique. Intermittent oxygen and CO_2 values, however, are less reliable; in part because of the wide range in values that are found in the dynamic fetal milieu, and also because of the potential for aerobic contamination of the sample which can alter the values (Saling, 1966; Willcourt & Queenan, 1981). Past experience has shown that there is a poor correlation between these values and the state of the fetus.

Fetal lactate measurement offers a chance to define the metabolic component of acidosis, and in conjunction with pH measurements should provide a better means of assessing the fetal acid–base state. It must be remembered that lactate will remain in the fetal circulation long after the hypoxaemic insult has occurred, using concomitant pH and hypoxanthine measurements because these will show a trend towards normal as the fetus recovers. The transcutaneous methods offer little practical promise but, in the investigative setting, have been illuminating. A combination electrode measuring Po_2, Pco_2, pH and lactate might provide more clinically useful information than either method alone. Advances in miniaturisation of components may make such an electrode possible. It is clear, however, that conventional electronic fetal monitoring will be the mainstay of good fetal surveillance with biochemically based enhancements being used only when it is unclear how the fetus is tolerating its intra-uterine environment. Ominous patterns, requiring action (stopping labour to allow intra-uterine resuscitation, abdominal delivery versus vaginal delivery, administration of oxygen or extra fluids) may be the areas most often helped by these techniques. As our knowledge of fetal physiology has expanded, showing the limitations of our current monitoring techniques, such an approach seems most worthy of pursuit.

REFERENCES

Bauer C, Ludwig M, Ludwig I, Bartels H 1969 Factors governing the oxygen affinity of human adult and foetal blood. Respiration Physiology 7: 271–277

Beard R W 1970 Fetal blood sampling. British Journal of Hospital Medicine 3: 523–534

Blechner J N, Stenger V G, Prystowsky H 1974 Uterine blood flow in women at term. American Journal of Obstetrics and Gynecology 120: 633–640

Boddy K 1976 Fetal circulation and breathing movements. In: Beard R W, Nathanielsz P W (eds) Fetal physiology and medicine. Saunders, London, pp. 302–328

Bonica J J, Figgs D C 1969 In: Bonica J J (ed) Principles and practice of obstetric analgesia and anesthesia. Davis, Philadelphia, pp 1127–1147

Brann A W, Myers RE 1975 Central nervous system findings in the newborn monkey following severe in utero partial asphyxia. Neurology 25: 327

Clark L C 1956 Monitor and control of blood and tissue oxygen tensions. Transactions of the American Society of Artificial Internal Organs 2: 41–45

Cohn H E, Sachs E J, Heymann M A, Rudolph A M 1974 Cardiovascular responses to hypoxemia and acidemia in fetal lambs. American Journal of Obstetrics and Gynecology 120: 817–824

Epstein M F, Nicholls E, Stubblefield P G 1973 Neonatal hypoglycemia after β-sympathomimetic tocolytic therapy. Journal of Pediatrics 94: 449

Fall O, Johnsson M, Nilsson B A, Rooth G 1979 A study of the correlation between the oxygen gas tension of the fetal scalp blood and the continuous, transcutaneous oxygen tension in human fetuses during labor. In: Huch A, Huch R, Lucey J F (eds) Continuous transcutaneous blood gas monitoring. Original article series—birth defects. National Foundation, March of Dimes, New York, A. R. Liss, Vol. 15(4), pp. 223–233

Flynn A M, Kelly J 1978 An evaluation of the continuous pH electrode (tpH) during labor in the human fetus. *Archives of Gynecology* 226: 105–113

Gauwerky J, Wernicke K, Boos R, Kubli F 1981 Heart rate variability, breathing and body movements in hypoxic fetal lambs. Journal of Perinatal Medicine 10: 113–114

Gillmer M D G, Combe D 1979 Intrapartum fetal monitoring practice in the United Kingdom. British Journal of Obstetrics and Gynaecology 86: 753–758

Harkness R A, Geirsson R T, McFadyen I R 1983 Concentrations of hypoxanthine, uridine and urate in the amniotic fluid at caesarean section and the association of raised levels with prenatal risk factors and fetal distress. British Journal of Obstetrics and Gynaecology 90: 815–820

Hon E H, Quilligan E J 1967 The classification of the fetal heart rate. II. A revised working classification. Connecticut Medical Journal 31: 779–784

Huch A, Huch R, Schneider H, Rooth G 1977 Continuous transcutaneous monitoring of fetal oxygen tension during labour. British Journal of Obstetrics and Gynaecology 84 (Suppl.) 1: 1–39

Ikenoue T, Martin C B, Murata Y, Ettinger B B, Lu P S 1981 Effect of acute hypoxemia and respiratory acidosis on the fetal heart rate in monkeys. American Journal of Obstetrics and Gynecology 141: 797–780

Itskovitz J, Goetzman B W, Rudolph A M 1982 The mechanism of late deceleration of the heart rate and its relationship to oxygenation in normoxemic and chronically hypoxemic fetal lambs. American Journal of Obstetrics and Gynecology 142: 66–73

Jacobson L, Rooth G 1971 Interpretive aspects on the acid–base composition and its variation in foetal scalp blood and maternal blood during labour. Journal of Obstetrics and Gynaecology of the British Commonwealth 78: 971–980

James L S, Morishima H O, Daniel S S, Bowe E T, et al 1972 Mechanism of late deceleration of the fetal heart rate. American Journal of Obstetrics and Gynecology 113: 578–582

Janecek P, Bossart H 1978 Clinical aspects of continuous tissular pH measurements of the newborn and the fetus. Archives of Gynecology 226: 121–127

Kunzel W, Wulf H 1970 Der Einfluss der maternen Ventilation auf die aktuellen Blutgase und den Saure-Base-Status des Feten. Zeitschrifte Fur Geburtschilfe und Gynaekologie 172: 1–24

Kurz C S, Fallenstein F, Schneider H, Huch R, Huch A 1981 The influence of maternal oxygen (O_2) administration on fetal heart rate (FHR) and long-term variability amplitude (LVA). Journal of Perinatal Medicine 10: 97

Lawrence G F, Brown V A, Parsons R J, Cooke I D 1982 Feto-maternal consequences of high-dose glucose infusion during labour. British Journal of Obstetrics and Gynaecology 89: 27–32

Lee S T, Hon E H 1963 Fetal hemodynamic response to umbilical cord compression. Obstetrics and Gynecology 22: 553–562

Low J A, Pancham S R, Worthington D N 1973 Intrapartum fetal heart rate profiles with and without fetal asphyxia. American Journal of Obstetrics and Gynecology 127: 729–737

Lumley J, Hammond J, Wood C 1969 Effects of maternal hypertension on fetal scalp blood pH, P_{CO_2} and P_{O_2}. Journal of Obstetrics and Gynaecology of the British Commonwealth 76: 512–517.

Lysikiewicz A, Vetter K, Huch R, Huch A 1981 Fetal transcutaneous P_{CO_2} during labor. Presented at The Second International Symposium on Continuous Transcutaneous Blood Gas Monitoring. Zurich, Switzerland

Makowski E L, Meschia G, Droegemueller W, Battaglia F C 1968 Measurement of umbilical arterial blood flow to the sheep placenta and fetus in utero. Distribution to cotyledons and the intercotyledonary chorion. Circulation Research 23: 623–631

O'Connor M C, Hytten F E, Zanelli G D 1979 Is the fetus 'scalped' in labour? Lancet 2: 947–948

Paul R H, Suidan A K, Yeh S-Y, Schifrin B S, Hon E H 1975 Clinical fetal monitoring. VII. The evaluation and significance of intrapartum baseline FHR variability. American Journal of Obstetrics and Gynecology 123: 206–210

Pearson J F 1976 Maternal and fetal acid–base balance. In: Beard R W, Nathanielsz P W (eds) Fetal physiology and medicine. Saunders, London, pp 492–509

Power G G, Hill E P, Longo L D 1971 A mathematical model of carbon dioxide transfer in the placenta; in respiratory gas exchange and bloodflow in the placenta. From: Longo D C, Bastels H (eds) Proceedings of a Symposium in Conjunction with the XXV International Congress of Physiological Sciences, Hanover, Germany. DHEW Publication, pp 395–416

Rankin J H C, Meschia G, Makowski E L, Battaglia F C 1971 Relationship between uterine and umbilical venous P_{O_2} in sheep. American Journal of Physiology 220: 1688–1692

Saling E 1964 Die Blutgasverhaultnisse und der Saure-Basen-Hanshalt des feten bei ungestortem Geburtsablauf. Zeitschrifte fur Geburtschilfe und Gynaekologie, 161: 262–292

Saling E 1966 Fetal blood gas and acid–base status. In: Saling E (ed) Fetal and neonatal hypoxia. Edward Arnold, London, pp 29–41

Saugstad O D, Gluck L 1982 Plasma hypoxanthine levels in newborn infants: a specific indicator of hypoxia. Journal of Perinatal Medicine 10: 266–272

Severinghaus J W 1981 Introduction to skin P_{CO_2} regulation and measurement. Presented at The Second International Symposium on Continuous Transcutaneous Blood Gas Monitoring. Zurich, Switzerland

Shelley H J 1973 The use of chronically catheterized foetal lambs for the study of foetal metabolism. In: Comline R S et al (eds) Foetal and neonatal physiology, Barcroft Centenary Symposium. Cambridge University Press, London, pp 360–381

Smith N C, Quinn M C, Soutter W P, Sharp F 1979 Rapid whole blood lactate measurement in the fetus and mother during labour. Early Human Development 3: 89–95

Smith N C, Soutter W P, Sharp F et al. 1983 Fetal scalp blood lactate as an indicator of intrapartum hypoxia. British Journal of Obstetrics and Gynaecology 90: 821

Soutter W P, Sharp F, Clark D M 1978 Bedside estimation of whole blood lacta. British Journal of Anaesthesia 50: 445–450

Stamm O, Latscha U, Janecek P, Campana A 1976 Development of a special electrode for continuous subcutaneous pH measurement in the infant scalp. American Journal of Obstetrics and Gynecology 124: 193–195

Stewart P, Hillan E, Calder A A 1983 A comparative assessment of an automated blood microprocessor for fetal blood pH measurements in a labor ward. British Journal of Obstetrics and Gynaecology 90 : 522

Sturbois G, Uzan S, Rotten D, Breart G, Sureau C 1977 Continuous subcutaneous pH measurement in human fetuses; correlations with scalp and umbilical blood pH. American Journal of Obstetrics and Gynecology 128 : 901–903

Swanstrom S, Bratteby L-E 1982 Hypoxanthine as a test of perinatal hypoxia as compared to lactate, base deficit, and pH. Pediatric Research 16 : 156–160

Tejani N, Mann L I, Bhakthavathsalan A 1976 Correlation of fetal heart rate patterns and fetal pH with neonatal outcome. Obstetrics and Gynecology 48 : 460–463

Thiringer K 1983 Cord Plasma hypoxanthine as a measure of foetal asphyxia. Acta Paediatrica Scandinavica 72 : 231

Weil M H, Afifi A A 1970 Experimental and clinical studies on lactate and pyruvate as indicators of the severity of acute circulatory failure (shock). Circulation 41 : 989–1001

Willcourt R J, Queenan J T 1981 Fetal scalp blood sampling and transcutaneous Po_2. Clinics in Perinatology 8 : 87

Willcourt R J, King J C, Indyk L, Queenan J T 1981 The relationship of the fetal heart rate patterns to the fetal transcutaneous Po_2. American Journal of Obstetrics and Gynecology 140 : 760

Willcourt R J, Paust J C, Queenan J T 1982 Changes in fetal tePo_2 valves occurring during labour in association with lumbar extra dural analgesia. British Journal of Anaesthesia 54 : 635

Wood C 1978 Fetal scalp sampling: its place in management. Seminars in Perinatology 8 : 87

Young B K, Katz M, Klein S A 1979 The relationship of heart rate patterns and tissue pH in the human fetus. American Journal of Obstetrics and Gynecology 134 : 685

Zalar R W, Quilligan E J 1978 The influence of scalp sampling on the cesarean section rate for fetal distress. American Journal of Obstetrics and Gynecology 135 : 239

Zanini B, Paul R H, Huey J R 1979 Intrapartum fetal heart rate: correlation with scalp pH in the preterm fetus. American Journal of Obstetrics and Gynecology 136 : 43

Implications of increasing rates of Caesarean section

Over the past decade there has been a gradual increase in the rates of Caesarean section in the Western world. It is questionable whether this rise, seen in all the Western countries, is in proportion to the benefits derived from it. This chapter is an attempt to assess the evolution of Caesarean births in Europe, to evaluate critically the benefits or otherwise to the mother and child, of the increasing Caesarean section rates, and to propose alternative measures to try and reduce the currently high Caesarean section rates.

The increasing maternal safety of the Caesarean section operation since the 1940s has made birth by Caesarean section a practical alternative to vaginal delivery. The initial rise in Caesarean section rates (mostly in the United States) was followed by the efforts of obstetricians and neonatologists to try and reduce the perinatal mortality rates. Limitations of family size, and the expectation of a healthy child at the end of each pregnancy, led to the development of new technologies, e.g. continuous fetal heart rate monitoring in labour and advances in neonatal intensive care. The increasing survival rates, particularly of the very small infant, led to further increase in Caesarean section rates. Whilst initially there might have been a concomitant decrease in perinatal mortality rate, this has not been substantiated. The unduly high Caesarean section rates may lead to increased maternal morbidity and mortality.

According to Chalmers (1985) the increasing Caesarean section rates explain why, in the United Kingdom, the maternal mortality rates failed to decrease significantly during the last decades. Chard & Richards (1977) have suggested that the rise in Caesarean section rate due to certain fetal problems, e.g. breech presentation, may, in the long run, prevent the transmission of traditional clinical skills to obstetricians in training, thus further reducing the chances of curtailing the Caesarean section rates in this group.

Since the late 1970s the rise in Caesarean section rates has led to both professional and public concern in several European countries (The Netherlands, U.K., France). It is therefore necessary to look critically at the current indications for Caesarean birth, and to suggest alternative options. In this respect it is encouraging to note that the U.S. Report on Caesarean section (Rosen, 1980) has already produced several studies assessing alternative approaches to Caesarean section (Demianczuk et al, 1982; Jarrell et al, 1985; Egliton et al, 1984).

EVOLUTION OF THE RATES OF CAESAREAN SECTION, PERINATAL MORTALITY AND MATERNAL MORTALITY

Caesarean section rates

Few countries have data available on national Caesarean section rates, particularly related to indications for the operation, and those published are generally extrapolated rates. Consequently we have to rely on regional and hospital data. The poor quality of the data available makes comparisons difficult.

National and international Caesarean section rates vary widely, but the upward trend is reflected in both North America and the European countries, signifying a change in obstetric practice (Gleicher, 1984). Figure 9.1 shows rate increases between 1970 and 1981 in selected countries (Chalmers, 1985). Current rates are: 18 per cent (1981) in the U.S.A. (Placek et al, 1983); 10·6 per cent (1982) in the U.K. (Maternity Alliance Report, Boyd et al, 1983).

The report of Bergsjø et al (1983) failed to detect a systematic trend between Caesarean section rates and other instrumental delivery procedures, indicating that the rise in Caesarean section rate did not show any reduction of other operative vaginal deliveries. The one exception to this was the experience in the Netherlands, but even here the current low rate (4·3 per cent in 1981) shows an increase of 60 per cent over the rate quoted from 1968 to 1975; particularly when the important changes in the obstetric population and its distribution that have occurred in this country are taken into account. This sort of data illustrates the importance of using standardised (age/parity/cause group) Caesarean section rates to assess the changes (Chalmers & Richards, 1977).

Only in the Republic of Ireland—and specifically in the National Maternity Hospital, Dublin—have mean Caesarean section rates remained virtually constant (4–5 per cent) in the period 1965 to 1980, during which more than 100 000 deliveries were performed (O'Driscoll & Foley, 1983).

Perinatal mortality rates

Whilst Caesarean section rates have been increasing in the Western countries, perinatal mortality rates have shown a steady and often steeper drop. All the developed countries have shown falling perinatal mortality rates during the last two decades. Figure 9.2 (left) shows the rates of perinatal mortality over the years in the United States (Bottoms et al, 1980)

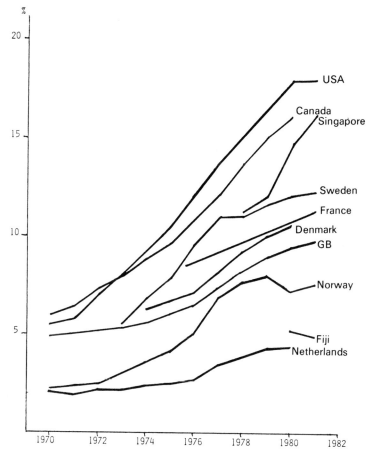

Fig. 9.1 Trends in the rate of Caesarean delivery in various countries, 1970–81 (Chalmers, 1985)

and Figure 9.3 gives data from selected countries in Europe (Rumeau-Rouquette, 1982) showing a similar fall in rates in all countries except for Greece.

Maternal mortality rates

The reporting of maternal mortality rates is not as good in all countries and under-reporting is often the case in some countries. Advances in anaesthetics and intensive care have also meant that the margin between mortality and severe morbidity is reduced, therefore making the maternal mortality rates an unreliable assessment of the effects of Caesarean section. Maternal mortality rates have decreased in the U.S.A. (Fig. 9.4) and Europe; however in certain countries, e.g. France, the decrease in maternal mortality was not as marked in women over the age of 35 (Chabaud et al, 1983). There are still important differences between countries, regions and hospitals.

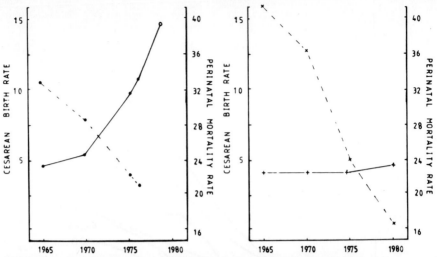

Fig. 9.2 Caesarean section and perinatal mortality (per hundred) rates in U.S.A. (left) (Bottoms et al, 1980) and in Dublin (right) (O'Driscoll & Foley, 1983). (Solid lines = Caesarean rates; broken lines = perinatal mortality rates; U.S.A. = circles; Dublin = crosses.)

IMPACT OF CAESAREAN SECTION ON PERINATAL MORTALITY AND MATERNAL MORTALITY RATES

Caesarean section and perinatal mortality rate

It is difficult to assess what, if any, has been the contribution of the increasing Caesarean section rate on the decreasing perinatal mortality rate.

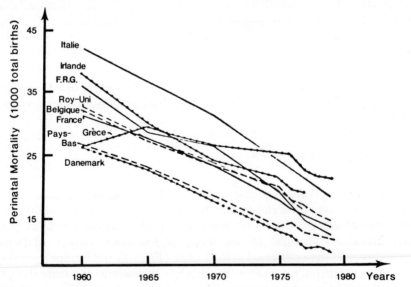

Fig. 9.3 Perinatal mortality rates in selected countries in Europe (Rumeau-Rouquette, 1982).

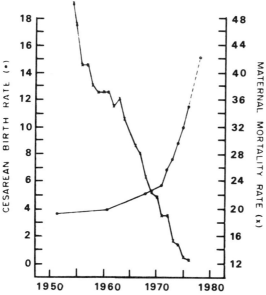

Fig. 9.4 Caesarean section rates (per 100 deliveries) and maternal mortality rates (per 100 000 deliveries) in the U.S.A. 1950–76 (Bottoms et al, 1980).

The reverse trends shown by the rates of perinatal mortality and Caesarean section are not uniform, nationally and internationally. Two extreme examples are the U.S.A. and Dublin (Fig. 9.2). In the U.S.A. and Dublin perinatal mortality rates have dropped between 1965 and 1980, although the drop has been steeper in Dublin than in the U.S.A. This has coincided with soaring Caesarean section rates in the U.S.A. and a virtually constant Caesarean section rate in Dublin. Bergsjø et al (1983) analysed the correlation between perinatal mortality and Caesarean section rates in 11 European countries (Fig. 9.5) during the same year, and the weak negative correlation ($r = -0.48$) found means that the frequencies of Caesarean section did not contribute much to the differences in perinatal mortality rates between countries assessed. Thus the increase in the number of Caesarean sections will, at best, have a very small impact on perinatal mortality, which suggests that perinatal mortality is more closely linked to other factors such as the rates of preterm birth, number of babies with intra-uterine growth retardation, and presumably other factors that differ between nations, e.g maternal age, parity and standard of obstetric and neonatal care.

Caesarean section and maternal mortality rate

Whilst Caesarean section operation is now safer than it has ever been, in terms of sophistication in anaesthesia and surgery, it can never be entirely safe and therefore is not an alternative to vaginal delivery. For this reason

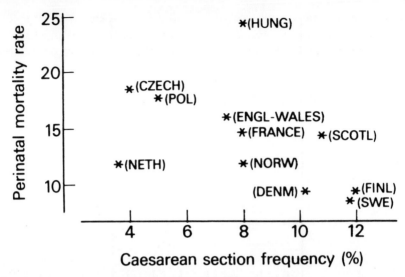

Fig. 9.5   Perinatal mortality rates against Caesarean section frequencies in some European countries (Bergsjø et al, 1983).

the two cannot be compared, and neither can mortality be an adequate yardstick to evaluate the risk of Caesarean section.

Caesarean section-related maternal mortality rates have decreased, but still form the major part of total maternal mortality rates. In both the U.S.A. and England and Wales, current Caesarean section-related maternal mortality rates are several times the mortality rates found in the mid-1960s. Apparently the decrease in maternal mortality rates has been greater than the Caesarean section-related maternal mortality rate (Chalmers, 1985).

Maternal mortality rates are believed to be under-reported in a number of industrialised countries, e.g. Belgium (Derom, 1986). High on the list of causes of death associated with Caesarean section are thromboembolism and anaesthesia accidents, both of which may be considered as related to the surgical procedure.

Conclusions

The available data make it doubtful that the current improvement in perinatal outcome is linked to the extended use of Caesarean section. To assess the intrinsic role of Caesarean section rates reliable national data are needed, including perinatal mortality rates related to indications for the Caesarean section operation. In the meantime we can wholly agree with the WHO recommendation: 'Countries with some of the lowest perinatal mortality rates in the world have Caesarean section rates of less than 10%. There is no justification for any region to have a rate higher than 10–15%.' We would prefer to put the limit at 10 rather than 15 per cent.

Caesarean section is, and will always remain, a potentially dangerous operation for the mother, and the added hazard of anaesthesia, of whatever form, should not be underestimated. The rates of maternal mortality related to Caesarean section are still unacceptably high.

POSSIBLE WAYS OF REDUCING CAESAREAN SECTION RATES ACCORDING TO INDICATION

Dystocia

The term dystocia (abnormal labour) is vague. It includes abnormalities related to the birth passages, the passenger, and the labour forces, the ultimate result being failure to progress in labour. In recent years a large divergence has become apparent in the diagnostic and therapeutic approaches taken to deal with failure to progress. Misinterpretation of the evolution of labour often leads to unwarranted Caesarean section: during the latent phase, lack of progress in cervical dilatation or fetal descent, two completely normal phenomena, are too readily interpreted as cephalopelvic disproportion (Lundy, 1983); during the active phase, contraction disorders which may be related to quite different reasons are often not treated causally (Friedman, 1981); and termination of labour simply because an arbitrary time is set for the duration of the second stage too often results in unnecessary Caesarean section (Cohen, 1977; Thatte, 1982; Apeldoorn et al, 1982; Cardozo et al, 1983).

The introduction of labour curves (Friedman, 1981; Philpott & Castle, 1972; Studd, 1973) has contributed to early identification of abnormal labour patterns and early intervention with oxytocin, thus decreasing the need for Caesarean section. In Dublin, adherence to a programme called Active Management of Labour (O'Driscoll & Meagher, 1980) has kept hospital Caesarean section rates consistently down (O'Driscoll & Foley, 1983). According to this programme, diagnosis of dystocia is based on trial and augmentation of labour. The philosophy and details of this management are so important that we wish to quote the authors (O'Driscoll & Foley, 1983):

> The essential nature of our practice is based on recognition of the fact that dystocia is a condition virtually confined to nulliparous women and that inefficient uterine contraction is by far the commonest cause. Furthermore, confident in the knowledge that the nulliparous uterus is almost immune to rupture, these observations have led to complete re-appraisal of traditional attitudes to the other two possible causes of dystocia: cephalo-pelvic disproportion and occipito posterior positions. At a clinical level, therefore, attention is focused on a correct initial diagnosis of labour, regular assessment of early progress, and effective stimulation with oxytocin whenever the pace of dilatation of the cervix is low in nulliparous women. A general commitment is given to the effect that the duration of labour (calculated from time of hospital admission), which is restricted to twelve hours, and the operative methods of delivery are confined to low forceps and Caesarean section, each at a very low level.

Other practices too may help to prevent dystocia. Minkoff & Schwarz (1980) at Downstate-Kings County Hospital, New York City, in an analysis of more than 100 000 deliveries between 1961 and 1977, concluded that the use of intra-uterine pressure monitoring had substantially lowered the Caesarean section rate in patients who initially were diagnosed to have failed to progress in labour. Fetal monitoring and fetal scalp sampling (FSS) are helpful for allowing labour to go on. Manual (Thatte, 1982) or forceps rotation (Cardozo et al, 1983) has significantly decreased the Caesarean section rate due to malposition of the fetal head in the second stage of labour in some hospitals. In some cases of overstimulation and dystocia, infusion with betamimetic drugs and change of maternal posture and ambulation may make vaginal delivery possible (Flynn et al, 1978). Thiery (1981) has shown that an infusion of prostaglandins instead of oxytocin could be more effective in cases of unfavourable cervix (low Bishop score) (Tables 9.1 and 9.2). In 58 nulliparae and 40 parae presenting with premature rupture of membranes and an unfavourable cervix (Bishop score <5) i.v. infusion of prostaglandin E2 was successful in as much as all but four women delivered vaginally with no increase in maternal or perinatal morbidity and mortality (Thiery et al, 1983).

Childbirth education has been reported to be associated with a decrease in Caesarean section rate for dystocia (Beck & Hall, 1978) and we have found that teaching women who elect to have continuous lumbar epidural anaesthesia (CLEA), antenatally how to bear down properly decreased the need for second-stage operative intervention significantly (unpublished

Table 9.1 Caesarean section rates (percentages) after (pre)induction of labour with extra-amniotic infusion of prostaglandin gel (500 µg PGE$_2$ in 8 ml 5 per cent aqueous Tylose® gel) (Thiery, unpublished data)

	Bishop score	
	0–2	*3–5*
Nulliparas	10·3	3·9
Parous women	4·4	1·2

Table 9.2 Results of the intravenous infusion of prostaglandin E$_2$ for the management of PROM in (near)-term gravidas (Thiery et al, 1983)

	Nulliparous cervix		Parous cervix	
	Unripe	*Ripe*	*Unripe*	*Ripe*
Number of patients	58	17	40	16
Mean Bishop score	3·7	7·5	3·5	6·8
Number of CS	2	0	2	0
Mean 5-min Apgar score	8·6	8·6	8·6	8·8
Mean umbilical-artery pH	7·29	7·31	7·31	7·29

data). Indeed, an effective block will prolong the second stage and delay rotation in a high proportion of cases, not because of any diminution of uterine performance but as the result of the sensory nerve block of the pelvic floor and the motor nerve block of the muscles of the lower abdomen and the pelvic floor (Crawford, 1982).

In summary, most obstetricians are now reasonably certain that changes in current practice can reduce Caesarean section rates for dystocia without affecting neonatal outcome. To assess the effectiveness and safety of alternative practices, randomised comparative trials are necessary.

Previous Caesarean section

In the U.S.A. previous Caesarean section emerges as a formidable (4·7 per cent of all Caesarean sections in 1978) and self-repeating cause of abdominal deliveries. Recent data, from the U.S.A. and other countries (Pauerstein, 1981; Meier & Porreco, 1982; Demianczuk et al, 1982; O'Driscoll & Foley, 1983) suggest trial of labour after a single previous low-segment transverse Caesarean section to be effective and of low risk to mother and fetus. Successful vaginal delivery occurred in 59 per cent (Merrill & Gibbs, 1978) to 95 per cent (Meier & Porreco, 1982) of cases. According to Demianczuk et al (1982) assessment of dilatation on admission in labour is the most significant predictor of success: 69 per cent when the cervix was more, and 27 per cent when it was less than 3 cm dilated.

Clearly doubt is cast on the validity of the dictum 'once a Caesarean section always a Caesarean section' (Craigin, 1916) and a change in policy must be seriously considered. The American College of Obstetricians and Gynaecologists has revised and liberalised its guidelines for vaginal birth after a Caesarean section:

> Women who have a low transverse scar on their uterus (the most common type of Caesarean incision) from a previous Caesarean delivery and without recurrent indication, can deliver vaginally with a high degree of safety, [provided there is] continuous electronic fetal heart rate and uterine activity monitoring throughout labour, as well as staff and facilities required to respond to acute obstetric emergencies.

One of the general recommendations at a recent WHO conference on appropriate technology for births reads 'There is no evidence that Caesarean section is required after a previous Caesarean section birth. Vaginal delivery after a Caesarean section should normally be encouraged wherever emergency surgical intervention is available.'

Breech

Several reasons have been put forward to perform an elective Caesarean section in the majority of, if not all, cases of breech presentation. Kubli et al (1976) were first to point out that fetal acidosis at the time of birth is much more common in breech presentation compared to cephalic presentation. On the basis of their findings they came to the logical conclusion that babies presenting by the breech should be delivered by Caesarean section.

Intra-uterine hypoxia and the resulting fetal acidosis are by no means the only risk. The other major fetal complication in breech presentation is traumatic birth injury. To reduce the incidence of birth injuries, abdominal delivery was advocated from the late 1950s onwards in the U.S.A. (Hall & Kohl, 1956) and from 1976 in continental Europe (Kubli et al, 1976). Most dreaded injuries are the tentorial tear and the resulting intracranial haemorrhage, fractures or dislocation of the cervical spine and occipital osteodiastasis so well described by Wigglesworth & Husemeyer (1977). Other injuries are: elongation of the plexus brachialis, laceration or even rupture of abdominal organs, e.g. the liver, and fractures of the bones of the extremities, especially the humerus. Finally, and this is a complication relating particularly to preterm births, entrapment of the aftercoming head by the insufficiently dilated cervix leads to hypoxia and trauma in the very vulnerable very-low-birthweight babies.

Do the advantages of the current obstetric practices outweigh the risks to the mother and the fetus? We should look separately at the management of full-term and the preterm breech presentation as each group has its own problems (Duignan, 1982).

Full-term breech presentation (singletons only)

A number of studies evaluate (compare) perinatal mortality and morbidity according to the mode of delivery. Recent ones are those of Schutte et al (1985), O'Driscoll & Foley (1983), Derom et al (1984), Collea et al (1980), Horovitz et al (1982), De Jong & Stolte (1982), and Jackson et al (1982). According to all of them, a variable number of term breeches may be allowed to deliver vaginally.

The U.S.A. Caesarean Birth Task Force (Rosen, 1980) espoused this selective vaginal birth policy, and in a special communication (1980) the experts concluded:

> Vaginal delivery of the term breech should remain an acceptable obstetric choice for delivery when the following conditions are present: 1. anticipated fetal weight of less than 3,584 gms; 2. normal pelvic dimensions and architecture; 3. frank breech presentation without extended head; 4. delivery conducted by a physician experienced in vaginal breech delivery.

To prevent litigation they cautiously added:

> Because all breech births have inherent risks that are often uncertain and unpredictable, the information should be shared with the family whenever possible as part of the decision-making process.

To assess the ideal Caesarean section rate for term breeches, Westgren et al (1982) analysed the effect of stricter selection on short- and long-term perinatal outcomes. The increase of Caesarean section rates in the two periods studied (from 16·9 per cent in 1971–74 to 37·1 per cent in 1974–77) was accompanied by a drop in the perinatal mortality rate (from 0·88 to 0·26 per cent) and neurologic handicaps at age 4 (5·3 against 2·4 per cent, the corresponding percentage for vaginal vertex delivery being 1·5 per cent). The frequency of visual and auditory disorders and behaviour problems did not differ in the two study periods, nor were these rates higher than in a vertex presentation group. At a Caesarean section rate of 37·1 per cent, the mortality and morbidity rates for vaginally delivered term breeches were not increased compared with those for vaginal vertex delivery, and the authors conclude that the acceptability of a further increase of the Caesarean section rate for this indication must be questioned. Faber-Nijholt et al (1983) performed a neurological follow-up study of all surviving breech children born (Caesarean section rate 20 per cent) in the Groningen University Hospital (The Netherlands) and compared them with matched controls (delivered vaginally in cephalic presentation). Significant differences between the study and control groups were found only for minor neurological dysfunction.

Preterm breech (singletons only)

Basically, the low-birthweight breech infant delivering by the vaginal route is exposed to the same types of hazard inherent in vaginal breech delivery as the mature infant, but is more vulnerable to mechanical trauma and hypoxia (including intraventricular haemorrhage). The dangers of cord prolapse and head entrapment (especially in the footling presentation) are increased and malformations are common. To this must be added the risks inherent in pulmonary immaturity resulting in the neonatal idiopathic respiratory distress syndrome (IRDS) and its sequelae.

The more liberal and sometimes routine use of abdominal delivery reflects the conviction of those authors who believe that they have proven that Caesarean section decreases the mortality and morbidity for very-low-birthweight breeches (Prichard et al, 1985; Quilligan & Zuspan, 1982).

Ingemarsson et al (1978) from a study based on a long-term follow-up of preterm breech births, concluded that the infants delivered by Caesarean section indeed had lower mortality rates, and that survivors had a lower rate of developmental anomalies at 12 months of age. In contrast, Karp et al (1979) found no significant difference in neonatal outcome related to the mode of delivery, and Kitchen et al (1982) reported that the mode of delivery did not significantly affect the handicap rate in survivors. Cox et al's (1982) report on an analysis of outcome of low-birthweight breeches during two periods (1973–74 and 1979–80) characterised by an increase in Caesarean section rate and continuing development of neonatal intensive care methods, runs in the same vein: although 'the neonatal mortality rate has fallen the increased survival rate was accounted for largely by the survival of handicapped infants', and the authors conclude that 'the value of routine Caesarean section in the absence of other obstetrical pathology for low birthweight breeches is unproven and may be deleterious to mother and baby'. From his study, Woods (1979) concluded that although Caesarean section might be safer for delivery of infants weighing between 1000 and 1499 g, evidence supporting the need for abdominal delivery in the group of heavier infants was lacking. In 1980, Crowley and Hawkins reviewed various studies on preterm breech delivery (Table 9.3) and concluded from the collected data that the survival rate of infants weighing 1500–2500 g was not affected by the mode of delivery, although Caesarean section did appear to provide an advantage to infants weighing between 1000 and 1500 g. However, the outcome for infants weighing less than 1000 g appeared to be strongly dependent on the quality of the neonatal care. On the basis of their own studies and the current literature, Kauppila et al (1981) offered the following principles for the management of low-birthweight breech delivery: 'vaginal delivery is justified from 32 weeks gestation (estimated weight 1,500 g onwards)' if continuous fetal monitoring and prompt operative intervention is possible when hypoxia is diagnosed or when there are signs that delivery may be prolonged; primary Caesarean section should be undertaken in footling breech presentation or in the presence of other obstetrical complications (toxaemia, hypertension, diabetes, IUGR, etc); for cases of less than 32 weeks gestation (estimated weight less than 1500 g) the higher incidence of cerebral haemorrhage compared with cephalic delivery suggests that primary Caesarean section be recommended. A randomised trial might answer the question whether elective Caesarean section in very-low-birthweight babies is justified, but we doubt, as others (Mentzel, 1984), that such an experiment is feasible.

External cephalic version

This procedure, which at one time was widely practised, came into disrepute because of the often-encountered complications of antepartum haemorrhage

Table 9.3 Neonatal mortality rates (percentages) for low-birthweight breeches, according to birthweight and mode of delivery: review of pertinent studies (Crowley & Hawkins, 1980)

Study	500–999 g		1000–1499 g		1500–1999 g		2000–2499 g	
	V	CS	V	CS	V	CS	V	CS
Bowes (1977)	88	36	37	16	—	—	—	—
Duenhoelter et al. (1979)[1]	—	—	55	0	0	9	8	0
Goldenberg & Nelson (1977)[1,2]	96	72	55	42	7	13	3	6
Karp et al. (1979)[1]	—	—	50	60	18	0	0	0
Mann & Gallant (1979)	93	80	47	30	9	11	—	—
Woods (1979)[1]	—	—	62	25	20	33	4	0

[1]Congenital malformations excluded.
[2]PM.
V = vaginal delivery, CS = Caesarean birth.

due to placental detachment. In the past decade, however, new interest has been shown in this procedure for two reasons: (1) the use of tocolytic drugs which allow for easier manipulation of the fetus through a relaxed uterine wall; and (2) the fact that it can be performed in late pregnancy and therefore reduces the incidence of breech presentation at the beginning of labour, and hence the Caesarean section rate. Saling & Muller-Holve (1975) were the first to report on the use of tocolytic drugs to aid external cephalic version.

The procedure is reported to be safe and effective: it should be done with the help of ultrasound, and the fetus monitored by cardiotocography (*Lancet* 1984—editorial). Three randomised controlled studies have been performed (Van Dorsten et al, 1981; Hofmeyer, 1983; Brocks et al, 1984); the number of cases was small: 48, 60 and 65, respectively. In each instance the incidence of cephalic presentations was higher and the Caesarean section rate was lower in the experimental group as compared to the controls; major fetal or maternal complications did not occur.

External cephalic version under tocolysis appears to be a worthwhile addition to the measures which can be taken in order to lower the Caesarean section rate. Our experience, though, is rather disappointing: out of 46 attempts, 22 primigravida and 24 parae, only 2 and 12 were successful, respectively (Parewijck et al, unpublished data, 1985). These disappointing results were obtained despite the intravenous administration of ritodrine, a tocolytic drug.

Management of labour

It is suggested, therefore, that a considerable number, indeed probably more than 50 per cent of full-term infants presenting by the breech, will deliver safely by the vaginal route, provided a number of conditions are fulfilled. However a strict adherence to them is a condition 'sine qua non', to achieve results which are comparable to those obtained by systematically resorting to Caesarean section. These conditions are:

1. At the beginning of labour, assess the case and look for contra-indications to vaginal delivery such as fetal macrosomia ($\geqslant$ 4 kg), contracted pelvis, hyperextension of the fetal head.
2. Make sure an experienced obstetrician is available for consultation during labour and delivery. Anaesthetic and paediatric cover is required in the delivery room at the time of the birth. Where needed, general anaesthesia should be available, for immediate administration.
3. Watch for regular progress of labour, particularly the descent of the presenting part. Deviation from normality both during the first and second stages means that safe delivery by the vaginal route will not be possible.

4. Use of electronic fetal monitoring: it is mandatory that this be carried out in all breech presentations.
5. Use of prostaglandin (see tables).

It is partly because of the strict requirements for vaginal breech delivery that some centres resort to elective Caesarean section in all breech presentations.

Fetal distress

'Fetal distress (read: fetal hypoxia) is an accepted indication for Caesarean section. The problem is to define fetal hypoxia and to identify the fetus at risk of ante and intrapartum distress, the reason for the distress, and measures for detection and modification of the distress' (Klein, 1982).

Although an accepted term, fetal distress is a misnomer and must be carefully distinguished from the real risk situation, i.e. fetal or intra-uterine hypoxia. Fetal stress is a clinical concept and is heralded mainly by alteration of the baseline fetal heart rate (FHR) and FHR pattern. Signs of fetal stress indicate only that the unborn baby is potentially endangered. Hypoxia, on the other hand, is a diagnosis based on changes of the acid–base (AB) equilibrium of the fetus assessed by scalp sampling or cord-blood analysis (gas levels and components of the AB and lactate–pyruvate equilibria), and the results must be compared with the values in the mother before the diagnosis of perinatal oxygen deprivation can be firmly established.

There can be no doubt that the introduction of uninterrupted FHR monitoring in labour has resulted in an increase of Caesarean section rates for 'fetal distress' in many hospitals (Antenatal Diagnosis, 1979). As experience increased, however, the overdiagnosis of intra-uterine hypoxia generally decreased, which in turn led to a concommitant drop of Caesarean section rates for this indication (Neutra et al, 1980). Nevertheless, overt overdiagnosis of fetal distress is apparent in some hospitals (Pontonnier et al, 1979). A study performed in Limoges, France (Peter et al, 1982) indicates that of all abdominal deliveries, one-quarter were performed for this indication, but the incidence of normal (8–10 per cent) 1-min (57 per cent) and 5-min (85 per cent) Apgar scores may point to overestimation of fetal hypoxia.

Concurrent use of fetal scalp blood sampling has enhanced the specificity of the diagnosis of fetal hypoxia (Haverkamp et al, 1979; Staudach & Lassmann, 1982; Pillai, 1984) and several authors have reported decreased Caesarean section rates after the institution of FSS programmes (Mann & Gallant, 1979; Ayromlooi & Garfinkel, 1980). In contrast, Zuspan et al (1979), who adopted an active programme of total surveillance with continuous FHR monitoring and FSS, found no change in their institutional Caesarean section rate for 'fetal distress' between 1970 (0·93 per cent) and 1976 (0·97 per cent). More demonstrative with regard to the proper rate of

Caesarean section for fetal distress is the large prospective randomised controlled trial in low-risk pregnancies conducted at the National Maternity Hospital, Dublin (MacDonald et al, 1985). The use of electronic fetal monitoring did not influence the number of Caesarean sections performed for fetal distress.

Future research should be directed at enhancement of the precision of electronic fetal monitoring. Several authors have made suggestions as to how this might be accomplished (Smyth, 1984; Chandler et al, 1984; Sawers, 1983). One of these is the analysis of fetal heart rate by computer (Sawers, 1983; Henry et al, 1979); if this method proved to be beneficial, microprocessors could profitably replace conventional (visual) interpretation of FHR patterns.

The European Economic Community sponsors an ambitious research programme which aims at a better understanding of interventions based upon cardiotocographic recording in a group of patients at high risk for fetal hypoxia (van Geijn et al, 1984; Thiery & Derom, 1986).

Very-low-birthweight babies

Improved neonatal results affect obstetrical practice. Whereas a decade ago few European obstetricians were ready to perform Caesarean sections for fetal reasons before the 32nd week (Kubli et al, 1976) a lot of units now view 28 weeks as a gestational age at which in certain circumstances, e.g. ruptured membranes, the infant does better outside than inside the uterus (Evaldson et al, 1982). To enhance further the chances of survival, with no long-term handicap, more and more Caesarean sections are performed. At the University Hospital of Lund, Sweden (Westgren et al, 1982, 1985) a quite rigid policy is applied: if the fetus is in presentation other than vertex, or if severe additional complications are involved, Caesarean section is performed for the delivery of very tiny infants. According to Haesslein & Goodlin (1979) the incidence of intraventricular haemorrhage in cephalic presentation is markedly reduced after Caesarean section. Mentzel (1984), a neonatologist, after a careful analysis of his results over a 7-year period, concluded that whenever a choice can be made in preterm birth, Caesarean section is the preferred mode of delivery. He admits, though, that it is difficult, if not impossible, to conclusively answer the question as to the advantages of Caesarean section.

The current trend of a liberalised policy of Caesarean section of the very-low-birthweight delivery is questioned by a number of authors. Lamont et al (1980) recommend Caesarean section only in breech presentation. According to Kitchen et al (1982) the mode of delivery does not significantly affect the handicap rate in the survivors of infants born before 29 weeks gestation. Barrett et al (1983), studying the effect of the type of delivery on neonatal outcome in singleton infants of a birthweight of 1000 g or less, concluded that in terms of morbidity and mortality there is no difference between neonates delivered by Caesarean section compared with those delivered vaginally.

One aspect of morbidity in the very-low-birthweight neonate merits separate discussion: the intraventricular haemorrhage. While some authors, e.g. Mentzel (1984), find a higher incidence in vaginal deliveries as compared to Caesarean section deliveries, others do not. Wulf et al (1984) conclude from their study, based on a review of the literature and the results of their own department, and results of the Bayern Perinatal Survey, that also considering the frequency of intraventricular haemorrhage, under certain circumstances (i.e. no other risk factors than preterm birth), a conservative approach to the delivery of the very-low-birthweight infant is warranted.

All this further emphasises the need for a good randomised study, but with the numbers involved in each individual centre, it may be that such a study is not possible.

Multiple gestation

Given the high incidence of preterm births and breech presentations in multiple gestation, both of which are considered by many authors as contraindications for vaginal delivery, it is not surprising that the Caesarean section rate is increasing in these patients (Rydhstrom & Ohrlander, 1985). The benefits of such a policy have not been clearly demonstrated, at least when the fetuses weigh 1500 g or more.

A number of North American authors consider or even recommend vaginal delivery in some instances. Acker et al (1982) reviewed retrospectively all twin deliveries in their hospital over a 3-year period: the corrected neonatal mortality rate was 0 for 74 babies in non-vertex presentation delivered by Caesarean section and 0 for 76 second-born babies weighing more than 1499 g, presenting by the breech and extracted vaginally. They conclude that 'vaginal delivery may be considered when the second twin, weighing more than 1500 to 2000 gms is in breech presentation'.

Loucopoulos & Jewelewicz (1982) analysed the management and outcome of 35 pregnancies involving triplets, quadruplets, and quintuplets. For 101 newborn infants the mortality rate, corrected for gestations of more than 28 weeks, was 7·5 per cent, 'one of the lowest reported in the literature'. The mode of delivery, in their hands, does not seem to play any particular role in so far as outcome is concerned. It appears again, as we have already stated, that proper training in vaginal operative obstetrics is a prerequisite for the proper management of breech presentations and preterm deliveries.

REFERENCES

Acker D, Lieberman M, Holbrook R H, James O, Philippe M, Edelin K C 1982 Delivery of the second twin. Obstetrics and Gynecology 59: 710–711
Apeldoorn Z, Kantz Z, Lancet M et al. 1982 A new approach to the treatment of inco-

ordinated uterine activity. Abstr. no. 1344. Xth World Congress of Gynecology and Obstetrics, San Francisco

Ayromlooi J, Garfinkel R 1980 Impact of fetal scalp blood pH on the incidence of Caesarean section performed for fetal distress. International Journal of Obstetrics and Gynecology 17(4): 391–392

Barrett J M, Boehm F M, Vaughn W K 1983 Effect of type of delivery on neonatal outcome in singleton infants of birthweight of 1,000 g or less. Journal of the American Medical Association 250: 625–629.

Beck N C, Hall D 1978 Natural childbirth. Obstetrics and Gynecology 52: 371

Bergsjø P, Schmidt E, Pusch D 1983 Difference in the reported frequencies of some obstetrical intervention in Europe. British Journal of Obstetrics and Gynaecology 90: 628

Bottoms S F, Rosen M G, Sokol R J 1980 The increase in the Caesarean section birth rate. New England Journal of Medicine 302: 559

Bowes W A 1977 Results of the intensive perinatal managements of very low birth weight infants. In: Pre-term labour. Proceedings of the Fifth Study Group of the Royal College of Obstetricians and Gynaecologists, London

Boyd C, Francome C, Bartley D et al 1983 One birth in nine. Caesarean section trends since 1978. The Maternity Alliance, London

Brocks V, Philipsen T, Secher N J 1984 A randomised trial of external cephalic version with tocolysis in late pregnancy. British Journal of Obstetrics and Gynaecology 91(7): 653–656

Cardozo L D, Gibb D M F, Studd J W W et al 1983. Should we abandon Kielland's forceps? British Medical Journal 287: 315

Chabaud F, Chaperon J, Brunet J B 1983 La mortalite maternelle en France. Revue Française de Gynécologie et d'Obstétrique 78: 15–33

Chalmers I 1985 Trends and variations in the use of Caesarean section. In: Clinch J, Matthews T (eds) Perinatal medicine MTP Press, Lancaster, pp 145–149.

Chalmers I, Richards M 1977 Intervention and causal inference in obstetric practice. In: Chard T, Richards M (eds) Benefits and hazards of the new obstetrics. Clinics in developmental medicine No. 64, Heinemann Medical Books, London, p 34

Chandler C J, Parsons R J, Palmer A 1984 Fetal monitoring during labour. British Medical Journal 288: 67

Chard T, Richards M (eds) 1977 Benefits and hazards of the new obstetrics. Heinemann Medical Books, London

Cohen W K 1977 Influence of the duration of second stage labour in perinatal outcome and pueperal morbidity. Obstetrics and Gynecology 49: 266

Collea J V, Chein C, Quilligan E J 1980 The randomised study of term frank breech presentation: a study of 208 cases. American Journal of Obstetrics and Gynecology 137: 235

Cox C, Kendall A C, Hommers M 1982 Changed prognosis of breech—presenting low-birthweight infants. British Journal of Obstetrics and Gynaecology 89: 881

Craigin C J 1916 Conservatism in obstetrics. New York Medical Journal 104: 1

Crawford J S 1982 The effect of epidural block on the progress of labour. In: Studd J (ed). Progress in obstetrics and gynaecology, vol. II. Churchill Livingstone, Edinburgh, p 85

Crowley P, Hawkins D F 1980 Premature breech delivery— the Caesarean section debate. Journal of Obstetrics and Gynaecology 1: 2

De Jong P A, Stolte L A M 1982 The influence of spontaneous breech delivery on the integrity of the CNS of the newborn: a prospective study. European Journal of Obstetrics, Gynecology and Reproductive Biology 13: 23

Demianczuk N, Hunter J S, Taylor D W 1982 Trial of labour after previous Caesarean section. American Journal of Obstetrics and Gynecology 142: 640

Derom R 1986 Maternal mortality (Dutch). Tijdschrift voor Geneeskunde 42: 619

Derom R, de Leeuw J Ph, van Geijn H P, Thiery M et al. 1984 Breech presentation: comparative description of populations, obstetrical care and outcome in three university hospitals of Belgium and the Netherlands. In: van Geijn H P (ed). Perinatal monitoring. 3rd Progress Report, EEC Concerted Action Project No I.1.1, Amsterdam

Duenhoelter J, Wells C E, Reisch J S, Santos-Ramos R, Jiminez J M 1979 A paired controlled study of vaginal and abdominal delivery of the low birth weight breech fetus. Obstetrics and Gynaecology 54: 310–313

Duignan N M 1982 The management of breech presentation. In: Studd J (ed) Progress in obstetrics and gynaecology. Churchill Livingstone, London, p 73

Egliton G S, Phelen J P, Yeh S Y et al 1984 Outcome of a trial of labour after prior Caesarean delivery. Journal of Reproductive Medicine 29 : 3–8

Evaldson G R, Malmborg A S, Nord C E 1982 Premature rupture of the membranes and ascending infection. British Journal of Obstetrics and Gynaecology 89 : 793

Faber-Nijholt R, Huisjes H J, Touwen B C, Fidler V J 1983 Neurological follow-up of 281 children born in the breech presentation : a controlled study. British Medical Journal 286 : 9–12

Flynn A M, Kelly J, Hollins G, Lynch P F 1978 Ambulation in labour. British Medical Journal 2 : 519–593

Friedman E A 1981 The labour curve. Clinical Perinatology 8 : 15

Gleicher N 1984 Caesarean section rates in the United States. The short-term failure of the National Consensus Development Conference in 1980. Journal of the American Medical Association 252 : 3273

Goldenberg R L, Nelson K G 1977 The premature breech. American Journal of Obstetrics and Gynecology 127 : 240–244

Haesslein H C, Goodlin R C 1979 Delivery of the tiny newborn. American Journal of Obstetrics and Gynecology 134 : 192

Hall J E, Kohl S 1956 Breech presentation. American Journal of Obstetrics and Gynecology 72 : 977–988

Haverkamp A D, Orleans M, Langendoefer S, et al 1979 A controlled trial of the differential effects of intrapartum fetal monitoring. American Journal of Obstetrics and Gynecology 134 : 399–412

Henry M J, McColl D D F, Crawford J W, Patel N B 1979 Computing techniques for intrapartum physiological data reduction. II : Fetal heart rate. Journal of Perinatal Medicine 7 : 215–228

Hofmeyer G J 1983 Effect of external cephalic version in late pregnancy on breech presentation and Caesarean section rate : a controlled trial. British Journal of Obstetrics and Gynaecology 90(5) : 392–399

Horovitz J, Dubecq J P, Sassin J R et al 1982 Breech presentation : 'Bordelaise' methods and results. Abstr. No. 1356. Xth World Congress of Gynecology and Obstetrics, San Francisco

Ingemarsson I, Westgren M, Svenningsen N W 1978 Long-term follow-up of pre-term infants in breech presentation delivered by Caesarean section. Lancet ii : 172

Jackson P, Ridley W J, Stewart J G 1982 The role of antenatal therapy in breech deliveries. Abstr. No. 1348. Xth World Congress of Gynecology and Obstetrics, San Francisco

Jarrell M A, Ashmead G G, Mann L I 1985 Vaginal delivery after Caesarean section : a five-year study. Obstetrics and Gynecology 65 : 628

Karp E, Doney J R, McCarthy T et al 1979 The premature breech ; trial of labour or Caesarean section ? Obstetrics and Gynecology 55 : 88

Kauppila O, Gronroos M, Aro P et al 1981 Management of low-birth-weight breech deliveries : should Caesarean section be routine ? Obstetrics and Gynecology 57(3) : 289–294

Kitchen W H, Yu V, Orgill A et al 1982 Infants born before 29 weeks gestation : survival and morbidity at 2 years of age. British Journal of Obstetrics and Gynaecology 89 : 887

Klein L 1983 Fetal distress as an indication for Caesarean section. 1982 Proceedings Xth World Congress of Gynaecology and Obstetrics, San Francisco, pp 161–165

Kubli F, Boss W, Ruttgers H 1976 Caesarean section in the management of singleton breech presentation. In : Rooth G, Bratteby L E (eds) Perinatal medicine. Almqvist & Wiksell, Stockholm, pp 69–75

Lamont R F, Dunlop P D M, Crowley P, Elder M G 1980 Spontaneous preterm labour and delivery at under 34 weeks gestation. British Medical Journal 286 : 454–457

Lancet editorial 1984 External cephalic version. Lancet ii : 385

Loucopoulos A, Jewelewicz R 1982 Management of multifetal pregnancies : sixteen years experience at the Sloan Hospital for Women. American Journal of Obstetrics and Gynecology 143(8) : 902–905

Lundy L 1983 Caesarean section. In : Cohen W R, Friedman E A (eds) Management of labour, University Park Press, Baltimore, p 263

MacDonald D, Grant A, Pereira M et al. 1985 The Dublin randomised controlled trial of intrapartum electronic fetal heart rate monitoring. American Journal of Obstetrics and Gynecology 154 : 524–539

Mann L I, Gallant J M 1979 Modern management of the breech delivery. American Journal of Obstetrics and Gynecology 134: 611–614

Meier P R, Porreco R P 1982 Trial of labour following Caesarean section: a two-year experience. American Journal of Obstetrics and Gynecology 144: 671

Mentzel H 1984 Sectio bei Frühgeburt aus der Sicht des Neonatologen. Gynäkologe 17: 243–249

Merrill B S, Gibbs C E 1978 Planned vaginal delivery following Caesarean section. Obstetrics and Gynaecology 52: 50

Minkoff H, Schwarz R 1980 The rising Caesarean section rate: can it safely be reversed? Obstetrics and Gynaecology 56: 135

Neutra R R, Greenland S et al 1980 Effect of fetal monitoring on Caesarean section rate. Obstetrics and Gynaecology 55: 175

O'Driscoll K, Foley M 1983 Correlation of decrease in perinatal mortality and increase in Caesarean section rates. Obstetrics and Gynaecology 61: 1

O'Driscoll K, Meagher D 1980 Active management of labour. Saunders, London.

Pauerstein C J 1981 Labour after Caesarean section. Journal of Reproductive Medicine 26: 409

Peter J, Martaille A, Ronayette D et al 1982 Les indications de la Césarienne. A propos de 1000 cas. Revue Française de Gynécologie et d'Obstétrique 77: 175–182

Philpott K, Castle W M 1972 Cervicographs in the management of primigravida. Journal of Obstetrics and Gynaecology of the British Commonwealth 79: 592

Pillai M 1984 Fetal monitoring during labour. British Medical Journal 288: 67

Placek P J, Taffel S, Moien M 1983 Caesarean section delivery rates: USA 1981. American Journal of Public Health 73: 861

Pontonnier G, Grandjean H et al 1979 Intérêt de la mesure du pH sanguin dans la surveillance foetale pendant l'accouchement. Journal de Gynécologie, Obstétrique et Biologie de la Reproduction (Paris) 7(6): 1065

Prichard J A, MacDonald P C, Gant N F 1985 Dystocia caused by abnormalities in presentation, position or development of the fetus. In: Pritchard J A, MacDonald P C, Gant N F (eds), Williams' Obstetrics, 17th edn. Appleton-Century-Crofts, pp 651–659

Quilligan E J, Zuspan F P (eds) 1982 Douglas-Stromme operative obstetrics. Appleton-Century-Crofts, New York

Rosen M G 1980 Draft Report of the Task Force on Caesarean Childbirth. US Dept. of Health and Human Sciences

Rumeau-Rouquette C 1982 Naître en France. INSERM, Paris

Rydhstrom H, Ohrlander S 1985 Twin deliveries in Sweden 1973-81: the value of an increasing Caesarean section rate. Archives of Gynecology 237 (suppl.): 168

Saling E, Muller-Holve W 1975 Die Aussere Wendung des Feten aus Beckenendlage in Schädellage unter Tokolyse. Geburtshilfe und Frauenheilkunde 35: 149–154

Sawers R S 1983 Fetal monitoring during labour. British Medical Journal 287: 1649–1650

Schutte M F, van Hemel O J C, van de Berg C, van de Pol A 1985 Perinatal mortality in breech presentations as compared to vertex presentations in singleton pregnancies: an analysis based upon 57819 computer-registered pregnancies in the Netherlands. European Journal of Obstetrics, Gynecology and Reproductive Biology 19: 391–400

Smyth C N 1984 Fetal monitoring during labour. British Medical Journal 288: 67

Staudach A, Lassmann R 1982 Intrapartum fetal monitoring and Caesarean section rate. Abstr. No. 1360, Xth World Congress of Gynecology and Obstetrics, San Francisco

Studd J W W 1973 Partograms and nomograms in the management of primigravid labour. British Medical Journal 4: 451

Thatte A 1982 Role of early manual rotation in occipito posterior position. Abstr. no 1354. Xth World Congress of Gynaecology and Obstetrics, San Francisco

Thiery M 1981 Induction of labour (Dutch). Stafleu, Brussels

Thiery M, Derom R 1986 Review of evaluative studies on Caesarean section: medical aspects. Presented at the ECC Workshop on Evaluative Research in Pre-, Peri, and Postnatal Care Delivery Systems, 14–16 March (to be published)

Thiery M, Parewijck W, Martens G 1983 Management of gravidae with PROM and unfavourable pelvic score with IV infusion of PGE2 (Dutch). Tijdschrift voor Geneeskunde 39: 1453–1455

van Dorsten J P, Shifrin B S, Wallace R I 1981 Randomised control trial of external cephalic version with tocolysis in late pregnancy. American Journal of Obstetrics and Gynecology 141 : 417

van Geijn H P, Duisterhout J S, Derom R 1984 Study of intervention based upon cardiotocographic recording in a group of patients at high risk for fetal hypoxia. In : van Geijn H P (ed) Perinatal monitoring. Concerted Action Project. I.1.1. of the Third Research Programme in the Field of Medical and Public Health Research. 3rd Progress Report, Commission of the European Communities, Brussels

Westgren M, Ingemarsson I, Ahlstrom H et al 1982 Delivery and long-term outcome of very-low-birth-weight infants. Acta Obstetrica et Gynecologica Scandinavica 61(1) : 25–30

Westgren M, Dolfin T, Halperin M et al 1985 Mode of delivery in the low-birth-weight fetus. Delivery by Caesarean section independent of fetal lie versus vaginal delivery in vertex presentation. Acta Obstetrica et Gynecologica Scandinavica 64 : 51–57

Wigglesworth J S, Husemyer R P 1977 Intracranial birth trauma in vaginal breech delivery : the continued importance of injury to the occipital bone. British Journal of Obstetrics and Gynaecology 84 : 684–691

Woods J R 1979 Effects of low birth rate breech delivery on neonatal mortality. Obstetrics and Gynaecology 53 : 735

Wulf K H, Kastendieck E, Seelbach-Gobel B 1984 Zum Geburtsmodus bei Frühgeborenen—abdominal oder vaginal. Zeitschrift fur Geburtshilfe und Perinatologie 188 : 249–255

Zuspan F P, Quilligan E J, Iams J D, van Geijn H P 1979 Predictors of intrapartum fetal distress : the role of electronic fetal monitoring. American Journal of Obstetrics and Gynecology 135 : 287–291

Caesarean and postpartum hysterectomy

HISTORICAL INTRODUCTION

The operation of Caesarean hysterectomy was originally proposed in 1768 by Joseph Cavallini in Florence. Based on animal experiments he suggested that such an operation was not only possible but might well be advantageous to the mother (Durfee, 1969). However, a further century was to pass before Horatio Storer performed and documented the first sub-total Caesarean hysterectomy in 1869. The patient had obstructed labour due to a large pelvic tumour and operation was proposed initially to excise the tumour per abdomen and then to deliver the baby per vaginam. However, on opening the abdomen the fibrocystic tumour was found to be firmly attached to the uterus and pelvic walls so he proceeded to open the uterus and deliver the mature fetus. The subsequent haemorrhage was so great that in order to save the woman he decided to attempt to remove the uterus and tumour. This was achieved by ligating the cervix, excising the uterus, cauterising the stump and attaching a clamp so that the stump could be fixed to the abdominal wound. Unfortunately the woman died after 68 hours.

If she had survived, the operation would most likely have been named after him rather than Eduardo Porro from Pavia whose first case in 1876 was successful. His patient was a 25-year-old primiparous dwarf, appropriately named Julia Cavallini, of only 57 inches in height, with a grossly distorted pelvis due to rickets which had an anteroposterior inlet diameter estimated at $1\frac{9}{16}$ inches. The operation was a sub-total amputation similar to that described by Storer. Porro observed her personally for 24 hours, feeding her with champagne and laudanum. She survived a turbulent 40-day postoperative course. He published the details in 1876 in a famous memoir entitled 'Della amputazione utero-ovarica complemento di taglio caesareo'.

As might be expected the news of such an operation stimulated widespread interest and immediately other surgeons, such as Hegar in Germany, Muller in Switzerland and Tarnier in France, reported cases (Durfee, 1969) but most of the mothers died. In the United Kingdom Professor Lawson Tait of Birmingham became a particular pioneer. By 1890 he had performed seven operations, six of which were successful, using a modification of Porro's amputation technique, and for a time it became commonly known as the Porro–Tait operation. After opening the abdomen a piece of rubber drainage tube about 18 inches long and held as a loop between the fore and middle finger of the left hand was slipped over the uterus and pulled down around the cervix as far as possible. This was tightened by a single hitch and the tension maintained by an assistant providing efficient clamping. A small hole was then made in the uterus, enlarged by fingers and the baby delivered by breech extraction. After delivery of the placenta the uterus was pulled out of the wound and the rubber tubing ligature tightened once more around the cervix and a second hitch applied. Two needles of steel wire were then passed through the flattened rubber tubing, through the uterus and out the other side forming a St Anthony cross or two parallel bars, to support the weight of the uterus and the stump and to keep it outside the wound. Following peritoneal toilet the abdominal wound was closed around the uterus. The uterus was then excised close to the tubing and needles, and the stump sprinkled with a little perchloride of iron—the whole operation taking about 6 minutes.

Lawson Tait urged that this procedure be seriously considered by obstetricians of his time as the most logical and satisfactory method of dealing with the not infrequent problem of impacted labour for which the maternal and fetal mortality associated with the existing methods of management was appalling (Table 10.1). The alternative of Caesarean section had a prohibitively high mortality (90–95 per cent), mainly due to sepsis and haemorrhage. His proposed management would almost always produce a live baby, a maternal mortality of about 5 per cent and the further reassurance for the mother that the complication could not be repeated (Lawson Tait, 1890). Initially his ideas received considerable criticism but gradually the number of operations increased and in the meantime the procedure became very popular in North America.

The first total Caesarean hysterectomy was described by Spencer Wells in 1881 and was performed because of invasive cervical carcinoma (Durfee, 1969).

Following the introduction of uterine closure with sutures, aseptic surgical techniques and later blood replacement and antibiotic therapy, the

Table 10.1 Mortality of impacted labour in nineteenth-century England (Lawson Tait, 1890) (percentages)

	Maternal	Fetal
Destructive procedures	20	100
Long forceps	15	14
Internal version	15	25–30
Induction premature labour	15	
Caesarean section	90–95	
Caesarean section with amputation of uterus	5–6	

indications for hysterectomy gradually diminished while the mortality and morbidity improved.

INDICATIONS FOR HYSTERECTOMY

In this century emergency hysterectomy in obstetric practice has become a relatively infrequent procedure (Table 10.2) with the indications still being mainly those where the life of the mother is threatened by uncontrollable haemorrhage. In addition elective Caesarean hysterectomy has been more widely practised as a means of sterilisation (Britton, 1980) and for those with coexisting ovarian or cervical malignancy. In many series from North America in particular rates of elective hysterectomy as high as 1 in 244 deliveries have been reported (Barclay, 1969). Much lower rates of 1 in 6509 and 1 in 5798 deliveries have been found in Australia and England (Hill & Beischer, 1980; Sturdee & Rushton, 1986) where, in the absence of life-threatening disease, opinion favours postponing hysterectomy until after the puerperium when the procedure is less hazardous.

Haemorrhage

Uncontrollable haemorrhage is the most common indication for emergency hysterectomy either at the time of Caesarean section or following a vaginal delivery (Table 10.3) and in most cases the bleeding will be from the placental site. Abruptio placentae with a Couvelaire uterus was the single most common indication in 96 of 200 cases reported by Barclay (1969) with ruptured uterus in 45, placenta praevia in 15 and placenta accreta in 3, whereas Sturdee & Rushton (1986) found a morbidly adherent placenta (MAP) was the cause of persistent haemorrhage in 16 of 35 cases and 8 of these were also placenta praevia (see below).

Other occasional causes of persistent haemorrhage include uterine atony, coagulopathy and uterine infection, some of which may present as secondary

Table 10.2   Series of emergency and elective Caesarean or postpartum hysterectomies with percentage of all deliveries and total and incidence of all Caesarean sections

Authors	Country	Emergency (%)		Elective (%)		Total deliveries	Total Caesarean sections (%)
Barclay (1969)	U.S.A.	200	(0·1)	800	(0·51)	195 512	6609 (3·4)
Patterson (1970)	U.S.A.	16	(0·02)	311	(0·34)	92 691	3368 (3·6)
Haynes & Martin (1979)	U.S.A.	26	(0·04)	123	(0·19)	63 259	2417 (3·8)
Hill & Beischer (1980)	Australia	25[1]	(0·07)	5	(0·02)	35 506	— (11·8)
Rachagan & Sivanesaratnam (1984)	Malaysia	21	(0·05)	—		45 045	3230 (7·19)
Sturdee & Rushton (1986)	U.K.	35	(0·05)	12	(0·02)	69 576	7937 (11·4)

[1] Excluding four cases of hysterectomy for trophoblastic disease in original publication.

Table 10.3 Clinical indications for emergency hysterectomy. Reproduced from Sturdee & Rushton (1986) by permission from the Editor, British Journal of Obstetrics and Gynaecology

	At or after Caesarean section	Following vaginal delivery
Primary haemorrhage	16	3
Secondary haemorrhage	3	3
Ruptured uterus		4
Lacerated cervix/vagina		2
Adherent placenta	3	
Retained placenta		1
Total	22	13

postpartum haemorrhage (PPH) many days after delivery (Sturdee & Rushton, 1986). Hill & Beischer (1980) found that 1 in 19 deliveries were followed by PPH and 1 in 219 of these required hysterectomy.

Rupture of uterus

Traumatic rupture of the lower uterine segment in labour may result from injudicious use of obstetric forceps, intra-uterine manipulation, attempted manual removal of a retained placenta or from unrecognised obstructed labour. In addition the scarred uterus is more vulnerable and rupture of a lower segment Caesarean section scar is reported to occur in 0·8–1·2 per cent of subsequent labours and vaginal deliveries, whereas the risk following classical Caesarean section is 8·9 per cent (Dewhurst, 1957). Ruptured uterus has been a common indication in some series, representing 22·5–38 per cent of emergency hysterectomies with an incidence of 1 in 4350–5900 of all deliveries (Barclay, 1969; Hill & Beischer, 1980; Rachagan & Sivaneseratnam, 1984). However, in our experience the incidence has been much lower at 11·4 per cent of emergency hysterectomies and 1 in 17 390 deliveries. There were four cases—one traumatic rupture, two lower segment and one classical Caesarean scar ruptures (Sturdee & Rushton, 1986). These differences may be due to many factors, but with modern policies of active management of labour, early recognition of obstruction and the avoidance of 'difficult forceps deliveries' or intra-uterine manipulations, this potentially fatal complication of labour should be rare.

OPERATIVE TECHNIQUE

Preliminary transfusion and resuscitation may often be necessary but undue delay in operating can also exacerbate the problem and increase the risk of a coagulation disorder. Furthermore in cases of uterine rupture and with a shocked patient it may be safer to attempt closure of the defect, perhaps accompanied by sterilisation rather than hysterectomy. At the time of Caesarean hysterectomy the tissues of the pelvis are very lax, highly vascularised and oedematous, especially after labour, and the ovarian and uterine vessels may be dilated up to six times their normal calibre (Park & Duff, 1980). Modification of the usual technique for abdominal hysterectomy is therefore necessary and special care is required in the clamping and ligation of each pedicle. In addition the increased vascularity and collateral circulations around the uterus result in more extensive 'back-bleeding' which can be limited by securing the uterine side of each pedicle as well.

For a Caesarean hysterectomy a vertical uterine incision may be quicker and more appropriate than a transverse, but either should be closed or adequately clamped prior to proceeding to hysterectomy. A major portion of operative blood loss can come from an atonic uterus for which intravenous oxytocic agents and uterine massage is helpful.

The most common surgical complication after haemorrhage and infection is injury to the bladder. Many patients will have had a previous Caesarean section causing adhesions of the bladder to the lower uterine segment, so that mobilisation of the bladder may be difficult. Injudicious pressure with a swab can easily result in a tear of the bladder wall that may not be recognised, especially in the presence of haemorrhage. However, when a bladder injury is identified at operation, repaired properly and the bladder drained post-operatively for 8–10 days, fistula formation is rare (Park & Duff, 1980). A sharp dissection technique using scissors to free the bladder is therefore recommended, keeping in the mid-line as far as possible so as to avoid the highly vascular bladder pillars. Initial dissection should be just far enough to allow safe ligation of the uterine arteries and veins, and further dissection, which can cause severe venous oozing, should be delayed until required to allow the ureters to fall away laterally prior to securing the transverse cervical ligaments and vaginal angles. The broad vaginal vault and cervix add to the risk of ureteric injury during the final stages of hysterectomy, thus identification of the ureters in the base of the broad ligament and palpation below the uterine vessels up to the bladder is particularly advisable. When there has been uterine rupture or extension of the Caesarean incision laterally to involve the uterine vessels the ureters may be difficult to visualise so that palpation is essential. However, in such circumstances the risk of bladder or ureteric injury is so much greater (Hayes & Martin, 1979; Mickal et al, 1969) that ligation of the internal iliac artery, which can control the haemorrhage, may be preferable to hysterectomy (Park & Duff, 1980; Pelosi et al, 1975).

In contrast to Porro's operation, opinion now favours a total hysterectomy where practicable, but identification of the lower margin of the cervix can be a limiting factor, especially when labour has resulted in effacement and dilatation of the cervix. For inexperienced surgeons a sub-total hysterectomy may therefore be the safest option, though the potential problems of a residual cervical stump must be appreciated. In practice many an intended total hysterectomy has subsequently been found not to be so because of failure to identify the cervix satisfactorily. Exploration of the cervical canal by a finger passed down through the uterine incision from above may help to identify the margin of the cervix and also avoid more extensive dissection of the bladder than is necessary from the very vascular vagina (Plauché et al, 1981).

In cases with infection, inadequate haemostasis or extensive haematoma formation the insertion of a corrugated drain for 12 hours may be advisable (Harley, 1980) and some would also advocate leaving the vagina open in the mid-line for this purpose (Myerscough, 1977).

The additional removal of either or both appendages may be appropriate in suspected malignant disease, and for carcinoma of the cervix a Wertheim Caesarean hysterectomy can be surprisingly easy because of the mobility of the tissues.

COMPLICATIONS

Intra-operative complications are reported to be about four times more common in emergency than elective cases (Plauché et al, 1981). The main complications are those related to haemorrhage, especially when there is extension of a uterine rupture or Caesarean incision into the uterine vessels with formation of a broad ligament haematoma. Determination of the volume of blood lost in obstetric procedures is notoriously difficult and is usually underestimated. In the report of the Confidential Enquiry into Maternal Deaths 1976–78 (DHSS, 1982) the number of deaths due to postpartum haemorrhage (26) and uterine rupture (14) increased from 10·9 to 14·9 per million maternities respectively. Among avoidable factors identified were underestimation of the total blood loss, inadequate transfusion and delay in performing life-saving surgery. Most emergency hysterectomies will require transfusion for the initial indication but the operation itself is inevitably accompanied by further haemorrhage. Many elective procedures will also require transfusion (Table 10.4). Reported transfusion rates in any series of Caesarean hysterectomies will depend on the proportion of elective to emergency cases and vary from 19 to 100 per cent (Park & Duff, 1980).

Urinary tract injuries occur more frequently than with either Caesarean section or total abdominal hysterectomy alone, and the rate of bladder injury is directly proportional to the number of previous caesarean sections (Park & Duff, 1980). Some other complications are shown in Table 10.5.

Table 10.4 Blood loss associated with hysterectomy assessed by total units of whole blood transfused. Reproduced from Sturdee & Rushton (1986) by permission from the Editor, British Journal of Obstetrics and Gynaecology

	No. transfused	Mean no. units	Range
Elective cases ($n=12$)	11	2·4	1–4
Emergency cases ($n=35$)	33	9·9	2–33

Table 10.5 Complications of caesarean hysterectomy compiled from 18 reported series from 1933–1977 (adapted from Park & Duff, 1980)

Complications in 3913 cases	No.	Percentage
Maternal death[1]	28	0·71
Bladder injury	118	3
Vesicovaginal fistula	18	0·4
Ureteric injury	10	0·25
Ureterovaginal fistula	4	0·1
Wound infection	126	3·2
Re-operation for intraperitoneal haemorrhage	35	0·97
Blood transfusion		19–100

[1] Includes cases of leukaemia and breast carcinoma.

A maternal death rate of 0·7 per cent has been reported in two large series (Mickal et al, 1969; Park & Duff, 1980) and of 1·3 per cent by Barclay (1969), but some of these include deaths from malignant disease and were also performed before modern transfusion facilities became available. More recent figures suggest a lower mortality with only one death (0·28 per cent) due to a pulmonary embolism reported from a combined total of 359 cases (Haynes & Martin, 1979; Hill & Beischer, 1980; Plauché et al, 1981; Rachagan & Sivanesaratnam, 1984; Sturdee & Rushton, 1986).

Rupture of the uterus may precipitate a rapid and massive internal haemorrhage, and the diagnosis may not become apparent until after cardiovascular collapse. Such cases will be associated with a higher maternal mortality rate and in one series of 64 patients there were six deaths (9·4 per cent) (Paydar & Hassanzadeh, 1978).

PATHOLOGY

Since haemorrhage may occur from relatively minor lesions or abnormalities of the postparum uterus careful pathological examination of hysterectomy specimens is essential. Even after thorough examination there will be no identifiable lesion in a significant proportion of cases.

In the authors' experience the initial examination of the uterus and adnexa is best performed on the fresh unfixed specimen. The lack of muscle tone allows the cavity to be opened and the lining of the uterus to be completely displayed. The examination should include careful inspection of any surgical incisions and the broad ligaments for torn or exposed blood vessels. The normal postpartum uterine lining is relatively smooth with little clot attached. Any loosely attached blood can be removed by a stream of cold water prior to detailed examination. The lining should be searched for protruding blood vessels (Fig. 10.1). Remnants of the placenta and decidua are usually readily identified. Suspicious vessels, attached placental remnants and decidua should be examined histologically in a block which includes the underlying myometrium. Tissue should also be sampled from the parametrium, to include uterine veins, since sublethal amniotic fluid embolism may

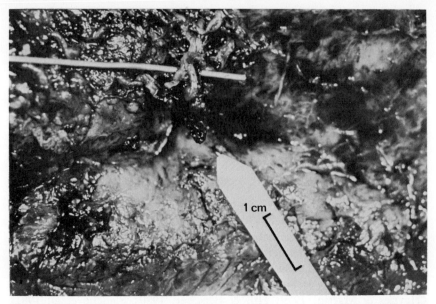

Fig. 10.1   Placental bed—an abnormal vessel forming a loop (over probe) with a bleeding point (at tip of arrow) with clot attached. In spite of a D and C, hysterectomy was required to control bleeding (× 1·5).

be confirmed by the demonstration of the constituents of amniotic fluid within the lumen of these vessels (Fig. 10.2).

The underlying pathology leading to emergency postpartum hysterectomy can be broadly classified into four categories:

1. abnormalities of placentation,
2. pre-existing uterine pathology,
3. cervical or uterine trauma,
4. disorders of haemostasis.

Abnormalities of placentation

The most common abnormality of placentation associated with life threatening haemorrhage after delivery is the morbidly adherent placenta (MAP). This may be subclassified into three clinical variants, placenta accreta (Fig. 10.3), placenta increta (Fig. 10.4) and placenta percreta, depending on the depth of penetration of the uterine wall. However, while these terms may be of some clinical value the underlying pathology is the same, being related to a failure of normal decidualisation in the placental bed either as the result of a primary or secondary deficiency in the endometrium.

The incidence of MAP reported in the literature is extremely variable (Fox, 1978) but our own experience (Sturdee & Rushton, 1986) and that of

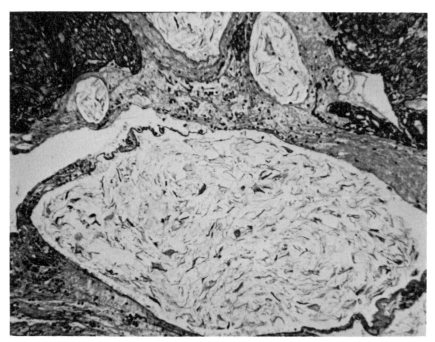

Fig. 10.2 Uterine veins containing amniotic squames. Following a transient hypotensive episode in labour massive postpartum haemorrhage necessitated hysterectomy (HVG × 112).

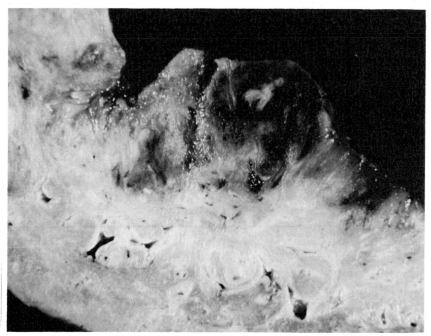

Fig. 10.3 Placenta accreta. Nodules of placental tissue interdigitating with the underlying myometrium (× 1·9).

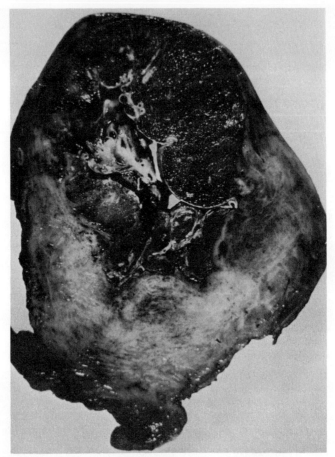

Fig. 10.4   Placenta increta. The placenta has produced eccentric thinning of the myometrium. At the top of the photograph there is almost complete penetration of the uterine fundus (× 1·1).

Hill & Beischer (1980) is consistent with an incidence of about 1 in 4500 pregnancies. This figure is inevitably an underestimate since minor degrees may go undetected or require only simple curettage. It is very uncommon in the primigravid patient, but in the multipara there have been several reports of an association with previous Caesarean section (Breen et al, 1977; Read et al, 1980), dilatation and curettage (Millar, 1959; Fox, 1972), Asherman's syndrome (Georgakopoulos, 1974; Cario et al, 1983) and manual removal of the placenta (Millar, 1959). The incidence would seem to reflect contemporary obstetric and gynaecological practice since there has been a considerable change in the frequency of associated pathology in recent years. Thus Fox (1972) found MAP was associated with placenta praevia in less than a third of cases, while in our series placenta praevia was present in half the cases (Fig. 10.5). There was twice the incidence of

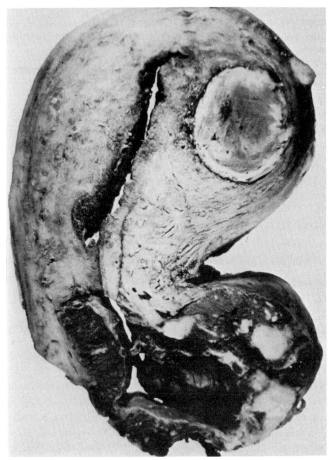

Fig. 10.5 Grade IV placenta praevia and placenta percreta. There is a degenerate fibroid in the myometrium. There are several pale infarcts in the placenta (× 1·1).

Caesarean section in an earlier pregnancy in our own series, and almost one-third of the cases had had a previous termination of pregnancy, an unlisted precursor in Fox's (1972) review. An association with previous termination of pregnancy is not surprising, and with the increasing number of terminations and the rising Caesarean section rate MAP may become more common. Only two of the 16 cases of MAP reported by Sturdee & Rushton (1986) had no history of instrumental or operative procedures involving the uterus, and several had a history of multiple procedures (Table 10.6). Our own experience suggests that a combination of a previous lower segment caesarean section scar and an anterior placenta praevia were particular risk factors. Placenta percreta (Fig. 10.6), the most severe form of MAP where the placental tissue penetrates the full thickness of the uterine wall, may be associated with uterine rupture, sometimes in early pregnancy (Hassim et al, 1968; Hornstein et al, 1984; Bevan et al, 1985; Bezdek, 1985).

Table 10.6 Morbidly adherent placentae and association of previous uterine surgery or instrumentation (emergency hysterectomies). Reproduced from Sturdee & Rushton (1986) by permission from the Editor, British Journal of Obstetrics and Gynaecology

Previous surgery					Placenta praevia (index pregnancy)	Type
CS	T	ID	MR	O		
1					+	accreta
1						increta
	1				+	accreta
1				1[1]	+	accreta
2		1			+	percreta
2	2				+	percreta
2	2					accreta
	1			1[2]		accreta
		1	1			increta
			2		+	increta
		1		1[2]		accreta
	1					accreta
					+	percreta
				2[2]		increta
						increta
						accreta

CS = Caesarean section; T = termination; ID = instrumental delivery; MR = manual removal of placenta; O = other.
[1] Repair of uterovesical fistula.
[2] Dilatation and curettage.

The diagnosis of MAP depends on the histological demonstration of the direct abuttment of villous tissue on uterine connective tissue or myometrium in the absence of intervening decidua. The finding of villi within uterine venous channels does not indicate MAP.

The process of placentation results in profound modification of the structure of the uterine spiral arteries with destruction of both the elastic and muscular components of the vessel walls (Brosens et al, 1967). The affected portions of these vessels are necessarily incapable of contraction either as the result of neural or humoral stimuli, and rarely such vascular remnants in the placental bed may be the source of torrential haemorrhage.

Pre-existing uterine pathology

Anatomical abnormalities of the uterus, uterine fibroids, vascular lesions and previous uterine surgery may all be associated with postpartum haemorrhage necessitating hysterectomy. The pathology is usually obvious though the mechanisms resulting in the haemorrhage are not always evident since many patients with apparently similar pathology may have uneventful pregnancies. It should therefore not be assumed that the demonstration of fibroids or a malformed uterus is the cause of the haemorrhage and other causes of haemorrhage should be sought and excluded whenever possible.

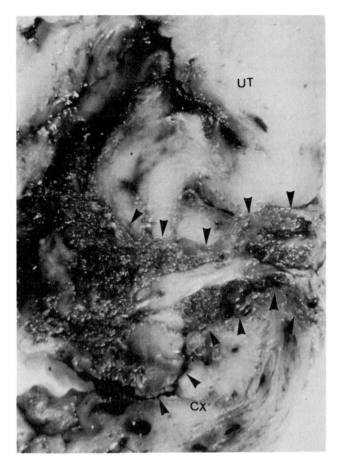

Fig. 10.6   Placenta percreta. Tongue of placenta (between arrows) extending through the site of a previous Caesarean section scar to invade the bladder wall. CX = cervix; UT = uterus (× 3).

Uterine and cervical trauma

The clinical history usually provides evidence of the traumatic nature of haemorrhage. From the pathological viewpoint it is frequently impossible to determine the site of major haemorrhage. Indeed the problems encountered by the surgeon in removal of the ruptured uterus may necessitate further uterine trauma and obscure the original lesion.

Disorders of haemostasis

These may be generalised, as in patients with known disorders of haemostasis, patients on anticoagulants and those with defibrination associated with complications of pregnancy such as missed abortion, amniotic fluid embolism and rarely fulminating pre-eclampsia. In many instances examination of the uterus by the pathologist is unrewarding, though evidence of missed abortion or histological lesions associated with pre-eclampsia may be demonstrated. Large amniotic fluid infusions may result in rapid and fatal defibrination, but smaller infusions may be clinically unsuspected until the surgically removed uterus is examined histologically. Evidence of infusion should be sought in all uteri removed as the result of haemorrhage associated with unexplained maternal defibrination.

Localised disorders of haemostasis may be the result of vascular adaptive changes (see above) or be due to local uterine pathology. It should not be forgotten that infection of the uterine cavity may result in haemorrhage and may be an occasional indication for emergency hysterectomy.

CONCLUSIONS

In current obstetric practice hysterectomy should be a rare event, and because few obstetricians will have much individual experience of the procedure it is advisable for all to be familiar with the factors that may precipitate the need for such life-saving surgery. Early involvement of experienced medical staff in high-risk cases should minimise the morbidity and mortality from shock and haemorrhage, and the operative complications of an often technically demanding procedure.

The association between previous uterine surgery and morbid adherence of the placenta may become more important with the rising incidences of termination and Caesarean sections.

A thorough histological examination of the uterus and placenta is important and will sometimes identify a previously unrecognised cause for the clinical events.

Elective Caesarean hysterectomy may be indicated for co-existing gynaecological disease but for sterilisation alone operation after the puerperium is safer.

REFERENCES

Barclay D L 1969 Cesarean hysterectomy at the Charity Hospital in New Orleans—1000 consecutive operations. Clinics in Obstetrics and Gynecology 12:635–651

Bevan J R, Marley N J E, Ozumba E N 1985 Uterine rupture, placenta percreta and curettage in early pregnancy. A case report. British Journal of Obstetrics and Gynaecology 92:642–644

Bezdek J 1985 Placenta percreta causing uterine rupture. Case report. British Journal of Obstetrics and Gynaecology 92:853–855

Breen J L, Neubecker R, Gregori C A, Franklin J E 1977 Placenta accreta, increta and percreta. A survey of 40 cases. Obstetrics and Gynaecology 49:43–47

Britton J J 1980 Sterilization by cesarean hysterectomy. American Journal of Obstetrics and Gynecology 137:887–890

Brosens I, Robertson W B, Dixon H G 1967 The physiological response of vessels of the placental bed to normal pregnancy. Journal of Pathology and Bacteriology 93:569–579

Cario G M, Adler A D, Morris N 1983 Placenta percreta presenting as intra-abdominal antepartum haemorrhage. Case report. British Journal of Obstetrics and Gynaecology 90:491–493

Dewhurst C J 1957 The ruptured caesarean section scar. Journal of Obstetrics and Gynaecology of the British Commonwealth 64:113–118

DHSS 1982 Report on confidential enquiries into maternal deaths in England and Wales 1976–1978. Report on Health and Social Subjects 26. Her Majesty's Stationery Office, London.

Durfee R B 1969 Evolution of cesarean hysterectomy. Clinics in Obstetrics and Gynecology 12:575–589

Fox H 1972 Placenta accreta 1945–1969. A review. Obstetrical and Gynecological Survey 27:475–490

Fox H (ed) 1978 Pathology of the placenta, vol 7: Major problems in pathology. W B Saunders Co, London, pp 64–69

Georgakopoulos P 1974 Placenta accreta following lysis of uterine synechiae (Asherman's syndrome). Journal of Obstetrics and Gynaecology of the British Commonwealth 81:730–733

Harley J M G 1980 Caesarean section. Clinics in Obstetrics and Gynaecology 7:529–559

Hassim A M, Lucas C, Elkabbani S A M 1968 Spontaneous uterine rupture caused by placenta percreta. British Medical Journal ii:97–98

Haynes D M, Martin B J Jr 1979 Cesarean hysterectomy: a twenty five year review. American Journal of Obstetrics and Gynecology 134:393–398

Hill D J, Beischer N A 1980 Hysterectomy in obstetric practice. Australian and New Zealand Journal of Obstetrics and Gynaecology 20:151–153

Hornstein M D, Niloff J M, Snyder P F, Frigoletto F D 1984 Placenta percreta associated with a second trimester pregnancy termination. American Journal of Obstetrics and Gynecology 150:1002–1003

Lawson-Tait J 1890 An address on the surgical aspect of impacted labour. British Medical Journal i:657–661

Mickal A, Begneaud W P, Hawes T P 1969 Pitfalls and complications of cesarean hysterectomy. Clinics in Obstetrics and Gynecology 3:660–675

Millar W G 1959 A clinical and pathological study of placenta accreta. Journal of Obstetrics and Gynaecology of the British Empire 66:353–364

Myerscough P R (ed) 1977 Munro Kerr's operative obstetrics, 9th edn. Baillière Tindall, London, p 547

Park R C, Duff W P 1980 Role of cesarean hysterectomy in modern obstetric practice. Clinics in Obstetrics and Gynecology 23:601–620

Patterson S P 1970 Cesarean hysterectomy. American Journal of Obstetrics and Gynecology 107:729–736

Paydar M, Hassanzadeh A 1978 Rupture of the uterus. International Journal of Gynaecology and Obstetrics 15:405–409

Pelosi M, Langer A, Hung C 1975 Prophylactic internal iliac artery ligation at cesarean hysterectomy. American Journal of Obstetrics and Gynecology 121:394–398

Plauché W C, Gruich F G, Bourgeois M O 1981 Hysterectomy at the time of cesarean section: analysis of 108 cases. Obstetrics and Gynecology 58:459–464

Rachagan S P, Sivanesaratnam V 1984 Caesarean hysterectomy—a review of 21 cases in the University Hospital, Kuala Lumpur. European Journal of Obstetrics, Gynaecology and Reproductive Biology 16:321–326

Read J A, Cotton D B, Miller F C 1980 Placenta accreta: changing clinical aspects and outcome. Obstetrics and Gynecology 56:31–34

Sturdee D W, Rushton D I 1986 Caesarean and postpartum hysterectomy 1968–1983. British Journal of Obstetrics and Gynaecology 93:270–274

Destructive operations

INTRODUCTION

When there is mechanical difficulty during labour, but the fetus is alive, the safest way to deliver the fetus is by Caesarean section. If labour has been prolonged and neglected and the fetus is dead, other considerations may come into play regarding the mode of delivery:

1. Sufficiently skilled staff to carry out Caesarean section at short notice, and in this sometimes difficult situation, may not be available.
2. The risk of overwhelming infection following Caesarean section in patients who invariably already have genital infection.
3. Obsession with having a vaginal delivery may make the patient or her relations refuse consent for abdominal delivery.
4. The patient may not have access to skilled supervision in her subsequent pregnancy or may choose not to avail herself of such skilled help because of (3) above.

In developed countries with high literacy rates, availability of a wide range of antibiotics, large numbers of skilled personnel and good communications, the circumstances summarised above no longer exist. It is, however, not far-fetched to envisage a situation in developed countries where a patient may choose to have a vaginal delivery when her attendants have advised abdominal delivery. In most developing countries there is a shortage of manpower, while health facilities and communication are poor. In Nigeria, for instance, a country with an estimated population of 90 million, a population growth rate of 3 per cent, there is a 70 per cent illiteracy rate, 80 per cent of the people live in the rural area, while only 25 per cent of births are supervised or attended by medical or nursing personnel. It is also not unusual for pregnant women to have to travel several hundred kilometres to hospital (Harrison, 1980). The evidence from most other developing countries is that Nigeria's experience is not unique (Brown, 1985). In view of this, it is obvious that most if not all of the considerations listed (1–4) apply in many developing countries. If this is so, the need to have an alternative method to Caesarean section for delivering the dead fetus, the result of neglected labour, exists even in the 1980s.

ASSESSMENT OF THE PATIENT WITH OBSTRUCTED LABOUR

In deciding whether to perform a destructive operation or a Caesarean section to deliver a dead fetus, it is important to be aware of the conditions that have led to fetal demise. Fetal death in these circumstances is caused by a combination of the following factors:

1. Interference with placental exchange by strong and continuous uterine contractions. The fetus will be even more susceptible where it is postmature.
2. Excessive moulding of the fetal head, in cephalic presentation, leading to intracranial bleeding. In breech presentation the unmoulded head may be trapped by an incompletely dilated cervix or may fail to enter the pelvis because of feto-pelvic disproportion.
3. Prolapse of the cord in shoulder and compound presentation.
4. Ascending genital infection, amnionitis and severe intra-uterine infection, the inevitable complication of prolonged labour and ruptured membranes in these cases.
5. Rupture of the uterus.

Assessment of the patient should detect the presence of dehydration and ketosis, evidence of infection, the relationship of the fetus to the pelvis, the presence of uterine rupture.

Most of the patients will have been in labour for 2 or more days in the rural area, although in some cases they will have been in labour in places not supervised by doctors or nurses, such as a herbal home or spiritualist church in the urban centres. Depending on the duration of the labour the patient may be anxious, dehydrated, ketotic, febrile and have tachycardia or may look quiet, exhausted and have laboured respiration. In some cases she may have been given various local concoctions to ingest in an attempt to expedite delivery while her perineum, vagina, cervix, urethra and bladder may have been severely lacerated by her untrained birth attendants. On abdominal and pelvic examination a variable amount of the fetal head will be palpable above the pelvic brim in a cephalic presenting fetus. There will be no fetal heart rate heard. The presenting part is usually jammed in the pelvis and the vulva and cervix may be oedemateous. The vagina is dry and warm and the liquor, when it is still present, is often foul-smelling from intra-uterine infection. The bladder may be distended with retained urine or thick or oedematous from compression, and may contain little urine. It may be necessary to displace the presenting part before a catheter can be passed.

The abdomen must be examined carefully to detect the presence of haemoperitoneum from ruptured uterus, as well as distended bowel from sepsis and ileus. The relationship of the fetus to the pelvis must be carefully assessed. By combining abdominal examination with a pelvic examination the amount of the fetal head palpable above the pelvic brim can be determined. In many of these patients it will be found that though a large caput succedaneum is visible at the introitus, there is still three-fifths or more of the fetal head palpable above the pelvic brim. The caput succedaneum and excessive moulding impede correct diagnosis of the position of the fetal head. In some cases the tamponade effect of an impacted head prevents bleeding per vaginam in cases of ruptured uterus. If the head is dislodged on vaginal examination, bleeding becomes obvious. Where there is rupture of the uterus, a destructive operation is contraindicated and laparotomy is mandatory.

PREOPERATIVE RESUSCITATION OF THE PATIENT

The patient is shaved, scrubbed and washed very quickly, and blood is sent for grouping and crossmatching of at least two units of blood. The haemoglobin, urea and electrolytes are tested, and also the blood-gases are studied if there is the facility to do this. An intravenous infusion is set up to correct dehydration, electrolyte deficiency and acidosis. One or two litres of 5 or 10 per cent dextrose alternating with dextrose/saline may be given rapidly, depending on the degree of dehydration, with 5 ml of buscopan (hyoscine-N-butylbromide 20 mg/ml) and 10 ml of calcium gluconate. A plasmolyte solution that contains sodium bicarbonate may be given separately. If a urinary catheter has not already been passed, this should be done, and an accurate record maintained. A urine sample should be examined by light microscopy for evidence of infection while a sample is obtained for culture and sensitivity. Parenteral ampicillin, and metronidazole with kanamycin, if available, are given. The combination is ideal but many hospitals cannot afford it and rely instead on intramuscular penicillin and streptomycin. Another alternative is ampicillin, gentamycin and metronidazole. A simple CVP manometer is set up if there is evidence of shock, and a CVP reading of between 5 and 8 cm of water is maintained. Having ruled out rupture of uterus the shock may be either hypovolaemic shock (corrected by fluids and blood transfusion) or septicaemic shock (treated with steroids and broad-spectrum antibiotics) or both. The blood pressure, pulse, CVP, temperature and urinary output must be charted frequently during the management. A Ryle's tube is passed to empty the stomach and magnesium trisilicate is poured in via the Ryle's tube and intramuscular atropine is given at the same time. It is sometimes necessary to continue to aspirate and inject the solution of magnesium trisilicate until the stomach content becomes clear, i.e. until all the green native medicine ingested has been removed. Philpott (1980) suggested a non-particulate oral antacid followed by cimetidine, metaclopramide and glycopyrrolate as ideal. These drugs reduce the acidity of gastric juice, empty the stomach downwards and reduce the production of gastric acid. Because they are expensive they may not be readily available in many centres in developing countries. In such circumstances magnesium trisilicate may be used alone as the antacid.

DESTRUCTIVE OPERATIONS

The incidence of destructive operations is a reflection of the standard of obstetric care in the community. If labour is properly supervised the need for destructive operation is rare. Destructive operations make up between 0·2 and 0·3 per cent of deliveries at Lagos University Teaching Hospital. At the University College Hospital, Ibadan, its incidence has varied from 1·65 per cent of deliveries (Aimakhu, 1975) to 0·48 per cent of deliveries more recently (Otolorin & Adelusi, 1981). In Zaria, Northern Nigeria, its incidence was 1·4 per cent of deliveries (Harrison, 1980). A lowering of the incidence of destructive operations may result from proliferation of maternity clinics and private hospitals in the areas served by each hospital and a greater diffusion of obstetric knowledge.

Before a destructive operation is performed it must be confirmed that the fetus is dead. The operator must be competent to do the procedure required, otherwise the patient will be safer having a Caesarean section or being transferred to a larger unit with more experienced staff and better facilities. Ruptured uterus must be excluded and resuscitation as previously described must be in progress. General anaesthesia, or regional anaesthesia combined with sedation with diazepam, is ideal for the procedure. Where these forms of anaesthesia are not available, or are unsuitable because of the state of the patient, an intravenous injection of 100 mg pethidine and 10 mg diazepam or a cocktail of pethidine, chlorpromazine and promethazine will provide sufficient analgesia and relaxation. Destructive operations are most safely performed at full dilatation of the cervix, although they may be performed by an experienced operator when the cervix is 7 cm or more dilated. Where there is hydrocephaly it is best to drain the cerebrospinal fluid before full dilatation because the uterus can rupture while the operator awaits full cervical dilatation. Craniotomy is the most commonly performed destructive operation (Lister, 1960; Otolorin & Adelusi, 1981). Table 11.1 summarises details of destructive operations performed at Lagos University Teaching Hospital between January 1970 and the end of December 1978.

Craniotomy

Craniotomy is indicated for the delivery of a dead fetus when labour is neglected and obstructed in a cephalic presentation. Usually the head has become impacted in the pelvic brim. If the head is more than three-fifths palpable above the pelvic brim, or if it is mobile, craniotomy may be difficult and dangerous and it is wiser to deliver the baby by Caesarean section. Old-fashioned crushing instruments such as the cephalotribe and cranioclast are now obsolete.

Of the various methods of craniotomy that have been described, the one by John St George (1975) is both simple and safe, and would appear to be suitable in virtually all situations where craniotomy is indicated for a cephalic

Table 11.1   Destructive operations at Lagos University Teaching
Hospital, January 1970 to December 1978

	No.	Percentage
Number of destructive operations	35	100
Craniotomy	20	57
Perforation of after-coming head	6	17·1
Decapitation	3	8·6
Cleidotomy	2	5·7
Craniotomy and cleidotomy	2	5·7
Embryotomy	1	2·9
Breech extraction and cleidotomy	1	2·9

presentation. For this operation the craniotomy trolley consists mainly of
the following instruments:

1. a Mayo curved sharp-pointed scissors;
2. two 7-inch Kocher's forceps;
3. swabs, lotions, bandage and sponge-holder;
4. weights (4, 5 and 7 lb) or sandbags or even bricks or stones wrapped in
   cloth;
5. two operating theatre stools, chairs or boxes will do;
6. an obstetric bed, but an ordinary bed or even a wooden chest with
   mattress will do as long as the patient can be moved to the edge.

After excluding rupture of the uterus and confirming that the fetus is dead
the patient is given an analgesic such as pethidine. By pushing the impacted
head, with two fingers, away from the back of the symphysis pubis, a
lubricated rubber catheter is passed into the bladder. It is vital to completely
empty the bladder before proceeding with craniotomy. After exposing the
large caput of the fetus by parting the labia, an incision of about 3 cm is
made on the posterior aspect of the scalp using a Mayo scissors. The index
finger of the left hand is inserted into this incision and moved around so as
to identify the suture and trace the fontanelle lying posteriorly. With the
index finger resting on the fontanelle, and the palmar surface facing
upwards, the Mayo scissors is now carefully directed along the palmar
surface of the left hand and index finger, and made to rest with the tip of the
scissors touching the fontanelle. The scissors is steadied and pushed through
the fontanelle into the cavity of the skull.

The scissors is then opened out in a cruciate direction and the brain is
evacuated with the fingers. A Kocher's forceps is now clamped on to each
lip of the incised scalp, making sure that a good bite is taken. The patient's
legs are now removed from the lithotomy stirrups and placed on two stools.
Two layers of bandage are now passed through the handles of the two
Kocher's forceps, the other end being attached to the chosen weight. When
the bandage has been firmly tied the weight is allowed to hang down gently.
Delivery takes from a few minutes to up to a few hours. The use of weights
may not be necessary. Post-delivery management includes continuous

drainage of the bladder for 5–10 days depending on the suspected state of the bladder, continuation of the antibiotic treatment, adequate intravenous fluids and correction of electrolytes. The advantages of this method of craniotomy over the other methods are its simplicity, the fact that the procedure takes only 10–15 minutes and requires no assistant, very little equipment is necessary and general anaesthesia is not required. This method can also be used when the cervix is only 7 cm dilated, unlike other methods of craniotomy that require full dilatation of the cervix. Lister (1960) also described a very simple and safe method of craniotomy.

Decapitation

In a case of neglected obstructed labour, with a shoulder presentation and dead fetus, the lower segment is very vulnerable. Decapitation is the treatment of choice and this must be carried out with considerable skill to avoid rupture of the uterus. Careful vaginal palpation will determine the exact position of the fetal neck, and if it is at all possible an arm is brought down and pulled by the assistant to give a better exposure of the fetal neck. If it is only a small fetus the neck can easily be severed with stout scissors. Sometimes when maceration has set in, pulling on the arm delivers the crumpled fetus or allows a hook to be passed round the neck of the fetus to facilitate delivery. In the larger fetus, or where the neck is not easily accessible, the Blond-Heidler decapitation saw modified by Mitra & John (1950) is probably the safest instrument. The saw is threaded around the fetal neck, and by keeping the handles attached to the ends of the saw close together, injury to the vagina is prevented and the neck is soon severed after a few firm strokes. By traction on the arm the trunk is easily delivered, care being taken to prevent the vagina from any injury. The after-coming head is then rotated in the uterus until the stump of the neck is pointing down the birth canal. The stump is then grasped with a heavy Volsellum and a finger is put in the fetal mouth to flex the head. By traction on the Volsellum, the head is delivered like the after-coming head of a breech. If an arm is left attached to the head during decapitation, this arm can be used as a handle to facilitate the delivery of the decapitated head (Philpott, 1980). Decapitation is also suitable treatment where there is obstructed labour and prolapsed arm. At times the arm may be oedematous, or it may naturally be so plump that access to the fetal neck is difficult. Amputation of the prolapsed arm usually allows access to the neck. If gross disproportion is suspected, a Caesarean section should be performed.

Cleidotomy

Cleidotomy is indicated when the shoulders are impacted in a dead fetus. A stout scissors is used to cut the clavicles, the most accessible clavicles being divided first. The reduction in size of the shoulder girdles following division of the clavicles facilitates delivery.

Embryotomy

This is rarely necessary, but is sometimes done for an abdominal tumour or a very large fetus following craniotomy and cleidotomy. An incision is made into the abdomen or thorax. The viscera are then evacuated manually. Once this has been performed the fetus is easily extracted now that its bulk is reduced. It is most easily performed if the breech is presenting, for then the abdomen is reached after the legs are brought down. In a cephalic presentation, if there is difficulty in reaching the abdomen after delivering the head, and performing a cleidotomy if necessary, a Caesarean section is advisable.

After-coming head of the breech:

Where there is obstruction to the after-coming head, this should be delivered by craniotomy, which is usually done by perforating the head through the occiput. The head can then be delivered with forceps or by the Mauriceau–Smellie–Veit manoeuvre. Lawson (1967a,b, 1982) described a method that reduces risk of damage to the anterior vaginal wall and neighbouring bladder.

Decompression of hydrocephalic head

In cephalic presentation the CSF is drained before full dilatation by perforating the head at its most accessible point on vaginal examination. Perforation can be performed using any sharp instrument such as a Simpson's perforator, a Drews–Smythe catheter, a spinal needle or a pair of scissors. Where there is an accompanying spina bifida in a breech presentation, CSF can be withdrawn by exposing the spinal canal and passing a catheter into the canal and up into the cranium. A hydrocephalic head can also be decompressed transabdominally using a spinal needle. Whichever procedure is adopted, the collapsed head is easily delivered vaginally, spontaneously or by forceps, once the cervix is fully dilated.

Symphysiotomy combined with a destructive operation

It has been demonstrated that symphysiotomy increases pelvic dimensions (Myerscough, 1977). Seedat & Crichton (1962), in a large series, described the operative procedure. Philpott (1980) states that symphysiotomy is only indicated if the fetus is alive. If a destructive operation is to be performed because the fetus is dead, and in order to avoid Caesarean section, a symphysiotomy can be combined with a destructive operation to make vaginal delivery of the fetus easier where there is borderline disproportion. Indeed, in some cases it may obviate the need for a destructive operation and a combination of symphysiotomy and an episiotomy may allow delivery of the dead fetus intact.

Complications associated with destructive operations

Where cases are carefully selected for destructive operation, complications should be few and minor. The complications of the operation are similar to those of the obstructed labour which necessitates its performance, and it may not be easy to differentiate the complications of one from the other. From the patient's point of view, however, such a differentiation is an academic exercise. Table 11.2 summarises the complications associated with 35 destructive operations performed at the Lagos University Teaching Hospital. The maternal death was in an unbooked eclamptic patient who was transferred in obstructed labour with a dead fetus. Craniotomy was performed on the fetus. Postpartum haemorrhage was the most common complication. This together with the complication of ruptured uterus emphasise the need to have blood available for transfusion in these patients. Apart from the risk of vesicovaginal fistula from pressure of the presenting part in obstructed labour, fistulae may be caused by the sharp instruments used for destructive operations or from bone spicules which are exposed during the procedure. The genital tract and rectum must be carefully examined after the procedure and continuous bladder drainage should continue for at least 5 days after a destructive operation. Urinary and genital tract infections are common in these patients. Chemoprophylaxis may prevent them, and when they are identified appropriate antibiotics should be given.

Table 11.2 Complications associated with destructive operations at Lagos University Teaching Hospital, January 1970 to December 1978

	No.	Percentage
Total number of destructive operations	35	100
Maternal death	1	2·8
Ruptured uterus	4	11
Postpartum haemorrhage	14	39
Cervical/vaginal/perineal tear	3	8·3
Vesicovaginal fistula	1	2·8

ALTERNATIVES TO DESTRUCTIVE OPERATIONS

The fact that the judicious performance of symphysiotomy combined with episiotomy sometimes averts the need for a destructive operation has been stated previously. Treatment must be individualised. The attendant must weigh all the options and if he decides on a destructive operation, he must decide which operation is needed after examining the patient. He must embark on it only if he is confident that he can safely perform it. If he is not sure what procedure to perform, and whether he can do it competently, it is wiser for the patient to have a Caesarean section. If one argument in favour of a destructive operation is that necessary expertise to perform a Caesarean section in the circumstances may not be available, it is important to remember that apart from destructive operations such as cleidotomy or decompression of a hydrocephalus, it is unlikely that a practioner who cannot safely perform a Caesarean section will be competent to do a destructive operation. People learn to do Caesarean sections earlier than they learn to do craniotomy, decapitation or embryotomy.

Some of the complications of Caesarean section in these cases are:

1. intraoperative haemorrhage from extension of the uterine incision;
2. severe postoperative shock;
3. generalised peritonitis;
4. the hazards of general anaesthesia, if general anaesthesia has been used;
5. rupture of the scar in a subsequent pregnancy.

In a series of 107 Caesarean sections performed in 156 patients with intrapartum infection, there was severe postoperative shock in 18 (16·8 per cent), generalised peritonitis in 70 (65·4 per cent), and 13 (12·1 per cent) patients died after Caesarean section (Gogoi, 1971). The mortality and morbidity can be reduced by active preoperative resuscitation and broad-spectrum antibiotic prophylaxis. The technique of extraperitoneal Caesarean section described by Crichton (1973) offers a method of reducing the incidence of peritonitis. Where there is established uterine infection and uterine rupture in a multipara a Caesarean hysterectomy may be the treatment of choice. Although Mogkokong & Marivate (1976) found total hysterectomy better than repair in the treatment of uterine rupture our experience in Nigeria has been that a repair is safer (Lawson, 1967a,b; Agboola 1972; Groen, 1974). Should a hysterectomy be necessary we find the mortality of the sub-total hysterectomy to be almost one-third of that of a total hysterectomy in these severely ill patients (Giwa-Osagie et al, 1983).

QUO VADIS?

Table 11.3 summarises some clinical situations where a destructive operation may be contemplated. An easy destructive operation should be the aim. If it is likely to be difficult it is best not to attempt it, for very serious injury can result from an ill-advised attempt. Medical officers going to practice in peripheral maternity centres must be taught to identify situations where a destructive operation is a safe alternative to Caesarean. Usually they will have been taught how to perform Caesarean section early in their training. In order to reduce mortality and morbidity preoperative resuscitation must

Table 11.3   A summary of the safest procedures in various clinical situations with a dead fetus

Clinical situation	Procedure
1. *Cephalic presentation*	
(a) Head not more than three-fifths palpable above brim	Craniotomy
(b) Head free or more than three-fifths palpable	Caesarean section
(c) Hydrocephalus	Perforation before full dilatation
(d) Obstruction due to abdominal tumour	Embryotomy if abdomen accessible, otherwise Caesarean section
(e) Impacted shoulders	Cleidotomy
2. *Breech presentation*	
(a) Obstruction due to after-coming head	Perforation of head
(b) Obstruction due to abdominal tumour	Embryotomy
(c) Impacted shoulders	Cleidotomy
3. *Transverse or oblique lie*	
(a) Shoulder presentation or arm prolapse	Decapitation
(b) Access to fetal neck difficult	Caesarean section
4. *Ruptured uterus*	Laparotomy
5. *Gross disproportion*	Caesarean section

be vigorous with rehydration, correction of acidosis and antibiotic prophylaxis being the tripod on which a good maternal outcome rests. Blood must be taken for crossmatching because of the risk of haemorrhage. Resuscitation must, however, not take too long and should not be allowed to delay for too long the delivery of the dead fetus. The availability of 'survival kits' comprising intravenous fluids, giving sets and needles, broad-spectrum antibiotics, sutures and ergometrine will facilitate resuscitation. Each maternity centre will have antibiotics depending on the most likely infective organisms and their known sensitivies.

The long-term solution lies in prophylaxis. Although distance from health facilities is a major problem for many patients, Harrison (1980) found that the reliance of patients on native doctors and untrained attendants was a major factor accounting for maternal and perinatal mortality among patients living not too far from the hospital. Education will eventually reduce this danger of ignorance. Philpott (1982) commends the use of waiting areas where mothers in early labour can live near the bigger health centres. This, combined with the adoption of a simple partographic record of labour which indicates to the attendant in the peripheral health centre when to refer to a bigger centre, will reduce the incidence of obstructed labour and the need for destructive operations.

REFERENCES

Agboola A 1972 Rupture of the uterus (a clinical study of 225 cases). Nigerian Medical Journal 1: 19–21
Aimakhu V E 1975 The place of craniotomy in obstetric practice. Nigerian Medical Journal 5(1): 38
Brown I M 1985 In: Studd J W (ed) The Management of Labour. Blackwell, Oxford

Crichton D 1973 A simple technique of extraperitoneal lower segment caesarean section. South African Medical Journal 47: 2011–2012

Giwa-Osagie O F, Uguru V, Akinla O 1983 Mortality and morbidity of emergency obstetric hysterectomy. Journal of Obstetrics and Gynaecology 4: 94–96

Gogoi M P 1971 Maternal mortality from Caesarean section in infected cases. Journal of Obstetrics and Gynaecology of the British Empire 78: 373–376

Groen G P 1974 Uterine rupture in Nigeria. Obstetrics and Gynaecology 44: 682–687

Harrison K A 1980 Approaches to reducing maternal and perinatal mortality in Africa. In: Philpott R H (ed) Maternity services in the developing world—what the community need. RCOG, London, pp 52–69

Lawson J B 1967a Ruptured uterus. In: Lawson J B, Stewart D B (eds) Obstetrics and gynaecology in the tropics and developing countries. Edward Arnold, London, p 189

Lawson J B 1967b Obstructed labour. In: Lawson J B and Stewart D B Obstetrics and gynaecology in the tropics and developing countries. Edward Arnold, London, p 196

Lawson J 1982 Delivery of the dead or malformed fetus. Clinics in Obstetrics and Gynaecology 9(3): 745–755

Lister U 1960 Obstructed labour. Journal of Obstetrics and Gynaecology of the British Commonwealth 67: 188–198

Mitra K N, John M P 1950 Decapitation by thread saw. Journal of Obstetrics and Gynaecology of India 1: 65–73

Mogkokong E T, Marivate M 1976 Treatment of the ruptured uterus. South Africa Medical Journal 50: 1621–1624

Myerscough P R 1977 9th edn Munro Kerr's operative obstetrics, Baillière Tindall, London, pp 550–563

Otolorin E O, Adelusi B 1981 Destructive operation in difficult labour. Tropical Journal of Obstetrics and Gynaecology 2(1): 73–79

Philpott R H 1980 Obstructed labour. Clinics in Obstetrics and Gynaecology 7(3): 601–619

Seedat E K, Crichton D 1962 Symphysiotomy technique: indications and limitations. Lancet i: 554–558

St George J 1975 A simple and safe method of vaginal delivery of cases of prolonged obstructed labour with head presentation. West African Medical Journal XXIII(2): 34–40

Sudden postpartum collapse

A 40-year-old multiparous woman with insulin-dependent diabetes is admitted to the hospital in labour at 38 weeks gestation. Intrapartum she develops mild pre-eclampsia and is treated with a continuous infusion of magnesium sulphate. Labour progresses rapidly, and under epidural anaesthesia she spontaneously delivers a 3100 gram neonate. Ten minutes after delivery, the patient suddenly develops apnoea, cyanosis, and hypotension. She then experiences a grand mal seizure, followed by cardiac arrest. Resuscitation efforts are unsuccessful.

As illustrated by this case history, sudden postpartum collapse can be a terrifying and frequently tragic experience for both patient and attending physician. It may occur as a consequence of several catastrophic events, notably amniotic fluid embolism, pulmonary venous embolism, anaesthetic toxicity, eclampsia, myocardial infarction and cardiac arrhythmia. Successful management of this acute emergency requires rapid diagnosis of the precipitating event and immediate institution of effective resuscitative measures.

The purpose of this chapter is to review the pathophysiology and management of the principal disorders responsible for postpartum collapse. Although all of these disorders are important, we will devote particular attention to a discussion of amniotic fluid embolism. We have chosen to do so for several reasons. First, because of its rare occurrence, amniotic fluid embolism is the condition with which clinicians are least likely to be familiar. Second, it is the disorder which is perhaps the most difficult to treat successfully. Finally, recent research has provided important new information concerning the pathophysiology and rapid diagnosis of amniotic fluid embolism. It is essential that the practising clinician be aware of these new developments.

AMNIOTIC FLUID EMBOLISM

Amniotic fluid embolism has been termed 'the most dangerous and untreatable condition in obstetrics'. The reported incidence ranges from 1 in 3360 to 1 in 80 000 pregnancies. The disorder is responsible for 4 to 10 per cent of all maternal deaths. Eighty-five per cent of women who experience amniotic fluid embolism die; one-fourth of these individuals expire within 1 hour of the acute event. Fetal mortality is approximately 40 per cent (Courtney, 1974; Duff, 1984; Morgan, 1979).

Pathophysiology

Amniotic fluid embolism has occurred in each trimester of pregnancy and has been associated with a variety of obstetric conditions (Table 12.1). The unifying feature of these clinical situations is that they are associated with disruption of the normal anatomic relationship between chorioamniotic membrane, placenta, and uterine wall and with disruption of uterine vascular integrity. These two derangements allow amniotic fluid to gain access to the systemic circulation. Figure 12.1 summarizes the pathophysiology of this unique disorder.

Once in the circulation, amniotic fluid elements are carried to the lung, where they lodge in the pulmonary capillary network. Deposition of these elements in the lung vasculature initially causes intense pulmonary vasoconstriction and a transient increase in pulmonary artery pressure. The vasoconstriction appears to be due to an anaphylactic-like reaction to one of several substances: prostaglandins, meconium, vernix caseosa, and particulate debris (Attwood & Downing, 1965; Courtney, 1974).

Amniotic fluid elements in the pulmonary vasculature also activate the complement cascade (Jacobs & Hammerschmidt, 1982). The C5a component of complement promotes leukocyte migration and aggregation within the small vessels of the lung. Leukocytes release a variety of inflammatory mediators that directly injure pulmonary capillary endothelium and disrupt normal alveolar architecture. This results in transudation of intravascular

Table 12.1 Obstetric conditions associated with amniotic fluid embolism (Duff, 1984)

First trimester abortion
Suction curettage
Sharp curettage
Second trimester abortion
Saline injection
Prostaglandin F2 alpha injection
Urea injection
Hysterotomy
Blunt abdominal trauma
Uterine rupture
Placental abruption
Insertion of uterine pressure catheter
Vaginal delivery
High parity
Tumultuous labour
Macrosomic fetus
Meconium-stained amniotic fluid
Caesarean delivery
Lower uterine segment laceration

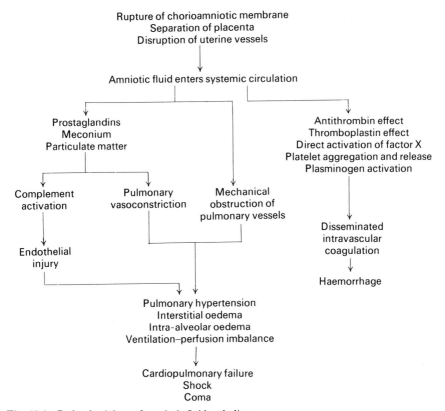

Fig. 12.1 Pathophysiology of amniotic fluid embolism.

fluid into the intra-alveolar and interstitial spaces. The net effect of these derangements is severe hypoxia, which then causes acute left ventricular failure, manifested by elevated pulmonary capillary wedge pressure (PCWP) and decreased cardiac output. Left ventricular dysfunction is, in fact, the most consistent haemodynamic finding in patients with amniotic fluid embolism (Clark et al, 1985).

Amniotic fluid infusion also disrupts the host's coagulation system. Disseminated intravascular coagulation develops in the majority of patients that survive the acute embolic event and is responsible for 40 per cent of the fatalities that ultimately result from amniotic fluid embolism.

The exact component of amniotic fluid responsible for the coagulopathy is not clear, but the functional derangements have been well documented in both laboratory and clinical studies (Courtney & Allington, 1971; Ratnoff & Vosburgh, 1952; Reid et al, 1953; Beller et al, 1963). Amniotic fluid has an antithrombin- and thromboplastin-like effect. It also stimulates platelet aggregation and release, and directly activates factor X. The coagulation cascade is intensified as a result of the activation of complement by amniotic fluid. Once activated, the coagulation system stimulates the fibrinolytic system. Fibrin degradation products, in turn, accelerate the consumption of coagulation factors.

Clinical manifestations

The clinical manifestations of amniotic fluid embolism develop with terrifying suddenness. At one moment the patient appears normal. Virtually without warning, she develops dyspnoea, cough productive of pink frothy sputum, and cyanosis. These changes are followed rapidly by apnoea, loss of consciousness, and profound shock. Ten to 20 per cent of women experience convulsions. Of those that survive the acute hypoxic episode, the majority develop a coagulopathy, manifested most prominently by uterine haemorrhage. Left ventricular failure also is a common complication in the immediate postembolic period.

Establishing the diagnosis

In patients who die of amniotic fluid embolism the diagnosis can be established definitively by postmortem examination of the lung. The principal histological findings are intra-alveolar oedema and haemorrhage, and intravascular emboli. The latter are composed of fetal squames, mucin, fat, and amorphous debris (Peterson & Taylor, 1970). Amniotic fluid elements may not be apparent in microscopic sections stained with haematoxylin and eosin. Therefore, special stains for acid mucopolysaccharide, keratin, and fat should be performed whenever the possibility of amniotic fluid embolism exists (Fig. 12.2).

Recent investigations have shown that the diagnosis also can be made antemortem. Wasser et al (1979) used open-lung biopsy to demonstrate the presence of amniotic fluid debris in alveoli and small pulmonary vessels. Stromme & Framke (1977) were able to isolate fetal squames from a sputum sample.

The principal technique for confirming the diagnosis, however, is cytologic examination of blood obtained from the central circulation via a central venous pressure or pulmonary artery balloon flotation catheter (Duff et al, 1983; Masson et al, 1979; Resnik et al, 1976; Schaerf et al, 1977). Special stains for fat, mucin, and keratin should be utilized to demonstrate the presence of substituents of amniotic fluid (Figs 12.3 and 12.4). These elements have been present in blood specimens obtained as long as 72 hours after the acute embolic event (Duff et al, 1983).

In a patient with clinical manifestations of amniotic fluid embolism, demonstration of amniotic fluid debris in the central circulation confirms the diagnosis. Recently, however, Plauche (1983) isolated fetal squamous cells from the pulmonary artery circulation in two patients who had right heart catheterization for management of pre-eclampsia. This finding raises

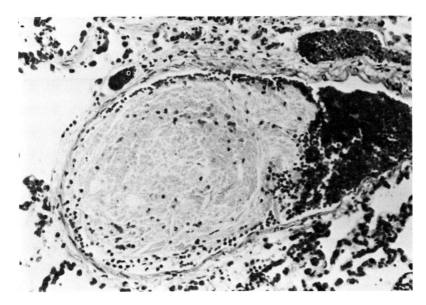

Fig. 12.2   Haematoxylin and eosin stain demonstrates occlusion of pulmonary vessel by mucin (light stain) and blood elements (dark stain).

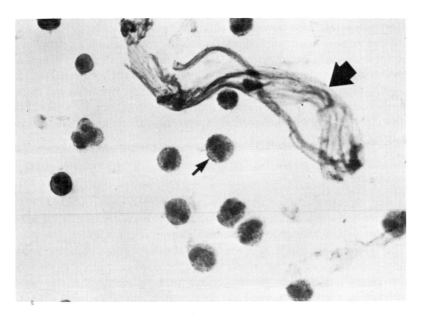

Fig. 12.3   Smear of buffy coat suspension was prepared from blood aspirated from pulmonary circulation. The large arrow denotes keratin and the small arrow a leukocyte (Ayoub-Shklar stain for keratin, × 65).

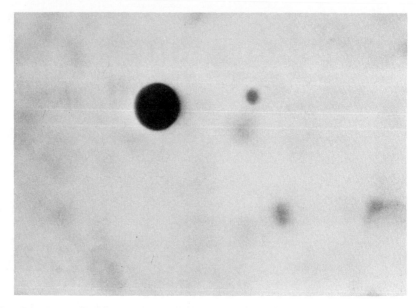

Fig. 12.4   Smear of buffy coat suspension demonstrates fat cell (Oil-red-O stain, × 65).

the intriguing possibility that the disorder is more common than previously suspected, but that only certain patients have a sufficient inoculum of amniotic fluid to produce clinical symptoms.

Haemodynamic measurements obtained by right heart catheterization also are of value in confirming the diagnosis (Clark et al, 1985). Immediately after the embolism, patients usually have an elevated pulmonary artery and central venous pressure and evidence of acute right ventricular dysfunction. The ECG may show right axis deviation. Pulmonary hypertension usually is transient, however. The haemodynamic abnormalities that persist are elevated pulmonary capillary wedge pressure and decreased cardiac output–reflecting left ventricular failure.

Management

The first objective is to secure the patient's airway and provide effective ventilation and oxygenation. In most instances this will require endotracheal intubation and mechanical ventilation with a volume-cycled respirator.

The second objective is to correct shock. Central haemodynamic monitoring is imperative to evaluate the degree of left ventricular dysfunction and to determine the rate of intravenous fluid replacement. If the patient has evidence of acute left ventricular dysfunction, digitalization is indicated. Infusion of a vasopressor such as dopamine or dobutamine also may be of value since these agents enhance myocardial contractility and improve perfusion of central organs. There is no conclusive evidence that corticosteroids are of value in improving haemodynamic function in this clinical setting.

Isotonic crystalloid solutions such as normal saline or Ringer's lactate should be used for fluid resuscitation. The rate and total amount of infusion should be guided by evaluation of the patient's sensorium, blood pressure, urine output, and PCWP. In order to prevent exacerbation of pulmonary oedema, infusion of fluids must be restricted if the PCWP rises above 14 to 16 mmHg.

The third objective of therapy is to anticipate the development of DIC and to treat it promptly if it occurs. Red cell deficits should be corrected by administration of red cell components. Thrombocytopenia should be corrected by infusion of platelets. Fresh whole blood or fresh frozen plasma should be utilized to replace clotting factors. If haemorrhage fails to resolve, use of heparin or fibrinolytic inhibitors should be considered. There is insufficient evidence at present, however, to justify routine use of these agents for treatment of amniotic fluid embolism.

The final goal of therapy is to provide optimal supportive care until the patient's haemodynamic and pulmonary dysfunction can be corrected. Thermal instability should be minimised. Metabolic and electrolyte abnormalities should be corrected promptly. Careful surveillance should be maintained for the development of infection.

MASSIVE PULMONARY VENOUS THROMBOEMBOLISM

The incidence of pulmonary embolism in pregnancy is approximately 1 per 2500 pregnancies. Seventy-five per cent occur in the immediate postpartum period. In the first 4 weeks after delivery the relative risk of pulmonary embolism is increased approximately 50 times above that in a control, non-pregnant population. Pulmonary thromboembolism remains one of the three leading causes of maternal death in industrialised nations (Aaro & Juergens, 1974; Bissell, 1977; Browse & Thomas, 1974).

Pathophysiology

Several of the physiological and anatomical changes associated with pregnancy predispose gravid patients to an increased risk of thromboembolism. First, increased hepatic synthesis of coagulation factors I, VII, VIII, IX and X creates a potential hypercoagulable state. Second, progressive uterine enlargement results in increased venous pressure and relative stasis of blood flow in the lower extremities. Third, the trauma associated with vaginal or Caesarean delivery results in injury to vascular endothelium which represents a stimulus for activation of the coagulation cascade. Finally, puerperal infection, a common complication of childbirth, increases the risk of venous thromboembolism because it, too, may result in injury and inflammation within the vascular endothelium.

The major source of pulmonary emboli are deep vein thromboses in the veins of the calf and iliofemoral system. Septic pulmonary emboli are most likely to arise from the veins of the pelvis. Factors that further increase the pregnant woman's risk of pulmonary embolism include advancing age, obesity, previous history of deep vein thrombosis, traumatic or operative delivery and prolonged inactivity.

Clinical manifestations

The principal clinical manifestations of massive pulmonary embolism are anxiety, retrosternal pain, tachycardia and dyspnaea. These alterations are followed rapidly by apnoea, cyanosis, loss of consciousness, and shock. Additional physical findings may include haemoptysis, pleural friction rub, fixed splitting of the second heart sound, accentuation of the sound of pulmonic valve closure, and an S-3 gallop. In many, but certainly not all, patients, evidence of deep vein thrombosis in one of the lower extremities is present (Humphries et al, 1976).

Establishing the diagnosis

Pulmonary embolization that is of sufficient magnitude to produce postpartum collapse is almost invariably associated with prominent hypoxemia. A normal aterial Po_2 effectively rules out the diagnosis of pulmonary embolism. The electrocardiogram may show P-pulmonale, right ventricular hypertrophy, incomplete right bundle branch block, or right axis deviation (Fig. 12.5). Although the chest X-ray may be normal,

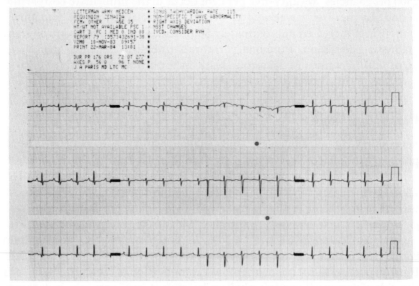

Fig. 12.5 Electrocardiogram demonstrates sinus tachycardia and right axis deviation. Note negative deflections in leads I, II, and aVL.

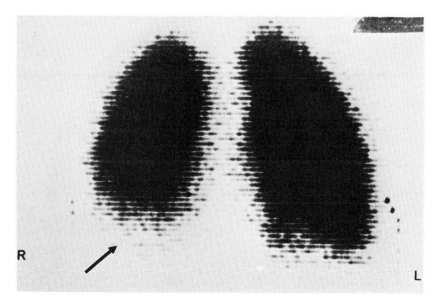

Fig. 12.6 Perfusion scan shows filling defects in lower lobe of right lung in a patient with acute pulmonary embolism.

abnormalities that support the diagnosis of embolism include discoid atelectasis, pleural effusion, pleural thickening, elevation of one hemidiaphragm, and oligaemia. The latter finding also is referred to as Westermark's sign. It is due to occlusion of the central branches of one or both pulmonary arteries. Wedge-shaped opacities within the lung parenchyma represent actual areas of infarction.

The ventilation–perfusion scan is the most accurate non-invasive means of establishing the diagnosis of pulmonary embolism. The typical findings of venous embolism are lobar or segmental perfusion defects in association with normal ventilation and a normal chest X-ray (Fig. 12.6). A normal scan reliably excludes the diagnosis of pulmonary embolism.

If the ventilation–perfusion scan is equivocal, pulmonary angiography should be performed. The typical angiographic findings associated with large emboli are filling defects and abrupt cut-offs (Fig. 12.7). Angiography may cause several life-threatening complications including cardiac arrest, acute cor pulmonale, and arrhythmia. Therefore it should be utilized only when the diagnosis cannot be established by less invasive means (Humphries et al, 1976).

Management

Medical therapy

Immediate management should be directed towards establishment of a patent airway and maintenance of ventilation and oxygenation. Hypotension should be corrected by administration of isotonic crystalloids. Once the

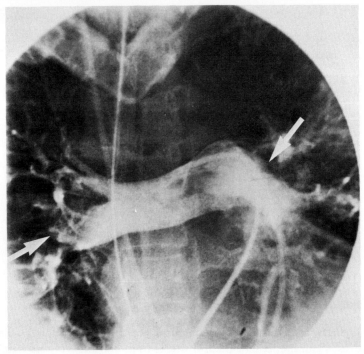

Fig. 12.7   Pulmonary angiogram demonstrates large emboli in the proximal portion of both the right and left pulmonary arteries (white arrows).

diagnosis of pulmonary venous thromboembolism is confirmed, anticoagulation is indicated. This is most effectively accomplished by administration of an initial intravenous bolus of 5000 to 10 000 units of heparin followed by a continuous infusion, adjusted to maintain the PTT at $1\frac{1}{2}$–2 times the control value or the serum heparin concentration at 0.2–0.7 iu/ml. Intravenous heparin should be continued for a minimum of 7–10 days, at which time oral anticoagulants may be administered. Anticoagulation with the latter agents should be continued for approximately 3 months.

There is minimal reported experience with the use of fibrinolytic agents in the immediate puerperium. The major complication associated with use of these drugs is haemorrhage; therefore they should not be used in patients who recently have had a major surgical procedure such as Caesarean section. Their safety in women who have had recent vaginal delivery also has not been established. Therefore their use should be restricted to exceptional cases where other therapy has failed to improve the patient's haemodynamic dysfunction (Bell & Meek, 1979; Sharma et al, 1982).

Surgery

Pulmonary embolectomy should be considered in the patient who has a massive embolism in the proximal portion of the main pulmonary arteries

(Fig. 12.7) and who experiences progressive deterioration in her condition despite institution of anticoagulation and cardiopulmonary resuscitation. In this situation surgical intervention may be the only way to stabilize the critically ill patient (Becker, 1983).

Surgery also must be considered in patients who develop recurrent embolization after an initial favourable response to anticoagulation and fluid resuscitation. In such a clinical situation continued embolization of thrombi from the lower extremities may be minimised and, hopefully, prevented, by plication of the inferior vena cava or by insertion of an umbrella filter (Bissell, 1977).

TOXICITY OF REGIONAL ANAESTHETICS

The frequency of serious toxicity in association with regional anaesthesia is approximately 1 in 1000 procedures. Pregnant patients are more susceptible than non-pregnant women to the toxic effects of local anaesthetics for several reasons. First, blood flow through the vessels surrounding the spinal cord and meninges is increased in pregnancy. Therefore there is a greater surface area for systemic absorption. Second, because these vessels are distended, the capacity of the epidural space is decreased. Third, during contractions, and particularly during voluntary expulsive efforts, there is a marked increase in pressures in the subarachnoid and epidural spaces. These alterations in pressure increase the probability that anaesthetic agents will be disseminated more widely.

Pathophysiology

Sudden postpartum collapse typically results from inadvertent intravascular injection of local anaesthetic or from administration of an excessive dose of drug. Factors that increase the duration of action of the local anaesthetic (high lipid solubility, high degree of protein binding, amide structure) also increase the likelihood of serious systemic reactions. Long-acting drugs such as bupivacaine and etidocaine, when used incorrectly, have a greater potential for systemic toxicity than shorter-acting agents such as chloroprocaine (Alper, 1976). Prolonged, irreversible myocardial depression, in fact, has been observed when a highly concentrated solution of bupivacaine (75 per cent) was used for regional anaesthesia (Albright, 1979).

Clinical manifestations

Signs and symptoms of systemic toxicity usually occur within 20 minutes of the time that the local anaesthetic is administered. Patients initially may note a metallic taste in the mouth, or ringing in the ears. They then may experience confusion and disorientation and have difficulty breathing. Ptosis and miosis may occur as a result of blockade of sympathetic B fibres that are present in the upper thoracic spinal nerves. Subsequently, respiratory muscle paralysis may be so marked that cyanosis and apnoea develop. Cardiac arrest may ensue either as the result of anoxia or as a result of the direct myocardial depressant effect of the drug. Generalized seizure activity also may develop in association with anoxia (Alper, 1976; Bonica, 1980).

Management

The most effective method of management of anaesthetic complications is to prevent them from occurring. This requires strict attention to anaesthetic technique, strict observance of altered dosage requirements for pregnant patients, and extended observation of the patient after administration of the drug. Local anaesthetics should be utilized only by individuals who are skilled in providing ventilatory assistance, and in a physical setting where resuscitative equipment is immediately available.

Once cardiorespiratory arrest has occurred, the first priority is to intubate and ventilate the patient. Fluid resuscitation should be initiated, and the circulation should be maintained. If seizure activity is present, small intravenous doses of a drug such as diazepam should be administered. Subsequent therapy is directed towards support of the airway and maintenance of effective ventilation and oxygenation until the effects of the local anaesthetic have dissipated. The prognosis for complete recovery of the patient is excellent provided that complications are recognized immediately and prolonged hypoxia and acidosis do not develop (Alper, 1976; Bonica, 1980).

ECLAMPSIA

In the Western countries of the world, eclampsia occurs with a frequency of 1/300 to 1/1500 pregnancies. Ten to 35 per cent of cases occur in the immediate puerperium. Despite improvements in obstetric care, the maternal mortality resulting from eclampsia still may be as high as 5 per cent in some institutions (Pritchard et al, 1985).

Predisposing risk factors

The risk factors for eclampsia are the same as those for pre-eclampsia. Such factors include young age, nulliparity, family history of pre-eclampsia or eclampsia, multiple gestation, diabetes, hydatidiform mole, fetal hydrops, and pre-existing chronic hypertension.

Most cases of eclampsia occur in women who initially have evidence of severe pre-eclampsia. It is important to recognize, however, that this may not always be true. Sibai and co-workers (1981) demonstrated that 20 per cent of eclamptic patients had diastolic blood pressures less than 90 mmHg, urine protein less than 2+, and normal deep tendon reflexes. Thirty-nine per cent of the women had no significant oedema.

Clinical manifestations

The clinical manifestations of eclampsia are familiar to all obstetricians. They include hypertension, hyperreflexia, headache, visual disturbances, and seizures. Seizure activity usually begins with involuntary twitching around the mouth and face. This is followed by generalized tonic–clonic movements. Seizure activity persists for approximately 1 minute, and the patient usually is apnoeic during this period. In the absence of treatment, convulsions may recur and may evolve into status epilepticus. Post-ictally, the patient demonstrates rapid, stertorous respirations. Rarely, patients will develop a central hyperthermia as a result of extended seizure activity. Temperatures may reach 39·5°C or higher.

Three of the most ominous complications of eclampsia are cerebrovascular accident, pulmonary oedema and coagulopathy. Lopez-Llera (1982) has shown that approximately 70 per cent of the maternal deaths that occur in eclamptic women are due to intracerebral haemorrhage. Ten to 15 per cent are the result of respiratory failure, and 6 to 10 per cent are due to haemorrhage. Another serious, but fortunately rare, complication of eclampsia is hepatic rupture.

Establishing the diagnosis

In women who are known to have pre-eclampsia, previous laboratory studies may be of value in confirming the diagnosis. Haemoconcentration usually is present, and the haematocrit is elevated. Some women, however, demonstrate a microangiopathic haemolytic anaemia. The serum concentration of uric acid, creatinine, and urea nitrogen is elevated, both as a consequence of haemoconcentration and as a result of renal dysfunction. Hepatic dysfunction is indicated by elevation of serum transaminase enzymes, alkaline phosphatase, and bilirubin. Creatinine clearance is decreased, and marked proteinurea is usually present. Some patients will also have evidence of coagulopathy, manifested by thrombocytopenia, hypofibrinogenaemia, and prolongation of the prothrombin time and partial thromboplastin time.

Management

As is true for the other disorders discussed in this review, the first priority in management of the critically ill patient is to provide a secure airway and to insure that ventilation and oxygenation are adequate. In the eclamptic patient the second priority is to administer medication that will limit the present seizure and prevent further convulsions. Small intravenous doses of diazepam are usually effective in abolishing seizure activity. Maintenance therapy should then be instituted with one of several agents.

In the United States the preferred drug for seizure prophylaxis is magnesium sulphate. The most commonly used dosage regimen employs a

4 gram loading dose, administered over 20–30 minutes, followed by a maintenance infusion of 2 to 3 grams per hour (Sibai, 1985; Sibai et al, 1983, 1984). Some investigators continue to achieve excellent clinical results with an intramuscular regimen of magnesium sulphate: 10 gram loading dose, followed by 5 grams every 4 hours (Pritchard et al, 1984). Magnesium sulphate clearly is not the only medication capable of providing effective seizure prophylaxis. In other countries diazepam, phenytoin and phenobarbital are used routinely for this purpose.

Marked elevations in blood pressure (> 110 mmHg diastolic, 170 mmHg systolic) must be treated promptly in order to reduce the risk of intracerebral haemorrhage, myocardial ischaemia, and pulmonary oedema. The two agents of most value in the clinical situation are hydralazine and nitroprusside. The former may be administered intravenously in small increments or by continuous infusion. The latter must be given by constant infusion (Sibai, 1985; Pritchard et al, 1985).

Patients with eclampsia should be followed carefully for evidence of a coagulopathy. In the presence of overt bleeding, severe thrombocytopenia (<50 000/mm³) and marked deficits in fibrinogen (<100 mg/dl) should be corrected by administration of platelets and cryoprecipitate. Deficiencies in other coagulation factors are most effectively treated by administration of fresh frozen plasma.

Finally, efforts must be made to prevent the development of pulmonary oedema and respiratory failure. The most common cause of this complication is excessive fluid replacement. Therefore fluid administration must be regulated precisely. Central haemodynamic monitoring is of great value in determining rates of fluid replacement.

MYOCARDIAL INFARCTION

Acute myocardial infarction is an unusual complication of pregnancy. The reported frequency is 1 in 10 000 to 1 in 42 000 pregnancies. The majority of cases occur in the third trimester and the immediate puerperium. The maternal mortality is approximately 35–45 per cent. Most of these deaths occur suddenly at the time of the initial infarction (Beary et al, 1979; Ginz, 1952; Hankins et al, 1985).

Predisposing risk factors

The principal risk factors for acute myocardial infarction are pre-existing atherosclerotic heart disease, hypertension, hyperlipidaemia, age greater than 35 years, and cigarette smoking. Other factors that appear to predispose to ischaemic events include insulin-dependent diabetes, obesity, and sedentary life style (Goldman & Meller, 1982; Hankins et al, 1985).

Clinical manifestations

The clinical presentation of acute myocardial infarction is similar in pregnant and non-pregnant patients. Most individuals experience severe crushing substernal pain associated with nausea, vomiting, diaphoresis, and dyspnoea. In many patients the pain radiates into the neck and down along the left arm. Shock, loss of consciousness, pulmonary oedema, and arrhythmia frequently develop as complications of the infarction.

Establishing the diagnosis

The two tests used most commonly to establish the diagnosis of acute myocardial infarction are the ECG and cardiac enzymes. Electrocardiographic findings consistent with acute infarction include ST-segment elevation, Q waves in leads II, III, and aVf (diaphragmatic infarction) or poor R wave progression in the precordial leads (anterior infarction) (Buckley et al, 1984).

Cardiac isoenzyme profiles initially demonstrate an elevation in creatine phosphokinase. Concentrations increase within 4–6 hours after the infarction, reach a maximum at 24 hours, and return to normal within 3 days. The amino acid transferase enzymes (SGPT and SGOT) begin to increase 6–8 hours after the acute event, peak at 24–48 hours, and return to baseline within 4 days. Lactic acid dehydrogenase (LDH) does not increase until approximately 12 hours after the infarction. The concentration reaches a maximum in 3–6 days and then decreases to normal within 14 days.

In clinical situations where the diagnosis of myocardial infarction is in doubt, radionuclide scans may be of value in resolving the uncertainty. Technetium pyrophosphate ^{99m}Tc) is a radioisotope with particular affinity for damaged myocardial tissue. It can be utilized to highlight a specific area of infarction. Thallium-201 (^{201}Tl), on the other hand, adheres only to normal myocardium, thus identifying infarcted tissue as a cold spot on scintiscan.

Complications

Over 90 per cent of patients develop some type of cardiac arrhythmia, most commonly ectopic atrial and ventricular beats. Thirty per cent of individuals experience life-threatening arrhythmia such as ventricular tachycardia, ventricular fibrillation, complete heart block, and asystole (Killip & Kimball 1967; Hankins et al, 1985).

In patients who have sustained large infarctions, left ventricular dysfunction may be so severe that congestive heart failure develops. Ten per cent of patients with acute infarctions develop cardiogenic shock. Eighty to 90 per cent of these individuals die (Karliner & Ross, 1971).

Management

The obstetrician's first objective is to identify antepartum the few women who are at risk for acute myocardial infarction. Special efforts should be made during labour to ensure that these patients are well oxygenated and relatively free of pain. Wide variations in blood pressure, heart rate, and cardiac output are most effectively prevented by utilisation of regional anaesthesia (Ueland & Hansen, 1969).

Should acute infarction develop in the immediate puerperium, emergency management by the delivery team is directed towards securing the patient's airway and providing effective ventilation. Closed cardiac massage may be necessary initially to support the circulation. If a vasopressor is needed to sustain perfusion pressure, dopamine and dobutamine are the preferred agents. These drugs enhance myocardial contractility and improve perfusion of the coronary circulation. They are less likely to cause arrhythmias than isoproterenol.

Life-threatening arrhythmias such as ventricular tachycardia and ventricular fibrillation must be treated immediately by countershock. Complete heart block should be treated initially with atropine until a cardiologist is available to insert a transvenous pacemaker. Once the patient is stabilised, she should be transferred to a coronary care unit for definitive management by medical specialists.

SUMMARY

Sudden postpartum collapse is a rare and terrifying obstetric complication that is caused by a limited number of disorders. The usual clinical manifestations are apnoea, cyanosis, shock, and generalised tonic–clonic seizures. The immediate objective in management is to provide ventilation and oxygenation and to initiate fluid resuscitation.

Coincident with these stabilisation measures, selected laboratory studies should be performed to determine the cause of cardiovascular collapse. The tests most likely to be of value in establishing the correct diagnosis are arterial blood gas analysis, ECG, evaluation of haemodynamic monitoring data, and examination of blood aspirated from the central circulation. Subsequent management should then be directed at the specific inciting event. Additional supportive therapy may include anticonvulsants, anticoagulants, antiarrhythmics, replacement of coagulation factors and continued support of the airway and circulation.

REFERENCES

Aaro L A, Juergens J L 1974 Thrombophlebitis and pulmonary embolism as complications of pregnancy. Medical Clinics of North America 58 : 829–834

Albright G A 1979 Cardiac arrest following regional anesthesia with etidocaine or bupivacaine. Anesthesiology 51 : 285–287

Alper M H 1976 Toxicity of local anesthetics. New England Journal of Medicine 295 : 1432–1433

Attwood H D, Downing S E 1965 Experimental amniotic fluid and meconium embolism. Surgery, Gynecology and Obstetrics 30 : 255–262

Beary J F, Summer W R, Buckley B H 1979 Postpartum acute myocardial infarction : a rare occurrence of uncertain etiology. American Journal of Cardiology 43 : 158–161

Becker R M 1983 Intracardiac surgery in pregnant women. Annals of Thoracic Surgery 36 : 453–458

Bell W, Meek A G 1979 Guidelines for the use of thrombolytic agents. New England Journal of Medicine 301 : 1266–1270

Beller F K, Douglas G W, Debrovner C H, Robinson R 1963 The fibrinolytic system in amniotic fluid embolism. American Journal of Obstetrics and Gynecology 87 : 48–55

Bissell S M 1977 Pulmonary thromboembolism associated with gynecologic surgery and pregnancy. American Journal of Obstetrics and Gynecology 128 : 418–423

Bonica J J 1980 Obstetric analgesia and anesthesia. World Federation of the Society of Anesthesiologists, Amsterdam

Browse N L, Thomas M L 1974 Source of non-lethal pulmonary emboli. Lancet 1 : 258–259

Buckley N B, Becker C L, Flaherty J T 1984 Myocardial infarction. In : Harvey A M, Johns R T, McKusick V A, Owens A H Jr, Ross R S (eds) The principles and practice of medicine, 21st edn. Appleton-Century Crofts, Norwalk

Clark S L, Montz F J, Phelan J P 1985 Hemodynamic alterations associated with amniotic fluid embolism. American Journal of Obstetrics and Gynecology 151 : 617–621

Courtney L D 1974 Amniotic fluid embolism. Obstetrical and Gynecological Survey 29 : 169–176

Courtney L D, Allington M 1971 Effect of amniotic fluid on blood coagulation. British Journal of Haematology 22 : 353–355

Duff P 1984 Defusing the dangers of amniotic fluid embolism. Contemporary Obstetrics and Gynecology, August : 127–149

Duff P, Engelsgjerd B, Zingery L W, Huff R W, Montiel M M 1983 Hemodynamic observations in a patient with intrapartum amniotic fluid embolism. American Journal of Obstetrics and Gynecology 146 : 112–115

Ginz B 1952 Myocardial infarction in pregnancy. Journal of Obstetrics and Gynaecology of the British Commonwealth 63 : 381–390

Goldman M E, Meller J 1982 Coronary artery disease in pregnancy. In : Elkayam U, Gleicher N (eds) Cardiac problems in pregnancy : diagnosis and management of maternal and fetal disease. Alan R Liss, New York

Hankins G D V, Wendel G D Jr, Leveno K J, Stoneham J 1985 Myocardial infarction during pregnancy : a review. Obstetrics and Gynecology 65 : 139–146

Humphries J O, Bell W R, White R I 1976 Criteria for the recognition of pulmonary emboli. Journal of the American Medical Association 235 : 2011–2012

Jacobs H S, Hammerschmidt D H 1982 Tissue damage caused by activated complement and granulocytes in shock lung, postperfusion lung, and after amniotic fluid embolism : ramifications for therapy. Annales Chirugiae et Gynaecologiae 71 : 3–9

Karliner J S, Ross J 1971 Left ventricular performance after acute myocardial infarction. Progress in Cardiovascular Disease 13 : 374–379

Killip T, Kimball J T 1967 Treatment of myocardial infarction in a coronary care unit. American Journal of Cardiology 20 : 457–461

Lopez-Llera M 1982 Complicated eclampsia. Fifteen years experience in a referral medical center. American Journal of Obstetrics and Gynecology 142 : 28–35

Masson R G, Ruggieri J, Siddiqui M M 1979 Amniotic fluid embolism : definitive diagnosis in a survivor. American Review of Respiratory Diseases 120 : 187–192

Morgan M 1979 Amniotic fluid embolism. Anesthesia 34 : 20–32

Peterson E P, Taylor H B 1970 Amniotic fluid embolism. An analysis of 40 cases. Obstetrics and Gynecology 35 : 787–793

Plauche W C 1983 Amniotic fluid embolism. American Journal of Obstetrics and Gynecology 147 : 982

Pritchard J A, Cunningham F G, Pritchard S A 1984 The Parkland Memorial Hospital protocol for treatment of eclampsia : evaluation of 245 cases. American Journal of Obstetrics and Gynecology 148 : 951–963

Pritchard J A, MacDonald P C, Gant N F (eds) 1985 Hypertensive disorders in pregnancy. In: Williams Obstetrics, 17 edn. Appleton Century Crofts, Norwalk

Ratnoff O D, Vosburgh G J 1952 Observations on the clotting defect in amniotic-fluid embolism. New England Journal of Medicine 247: 970–973

Reid D E, Wiener A E, Roby C C 1953 Intravascular clotting and afibrinogenemia, the presumptive lethal factors in the syndrome of amniotic fluid embolism. American Journal of Obstetrics and Gynecology 66: 465–474

Resnik R, Swartz W H, Plumer M H, Benirschke K, Stratthaus M E 1976 Amniotic fluid embolism with survival. Obstetrics and Gynecology 47: 295–298

Schaerf R H M, deCampo T, Civetta J M 1977 Hemodynamic alterations and rapid diagnosis in a case of amniotic fluid embolus. Anesthesiology 46: 155–157

Sharma G V R K, Cella G, Parisi A F, Sasahara A A 1982 Thrombolytic therapy. New England Journal of Medicine 306: 1268–1276

Sibai B M 1985 Preeclampsia–eclampsia. In: Sciarra J J (ed) Gynecology and obstetrics, revised edn, volume 2, chapter 51. Harper and Row, New York

Sibai B M, McCubbin J H, Anderson G D, Lishitz J, Diltz P V Jr 1981 Eclampsia. I. Observations from 67 recent cases. Obstetrics and Gynecology 58: 609–613

Sibai B M, Spinnato J A, Watson D L, Lewis J A, Anderson G D 1984 Effect of magnesium sulfate on electroencephalographic findings in preeclampsia–eclampsia. Obstetrics and Gynecology 64: 261–266

Stromme W B, Fromke V L 1977 Amniotic fluid embolism and disseminated intravascular coagulation after evacuation of missed abortion. Obstetrics and Gynecology 52: 76S–80S

Ueland K, Hansen J M 1969 Material cardiovascular dynamics. III. Labor and delivery under local and caudal analgesia. American Journal of Obstetrics and Gynecology 103: 8–11

Viamonte M, Koolpe H, Janowitz W, Hildner F 1980 Pulmonary thromboembolism–update. Journal of the American Medical Association 243: 2229–2234

Wasser W G, Tessler S, Kamath C P, Sackin A J 1979 Nonfatal amniotic fluid embolism: a case report of postpartum respiratory distress with histopathologic studies. Mt Sinai Journal of Medicine 46: 388–391

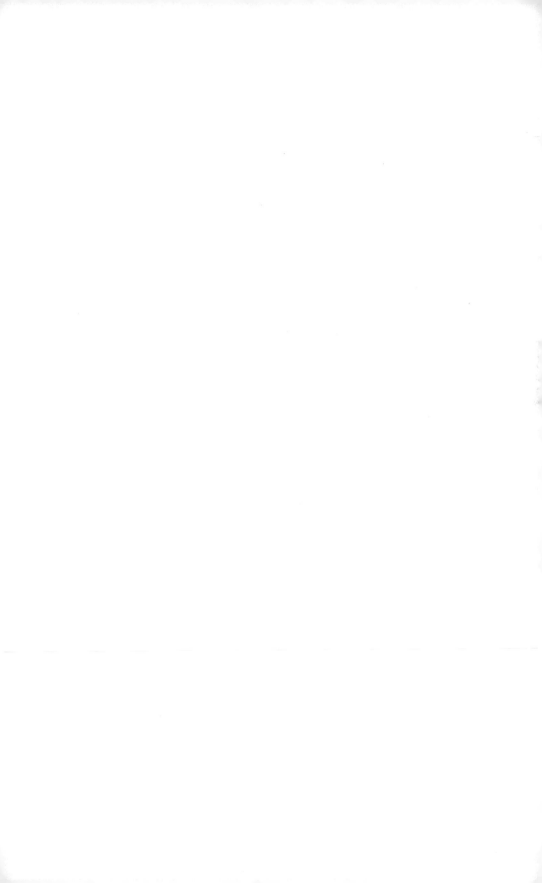

PART TWO

Gynaecology

The new ethical problems in infertility

The concept of the 'artificial family' is becoming increasingly familiar, and is increasingly widely discussed. One consequence of this is that infertile couples are less likely to put up with their own childlessness without a determined effort to remedy it. It is to be presumed that gynaecologists come under greater pressure than ever before to take action on behalf of infertile couples; and this is in itself a great advance.

There is one perfectly general problem that arises out of these, or indeed any other, advances in medicine, and that is the problem of finance. I do not intend to tangle with this in the following pages. For the question of 'priorities', as it is called, cannot be entirely for the individual doctor to decide. Regional Health Authorities will decide where to put money according, partly, to their own strengths, and the pressures they are under: charity will continue to come up with money, but unpredictably. One thing only is certain. The problem of infertility has now entered the mainstream of medicine, as far as the perception of the general public goes, and it will not go away.

If I turn then to more narrowly ethical problems, my concern as a philosopher ought to be not to point out what these problems are (for the medical profession, it may be thought, is perfectly capable of identifying these itself) but to examine the methods or principles according to which the problems should be solved. I should, that is, speak of methodology, not of moral content. Nevertheless there are a few preliminary points about the nature of the problems themselves which, though obvious enough, are perhaps worth restating; and in the stating of them, questions of method inevitably arise.

Treatments for infertility may be divided into those which involve, beside the gynaecologist, none but the infertile couple; and those which involve a third party, as donor of egg, sperm or embryo, or as surrogate mother.

On the whole the strictly ethical problems peculiar to the first kind of treatment are few. People who raise ethical objections to the use, for example, of IVF treatment do so either because they fear the wider consequences of the fertilising of egg and sperm in the laboratory, or because they regard the technique as excessively expensive, given the comparatively few people who

243

benefit from it. (There are also those who have specifically religious objections; but these people will, presumably, not seek the treatment for themselves.) I shall return to the first of these objections later. The second, as I have said, I do not believe is a moral problem peculiar to this kind of procedure, but such as may arise from any medical advance whatever.

There may, of course, be technical decisions that have to be made. Is superovulation necessary to the success of IVF? How many embryos is the optimum number to insert in the uterus, with the best hope of successful implantation? These are questions on which lay people and moral philosophers are not entitled to have views. Even questions about the risk of multiple births may be thought to be more properly a matter for medical than for moral or social debate.

If we turn to the second set of treatments, however, the picture is very different. Here the gynaecologist is likely to find himself beset by moral advice, if not by actual commands and prohibitions. A doctor's normal duty is to take into account the good of his patient. In this case there must enter into his consideration both the good of any child born as a result of the procedures, and the good of the third party who is involved. At once new and wider moral problems present themselves, all of them interlocking. Some methods of alleviating the distress of infertility might have to be ruled out, on moral grounds.

I presume as a start that any gynaecologist, confronted by a case of infertility, will regard this as a condition that merits treatment (a view, incidentally, not shared by all of the lay public). Nevertheless, a gynaecologist might find himself in a position of saying to a particular couple that in their case there was nothing that it would be morally right to do.

There are, I believe, fairly acute problems that may arise from AID, not from the point of view of the donor, but from the point of view of the child and his nurturing parents. I shall return to these below. These family-centred problems are identical in the case of surrogacy using AID; but they are compounded by ethical problems relating to the woman who goes through the pregnancy and gives birth to the child. In the case of a surrogacy using IVF, where the child is genetically the child of the commissioning couple, and where the surrogate is simply acting as a living incubator, ethical problems are confined to those relating to the surrogate. What then are these problems? Are they capable of clear statement and of resolution?

It is here perhaps above all that it becomes impossible to separate the nature of the problem from its method of solution, in so far as solution is possible. At the centre of the ethical question is the question whether it is ever right to use one person as a means to the ends of another, however estimable these ends may seem. Does this not constitute exploitation in the bad sense of that word, whether or not the person used has expressed herself willing? The *Report on Human Fertilisation and Embryology* was, I believe, too vague and general on this point. In citing the argument that any use of a surrogate must constitute exploitation in the bad sense (an argument strongly canvassed in many quarters), we did not, I now think, take time enough to separate different strands within it. The word 'exploitation' is of course slippery and this is why, in using it as part of an argument against surrogacy, or, say, prostitution, one has to be careful to talk about 'bad' exploitation. But if this qualification has to be put in, one has to be prepared to specify what is 'bad' about it, in a given case. It is generally deemed ethically tolerable to exploit the particular skills of, say, an underwater diver, or a steeplejack, for ends not his own, provided that he understands the risks he is taking, chooses to use his skills in this way, and is properly rewarded for doing so. Indeed the charge of exploitation is generally withdrawn if the reward for the service is high enough. Yet in the case of the surrogate undertaking to become pregnant for another, if anything the argument goes the other way. Surrogacy is thought to approach nearer to moral respectability the less the surrogate is to be paid. (Equally, in the case of AID, it is thought to be morally better if the donor is not paid, and the recommendation of the Inquiry was that we should move towards non-payment of donors.) What accounts for this difference? No-one would say 'if we pay deep-sea divers a lot we shall get the wrong kind of divers, who go in for it only for the money'. Yet this is the kind of thing people say about sperm donors, and with even more passion about surrogate mothers. The disparity must be accounted for then by our special attitude towards the birth of children. Those who regard surrogacy in any form as bad exploitation do so not on the grounds that it is the using of one person as a means to the ends of another, nor even on the grounds that one person must not be put at risk for the sake of another, but on the grounds that pregnancy itself is intrinsically different from other kinds of risks or of service undertakings.

It is very difficult then to frame this argument in terms of principles of a general kind since pregnancy is its *particular* content. Nor do things go better if one tries to frame it in terms of the principle of utility. On the latter principle an act is deemed to be right if the benefits it brings outweigh the harms; wrong if the balance is the other way. And, it may be said, where a surrogate offers her services willingly, enjoys being pregnant, is in good health, and is psychologically tough enough not to be more than momentarily put out, or not put out at all, by handing her baby over when she has given birth to it; when moreover she needs the money she is paid and will enjoy its use; and when the commissioning couple have been desperate perhaps for years to have a child which they will now in some sense have . . . then all the balance is on the side of benefit, none on the side of harm. To introduce harm into this rosy picture is purely speculative. An opponent of surrogacy may say 'you cannot tell whether or not a woman will suffer harm from being a surrogate until years after the event'. He will quote, for example, the case of a woman who recently appeared on television and who claimed that after 5 years she still bitterly reproached herself for having acted as a surrogate, not knowing whether it was worse to have sold her own body, or sold her own son, though she had entered the agreement willingly, thinking that it would produce nothing but good. The same opponent, perhaps more plausibly, may say that we cannot weigh up the whole cost/benefit balance of surrogacy transactions, or indeed AID, until we have far more evidence than we have at present about the final outcome, the effect on the child and his commissioning parents. But, on the whole, utilitarian arguments seem to favour surrogacy; and its opponents must, if they are to express their views, express them in less rational terms, in terms that is to say of a 'guts reaction' or a sentiment.

To introduce sentiment as a factor in moral arguments may seem dangerous. Reason, or the weighing up of consequences which in moral arguments seem to be the same thing, is after all common to all circumstances and shared by everyone. It may produce definite answers to problems, correct solutions to dilemmas which can be universally accepted. Feelings, on the other hand, are notoriously diverse, changeable, incapable of justification, and certainly not of universal currency. Should they not be as far as possible eliminated from the decision-making process? We would all condemn a doctor who refused treatment to someone because he felt an antipathy towards him, or even because he was too squeamish to carry out the treatment. All such feelings should be put aside under the demand of his plain duty to treat. How can it be proper therefore to base a judgement about surrogacy as a possible treatment on so flimsy a foundation as sentiment?

There is a great deal of force in such arguments. It has to be said, however, that to attempt a description of a moral, as opposed to a prudential, argument which contains no reference to feelings or sentiment is to attempt the impossible. If no-one had any feeling that something was wrong, or that something was demanded, despite all difficulties, then there would be no such thing as morality. Moral ideals, after all, are embraced because they are attractive, because we would love to live up to them, not because they are thought to have, overall, the best practical outcome. If someone says, then, that there is an ideal of pregnancy where the woman becomes pregnant as a result of sexual intercourse which she has enjoyed with someone she loves, where the child is loved even before he is born, and where the birth is eagerly awaited because both of the partners look forward to welcoming this new baby into the family . . . if this is the ideal of pregnancy, then it is easy to see in how many respects the surrogate pregnancy departs from this ideal. Now it is plain to everyone that not all pregnancies satisfy these ideal conditions. There are many pregnancies as a result of rape; there are other forms of unwelcome pregnancies, and in some cases to put the resulting child out for adoption may seem the only right solution, or an abortion may be preferable to carrying the child to term. But that these kinds of disastrous pregnancies occur does not entail that departures from the ideal should be positively encouraged. And I suspect that those who are opposed to permitting surrogacy are really relying, in their opposition, not on reason but on a kind of regret that an ideal should be deliberately abandoned.

At the time of writing, to set up an agency to provide surrogate mothers for commissioning couples on a commercial basis is about to become a criminal offence. Such a ban on commercial surrogacy appears to have very wide support, both in parliament and among the general public. Here there is a widely perceived risk of bad exploitation, both of the potential surrogate and of the commissioning couples themselves. Moreover the legal tangles that might result from the kinds of contract drawn up by such agencies constitute a further reason against allowing the agencies to operate. The BMA, on the other hand, has recommended that gynaecologists should be permitted to provide the possibility of carefully regulated surrogacy for some of their infertile patients, without thereby putting themselves at risk as 'agents'. It may well be that the moral feelings of the members of the BMA are in fact a better reflection of the moral feelings of the general public than the Report of the Inquiry. And it is also possible that feelings about surrogacy may change fairly rapidly in the new climate of opinion about infertility treatment as a whole. Nevertheless it remains true that a gynaecologist who recommends surrogacy has a tremendously difficult moral decision to make, and he has to take responsibility for four people: the infertile couple, the surrogate and the resulting child.

If the gynaecologist has decided that surrogacy is, in general, a tolerable option, and in this he will be guided by the received wisdom among members of the profession, then he has to exercise his judgement as to whether in a particular case a surrogate can be found who will not suffer harm. But in addition in this and all other cases he has to consider the good of the child. Here we enter a moral minefield. I do not believe that gynaecologists should be asked to decide whether or not a particular couple will make good parents. It is true that the social services or the adoption societies are required to make such assessments in the case of every adoption. But this, at first a means of protecting the interest of an existing child, has now become the more stringent a requirement as the number of children for adoption becomes smaller. The position is not strictly comparable to the case of an infertile couple seeking treatment from a gynaecologist. Obviously in the case of IVF, or indeed tubal surgery, the doctor will have to make a professional decision about the fitness of the woman for surgery and the likelihood of success. But this sort of decision should not be confused with purely social screening; nor should one kind of reason for giving or withholding treatment be disguised as the other. This would seem almost too obvious a point to make were it not for the fact that doctors quite often slide in their discussion from one kind of 'screening' to the other, with or without the slippery intermediate step of 'psychological screening'. The word 'fit' is conveniently ambiguous for those who want surreptitiously to withhold treatment from some patients. These patients could be described as 'unfit' in a variety of senses.

In this connection it is sometimes asked what decision doctors ought to make if they are asked for treatments, normally used for infertile couples, for those who are not, or not known to be, infertile, but who for various reasons want to make use of surrogacy or of AID. It may be that, at least in the foreseeable future, gynaecologists will feel able to embark on the producing of an 'artificial' family only where there is evidence of some malfunction (infertility) or where the risk of passing on an inheritable disease is so great that IVF could be recommended (and as the success rate of IVF gradually improves, this is more likely to become an option). In practice this will probably be what happens. But a doctor must make up his mind what to say if a woman comes to him saying she wants AID, and when asked whether her partner is infertile, and by whom the tests were carried out, says 'I have no partner; but I want a baby all the same.' To make the decisions involved in this kind of case must always be very hard for a gynaecologist. He may say 'There's nothing wrong with you, so I won't treat you.' But to say this may simply be refusing to face the problem. I believe that it will be easier if clinics for the provision of AID (and perhaps surrogacy of a non-commercial kind) are established which have a consistent policy. Individual doctors will not then be called on to make difficult decisions about whom they will treat, and whom they will not. I very much hope that, one day, such clinics may be established within every regional health authority.

Apart from questions about whether an individual or a couple will make good parents, there are further, perhaps more general, questions about the good of the child that arise in all 'third-party' kinds of family. It is often said by proponents of surrogacy that at least we can be sure of one thing: the child who results from a surrogacy arrangement will be well-looked after and will have a good life, because the commissioning parents wanted him very much and were even prepared to pay large sums of money for him. I believe that this is a false conclusion. If you had very badly wanted a dog, you might, when you got it, be supposed to be about to look after it well and give it a good life. But the analogous argument does not hold, in the case of children. You may indeed look after the wanted child well; but it is possible that you will look after him too well. If this much-wanted child is the only child (and this is very likely to be the case, if he was the outcome of an expensive and difficult surrogate arrangement) then the pressures on that child may be extreme. Unlike a dog, he may suffer not from neglect, but from over-attention, or excessive expectations. If he turns out a mediocre child, or if he rebels against his parents, those parents may feel as they would if they had spent huge sums on a racehorse of impeccable origins, who nevertheless did not show form. But there would be no selling the child as they could the dud racehorse. Reproaches, though doubtless illogical, would be difficult to avoid.

Again, there are questions of secrecy or openness which, though not the gynaecologist's direct concern, may yet come into his mind when he thinks about the wider implications of what he is doing, and the advice he may be called upon to give his patients. Fortunately to pursue these questions in the present context would take too long, and would in any case probably lead us rather far from the ethical problems of gynaecology itself. Nevertheless it has to be said that there are problems, and they are thorny and difficult, as well as controversial.

It is time to turn now, though fairly briefly, to the whole range of ethical problems arising indirectly from IVF treatment. I refer to the problems concerned with research. Even though a gynaecologist may not himself work in a research laboratory, he cannot dissociate himself from the problems involved, since the continued use of the techniques such as IVF depends on prior and continuing research. No-one could conscientiously recommend or practice IVF, unless research were to continue, to improve its success rate; and such research inevitably involves the use of human embryos which are not going to be implanted, and are known from the start not even to be intended for replacement in the uterus. There may be gynaecologists who would regard all such research as morally repugnant. If they embarked on IVF treatment at all, these gynaecologists would presumably insist on inserting all available embryos into the uterus, or if there were any spares, would immediately destroy them. But it is hard to envisage many gynaecologists holding such views. For most of them, continued research, either using spare embryos or embryos fertilised specially for the purposes of research, must seem an essential concomitant of IVF itself. And it is this view, this relatively uncritical acceptance of research as something that has been going on unimpeded for years, which it is hard to get the general public to accept or even understand. For the public, the problems of embryo research are new: they have heard about such research only in the past few years. Gynaecologists are as familiar with it as they are with other research, the foundation upon which medical practice is founded.

Nevertheless there may be a few gynaecologists who accept the fundamentalist view that the embryo immediately after fertilisation is a human *person*; and must therefore be granted the full protection of the law, and not used for research even with parental permission. (I doubt whether even these gynaecologists would be fully happy with the title of the Enoch Powell Bill, talked out of Parliament in the Spring of 1985: The Protection of the Unborn Child Bill. Whatever his moral views, a professional is likely to insist on the distinction between an embryo consisting of sixteen cells and a 'child'.) The moral problem such anti-research gynaecologists have to face is this: if they are convinced of the moral rightness of their own views, should they campaign to make it illegal for anyone to act against them? If a doctor dislikes or disapproves of a certain treatment, or a procedure consequent on such treatment, should he be content simply to abstain from the practices he disapproves of; or should he attempt to get a law passed which makes such practices illegal? This question goes to the very heart of the vexed matter of the relation between morality and the law, a question that has occupied philosophers and jurists for years. Although the medical profession has no direct access to Parliament, no special relation with legislators, yet the profession as a whole is influential. What the profession introduces as guidelines for their colleagues may well have influence on what Parliament decides in due course. If this is so then the deliverances of the individual medical conscience may, though perhaps only after a long time, influence the future state of the law. If the majority of doctors morally disapproved of abortion, for example, and individually refused abortions to their patients, then in the end it is likely that the law would be changed. Gynaecologists as a profession cannot evade the responsibility of deciding what should and what should not be permitted, even though their influence on the course of legislation is only indirect.

As far as I know, a majority of gynaecologists are in favour of research using human embryos, provided that it is subject to controls and monitoring. Certainly the voluntary body set up to examine and control research, and establish guidelines, has been widely welcomed within the profession and can at the time of writing be deemed a success. If this is so, then it is of the utmost importance that gynaecologists should explain the basis of their opinion, and justify it. And so we return to the question of method. *How* is the continuation of research to be justified? How are Members of Parliament, or of the pro-life organisations, to be persuaded that research is not only all right, but actually *right*? Utilitarian arguments must have their place here. For law must be based on a crude utilitarianism, among other considerations. Nothing should become law which is not broadly seen to be beneficial to a substantial number of people, without penalising too many people on the way.

But besides reciting the benefits that would accrue from research, the medical profession has also to face the irrational and necessarily unargued position of those who, relying on their feelings (and we have seen that their feelings are indeed relevant to the morality of the practices) say that, benefits notwithstanding, they hold that such research is wrong. Here I believe that gynaecologists have an important role to play. For they more than anyone, being experts, can persuade people that the embryo immediately after fertilisation is not identical with a child, is not indeed even a potential child unless certain elaborate conditions are fulfilled to allow it to develop into a child and is not therefore a human *person*, whose life must be protected. The difference between the collection of four or eight or sixteen cells and the curled-up fetus in the womb needs to be emphasised so that people get used to the idea. I have heard it suggested that a different name ought to be used to refer to the pre-14-day embryo, in order to make research more acceptable. I do not think that such a transparent semantic trick would work; nevertheless I believe that there is a lot to be done in the way of educating those members of the public who are, in principle, in favour of research, and its fruits, but who yet jib at what they regard as the misuse of humans. No-one is better placed to carry out this education than gynaecologists; and they have a duty to seize every opportunity to do it. It is not that they need to give people new *reasons* for accepting research, or not this alone. The aim must be to produce a change in attitude which enables people to recognise distinctions where these exist. A gynaecologist is professionally committed to caring for women and to enabling them to have children. If gynaecologists are prepared to use the four-cell embryo in research, then this fact will, in the end, change people's moral feelings. Without such change not only is research in jeopardy, but all kinds of desirable improvements in the treatment of infertility are at risk. Perhaps the greatest moral problem that gynaecologists have is the problem of explaining their own moral views, and persuading people that they are to be trusted. The reaction of the public to the medical profession is a strange mixture. On the one hand we treat doctors as gods, in those hands we are ready to place ourselves in moments of crisis and despair : on the other hand doctors are confused with the Mad Scientist, whose passion for knowledge will in the end undermine our moral certainties, and our security. Gynaecologists must use their powers of persuasion, and, at the same time, allay some of these ignorant and alarmist fears.

Male infertility and *in vitro* fertilisation

It is estimated that in approximately 30–50 per cent of infertile couples the cause lies wholly or partly with the male partner (Gottesman & Bain, 1980). The vast majority of these men are physiologically and anatomically normal, with only a small proportion having detectable abnormalities such as endocrinological disorders, varicocele, antisperm antibodies or scrotal hyperthermia. To date the treatments given to these men have been legion, with largely disappointing results, and where an improvement in semen quality has been achieved it has not necessarily been accompanied by an increased incidence of pregnancy. Many of the 'conventional' therapies for male infertility are empirically based, reflecting our poor understanding of the physiological processes involved in spermatogenesis and sperm maturation.

Until this gap in our knowledge is filled, real advances in the treatment or prevention of male infertility are unlikely. However, theoretically, less spermatozoa are required to achieve fertilization of oocytes *in vitro* than *in vivo* and the fact that this process could be assessed and manipulated under laboratory conditions led Edwards and Steptoe some 15 years ago to believe that fertilization *in vitro* could be established using subnormal semen from infertile men for the insemination of their wives' oocytes (Edwards & Steptoe, 1980). Although the incidence of fertilization in these cases was low, and pregnancies were not established, the assumption that IVF could be a treatment for the infertile male was reintroduced 4 years ago in Bourn Hall Clinic (Cohen et al, 1984a), and an effective treatment for the infertile male has since been developed.

By utilising IVF procedures for the treatment of male infertility it is now possible to by-pass to a certain extent the lack of effective pharmacological and surgical methods presently available. IVF therefore offers treatment for those men presently afflicted by infertility problems and, by opening the door for further research, will undoubtedly enable future generations of infertile men to be treated more successfully.

ASSESSMENT OF MALE INFERTILITY TREATMENTS

As already stated, most infertile men have no detectable abnormalities other than a poor semen analysis, and it is to this 'idiopathic' group that the widest range of treatments have been applied. The critical evaluation of such therapies presents many problems for a number of reasons, including disagreements about the normality of semen, variable patient selection criteria, the lack in many instances of properly controlled (placebo or non-treatment) studies, the necessity to assess the female partner's reproductive capability in depth, and the failure of many studies to take into account the duration of a couple's infertility at the time of treatment. Most published work on male infertility therapies can be criticised on some, if not all, of these grounds.

The duration of infertility is of critical importance, since it has been shown that approximately 20 per cent of couples with a 2-year history of male-related infertility, achieve a pregnancy over the subsequent 3 years without any treatment (Aafjes et al, 1978). This 'spontaneous' pregnancy rate is reduced to 5 per cent after 6 years of infertility. Consequently care must be taken when interpreting results of treatment which have been applied to men with only a short duration of infertility, especially when control studies are not performed.

SUMMARY OF 'CONVENTIONAL' MALE INFERTILITY TREATMENTS

Men with varicocele

Varicocele has been estimated to be present in as many as 30 per cent of infertile men (Dubin & Amelar, 1971) compared with an incidence of 10–23 per cent in normal males (Verstoppen & Steeno, 1977). The relationship between varicocele and male infertility was generally accepted up until the mid-1970s, when several authors began to question the role of varicocele correction (Nilsson et al, 1979; Rodriguez-Rigau et al, 1978). Pregnancy rates as high as 70 per cent have been reported following surgical repair (Ferrie et al, 1982; Abdelmassih et al, 1982; Lome & Ross, 1977; Dubin & Amelar, 1975). However, Vermeulen and Vanderweghe (1984) could not demonstrate any increase in the incidence of pregnancy following surgery when a comparison was made with similar patients who were not treated. Other authors have also noted no increase in either semen quality or pregnancy rates following varicocele correction (Nilsson et al, 1979). However the evaluation of the efficacy of varicolectomy is difficult, since the severity of the varicocele varies between patients and the interpretations of the diagnostic tests differ from clinic to clinic (Getzoff, 1975).

Men with antisperm antibodies

Sperm-agglutinating or immobilising antibodies have been estimated to occur in 3–13 per cent of infertile men (Hargreave et al, 1980; Aafjes & Van der Vijver, 1976). The use of corticosteroids has produced good results with regard to decreasing antibody titres but an increase in pregnancy rates could only occasionally be demonstrated (Dondero et al, 1979; Baker et al, 1983; Hendry et al, 1981; Hargreave & Elton, 1982). The incidence of serious side-effects with this form of therapy has been rather high, ranging from 2 to 6 per cent (Schulman & Schulman, 1982; Hendry et al, 1981).

Men with scrotal hyperthermia

Increased testicular temperature is known to have a detrimental effect on spermatogenesis and a variety of cooling devices have been designed in order to achieve a long-term reduction in scrotal temperature (Zorgniotti & Sealfon, 1984). Using ice-packs, jockey shorts or special evaporative devices for oligospermic men, may increase sperm density in patients with proven scrotal hyperthermia, irrespective of whether the men have a varicocele or not (Zorgniotti et al, 1982; Mulcahy, 1984).

Men with endocrinological abnormalities

These patients account for only 1–3 per cent of the total population of infertile men (Aafjes & Van der Vijver, 1976).

Hypogonadotrophic males

There are numerous causes of this condition (chromosomal, infective, metabolic, traumatic and neoplastic), and understandably the efficacy of gonadotrophin and/or testosterone replacement therapy for these patients is related to the individual aetiology. Because of the rare nature of these conditions there have been no large-scale studies published. However several authors have reported single cases in which such patients have achieved a pregnancy following gonadotrophin replacement therapy (Paulsen et al, 1970; Johnson, 1978; Schrofner, 1978).

Hyperprolactinaemic males

This is also an uncommon condition with consistently elevated prolactin levels being demonstrated in only 2/68 hypogonadotrophic males (del Pozo, 1982). The hyperprolactinaemia may be associated with hypothalamic, pituitary, renal or liver disorders and may result in reduced androgen production. Treatment of affected males with either testosterone or bromocryptine therapy has been reported to increase androgen levels and sexual potency (Carter et al, 1978; Franks et al, 1978), however there is little evidence that there is any corresponding increase in semen quality or pregnancy rates (Hovatta et al, 1979).

Men with idiopathic infertility

Antioestrogens

These compounds increase gonadotrophin secretion by blocking the negative feedback of the testicular–hypothalamic–pituitary pathway. Originally used for follicular stimulation in the female, they have been applied to male infertility with largely disappointing results. Clomiphene citrate was the first to be used; however the outcome has generally been unsatisfactory, with no increase in seminal or histological parameters being demonstrated (Schellen, 1982; Charny, 1979). Ronnberg (1980) performed a double-blind, cross-over, placebo-controlled study on a small group of infertile males, and whilst significant increases in sperm density, FSH, LH and testosterone levels were reported following the administration of clomiphene, there was no corresponding increase in pregnancy rates.

Another antioestrogen, tamoxifen, has less intrinsic oestrogenic activity than clomiphene, and should therefore be theoretically more suitable for the treatment of the infertile male. It has been shown to produce a two-fold increase in sperm density, and promising results have been reported following its use (Comhaire, 1976; Schill & Landthaler, 1981), although Buvat et al (1983) could not rule out the possibility of a placebo effect.

Gonadotrophins

Apart from its use in hypogonadotrophic males, parenteral gonadotrophin therapy has been administered to men with idiopathic infertility for the past 15 years with inconclusive results, both human menopausal gonadotrophin and human chorionic gonadotrophin being used singularly or in combination (Lunenfeld et al, 1967; Homonnai et al, 1978).

Androgens

The administration of large amounts of testosterone suppresses the hypothalamic–pituitary axis, thereby producing severe oligospermia or even azoospermia. On cessation of therapy large amounts of FSH and LH are secreted, and a corresponding overproduction of spermatozoa is sometimes seen (rebound therapy), but results have been inconclusive (Getzoff, 1955; Lamensdorf et al, 1975). The androgen mesterolone (Pro-viron) lacks the hypothalamic inhibitory effect of testosterone and cannot be aromatised to oestrogens. Promising results have been reported (Hendry et al, 1973; Schellen, 1970); however in a double-blind, cross-over, placebo-controlled study of oligospermic men, no significant influence of mesterolone was found (Aafjes et al, 1983).

Other agents

Many other therapies for male infertility have been administered over the past 30 years. Kallikrein (a kinin-releasing proteinase) has been used both systemically and as an additive to ejaculated semen (Schill, 1979), which has then been prepared and instrumentally inseminated. No consistent results have been found following such therapy (Batterinck et al, 1983; Comhaire & Vermeulen, 1983).

Artificial insemination of husbands' semen

Artificial insemination with husbands' semen (AIH) is largely unsuccessful when applied to the oligoasthenospermic male (Russel, 1960), with the pregnancy rate per cycle following intra-uterine AIH being only 2 per cent (Hewitt et al, 1985). Additives such as caffeine have been shown to increase the percentage motility of ejaculated semen (Schoenfield et al, 1973) and this therapy may be applicable for men with borderline semen. Filtration methods and proteolytic agents may be useful for men with specific disorders such as seminal plasma debris and high-viscosity semen (Cohen & Aafjes, 1982). Two special groups of men for whom AIH may be particularly successful are those patients with relative oligospermia due to a high semen volume (dilution oligospermia), and patients with retrograde ejaculation.

RESULTS OF IN VITRO FERTILISATION THERAPY

Three centres to date have published data on the outcome of the application of IVF for exclusively male or combined male and female infertility (Cohen et al, 1985a; Yovich & Stanger, 1984; Mahadevan & Trounson, 1984). A summary of the results from these three groups is given in Table 14.1. It can be seen that the criteria for male infertility varied slightly from centre to centre; however all three groups have restricted treatment to patients with a long history of infertility and who were either unsuitable for, or had had an unsuccessful outcome following, conventional treatments.

The incidence of fertilisation, and therefore the proportion of cycles resulting in embryo replacement and subsequent pregnancy, varied from centre to centre (Table 14.1). This is to be expected since the same centres report varying success following IVF in cases of tubal infertility, when normospermic samples are used. This variation is due to differences in follicular stimulation regimes, follicular phase monitoring (endocrinological and/or ultrasonic), methods of oocyte recovery (laparoscopic or ultrasound-directed) as well as embryo culture and replacement techniques.

In order to achieve success by the application of IVF in cases of male infertility, modified semen collection, preparation and insemination techniques are required. These also vary from one centre to another and it is therefore unlikely that centres will produce identical results in such cases. Despite this, the incidence of fertilisation (percentage of oocytes fertilised) was as high as 51–79 per cent when semen from infertile men was used for insemination. The proportion of cycles resulting in an embryo replacement was reasonably similar in all three groups (60–76 per cent); however the

Table 14.1 Summary of results from three centres where IVF was applied to infertile men

Infertility centres	Cause of infertility	Duration of infertility (years) mean range	No. of treatment cycles	Proportion of oocytes fertilised (%)	Proportion of cycles resulting in embryo re-placement (%)	Proportion of cycles resulting in pregnancy (%)	Criteria for male infertility		
							Oligospermia	Asthenospermia	Teratospermia
Bourn Hall (UK) (Cohen et al, 1985a)	Male only	6 (3–16)	62	98/193 (51)	42/62 (68)	14/62 (23)	$\leqslant 10 \times 10^6$/ml	and $\leqslant 20\%$ motile	and $\geqslant 80\%$ abnormal forms
	Male plus female	8 (2–15)	102	167/283 (59)	77/102 (76)	16/102 (16)		or	or
Melbourne (Australia) (Trounson & Wood, 1984)	Male only	?	134	101/172 (59)	81/134 (60)	15/134 (11)	$< 20 \times 10^6$/ml	and $< 50\%$ motile	and $> 40\%$ abnormal forms
Perth (Australia) (Yovich & Stanger, 1984)	Male only	'Prolonged'	21	39/66 (59)	?	6/31 (19)	$< 20 \times 10^6$/ml	and $< 60\%$ motile	and $> 60\%$ abnormal forms
	Male plus female	'Prolonged'	10	30/38 (79)	?				

incidence of pregnancy (per treatment cycle) ranged from 11 to 23 per cent, possibly reflecting differences in embryo quality and replacement techniques.

When it is remembered that these pregnancy rates are *per treatment cycle* rather than per year, and *include* cases of failure of fertilisation (where embryo replacement could not be performed), then the results are particularly promising, bearing in mind that the spontaneous incidence of pregnancy in couples with a similar duration of infertility is less than 1 per cent per cycle (Aafjes et al, 1978).

Outcome according to semen abnormality

One group (Bourn Hall) has presented its data according to both the type of semen abnormality encountered and whether the couple's infertility was due to exclusively male, or combined male and female, factors. The outcome of treatment using these parameters is shown in Table 14.2.

Pregnancies were established in couples where the men had a variety of abnormalities, all these patients having a long duration of infertility (mean 6 and 8 years for the exclusively male and combined male and female groups respectively). The proportion of oocytes fertilised *in vitro* was lowest in cases of exclusively male infertility due to combined oligoasthenospermia (30 per cent), these patients also having the lowest proportion of cycles resulting in embryo replacement (39 per cent). However, for the patients in this category who had embryos replaced the pregnancy rate per cycle was 33 per cent,

Table 14.2   Results of IVF Therapy for male and 'combined' infertility—Bourn Hall, 1982–84

Type of male infertility	Infertility caused by man only (A) or by both partners (B)	No. of patients (no. of cycles)	Proportion of oocytes fertilised (%)	Proportion of cycles resulting in embryo replacement (%)	Proportion of pregnancies per oocyte recovery (%)	Proportion of pregnancies per embryo replacement (%)
Oligo-spermia	A	11 (20)	33/54 (61)	16/20 (80)	2/20 (10)	2/16 (13)
	B	16 (32)	40/88 (46)	20/32 (63)	3/32 (9)	3/20 (15)
Astheno-spermia	A	9 (12)	28/40 (70)	10/12 (83)	6/12 (50)	6/10 (60)
	B	27 (47)	101/138 (73)	40/47 (85)	8/47 (17)	8/40 (20)
Oligo- & astheno-spermia	A	15 (23)	21/70 (30)	9/23 (39)	3/23 (13)	3/9 (33)
	B	13 (18)	21/45 (47)	14/18 (78)	4/18 (22)	4/14 (29)
Autoanti-bodies	A	3 (3)	8/11 (73)	3/3 (100)	1/3 (33)	1/3 (33)
	B	4 (4)	5/11 (46)	3/4 (75)	1/4 (25)	1/3 (33)
Terato-spermia	A	3 (4)	8/18 (44)	4/4 (100)	2/4 (50)	2/4 (50)
	B	1 (1)	0/1 (–)	0/1 (–)	0/1 (–)	0/1 (–)
All patients	A	41 (62)	98/193 (51)	42/62 (68)	14/62 (23)	14/42 (33)
	B	61 (102)	167/283 (59)	77/102 (76)	16/102 (16)	16/77 (21)

which is comparable to that of tubal infertility patients (Edwards et al, 1984).

The highest incidence of fertilisation was found in couples with exclusively male infertility due to asthenospermia only (70 per cent), reflected in the highest proportion of embryo replacement cycles (83 per cent) and a 50 per cent pregnancy rate per treatment cycle (60 per cent) pregnancy rate per embryo replacement). Although good sperm motility is considered necessary for *in vivo* fertilisation (in order for sufficient numbers of spermatozoa to reach the ampulla and therefore be in a position to fertilise an oocyte), it may well be that asthenospermic spermatozoa are perfectly able to achieve fertilisation once they are brought into close proximity with a mature oocyte.

Slow spermatozoal progression may be an asset rather than a hindrance to *in vitro* fertility since the incidence of fertilisation is not reduced when freeze–thaw spermatozoa are used for *in vitro* insemination (Cohen et al, 1985b). Moreover it was shown that 'cold' exposed and other physiologically slow spermatozoa have a higher hamster egg penetration rate than spermatozoa with normal progression (Cohen et al, 1982a, 1985c).

The overall incidence of fertilisation in cases of exclusively male and combined male and female infertility was 51 and 59 per cent respectively, which is a reduction from the 80 per cent overall fertilisation rate of oocytes achieved with normospermic specimens in cases of exclusively tubal infertility at Bourn Hall (Edwards et al, 1984). However, despite this fact, the incidence of pregnancy per embryo replacement was high, and as it was different in the two groups (33 and 21 per cent for male and 'combined' infertility respectively), this raises the interesting possibility already noted (Cohen et al, 1985a) that the reduced incidence of fertilisation in cases of male infertility may be balanced by a more receptive endometrium in couples where the female partner is reproductively normal. Cases involving an element of tubal infertility due to a proven previous infective process appear to have a reduced incidence of embryo implantation, with residual uterine effects of chlamydial infection possibly being responsible (Rowland et al, 1985).

Factors influencing the outcome of IVF therapy for male infertility

As already stated, the utilisation of IVF therapy for cases of male infertility necessitates modifications of some of the standard techniques that are employed in IVF practice when normospermic specimens are being handled.

(a) The number of embryos replaced

As is the case with tubal infertility patients, the replacement of more than one embryo per cycle will produce better results (Edwards et al, 1984; Cohen et al, 1984b).

(b) Number of oocytes recovered

It is absolutely essential to recover adequate numbers of oocytes per cycle in cases of male infertility, bearing in mind the reduced fertilisation rate in such couples. At Bourn Hall the proportion of such patients having an embryo replacement was 52 per cent when only one oocyte had been recovered, this figure rising to 80 per cent when two or more oocytes were recovered (Cohen et al, 1984b).

(c) Collection methods

The use of split ejaculates, thereby producing a relatively spermatozoal-rich first fraction and improving the chance of fertilisation even in cases of poor semen, is mandatory in most of these cases (Cohen et al, 1984b). Specimens can also be collected into a variety of solutions (culture medium or donor serum) for special cases such as highly viscous semen or seminal plasma antisperm antibodies (Cohen et al, 1982b; Fishel & Edwards, 1982). In cases of severe oligoasthenospermia a series of specimens can be collected, prepared, stored at room temperature and aggregated in order to allow sufficient spermatozoa to be available at the time of insemination (Cohen et al, 1985c).

(d) Semen preparation

Once collected, the actual preparation of the semen is of vital importance. In cases with normal semen standard centrifugation is adequate; however merely centrifuging oligoasthenospermic semen does not always produce sufficient motile spermatozoa in the insemination pellet.

The aim of semen preparation for IVF in cases of male infertility is to produce a final suspension containing 50 000 active spermatozoa per ml, which is free of contaminating debris and cells. Simple centrifugation tends not to rid the insemination droplet of these latter two problems.

In some cases as little as 0·2 ml of such a suspension is actually needed to achieve successful *in vitro* fertilisation of oocytes, which means that even severely oligospermic patients can be successfully treated. All the modifications of semen preparation employed in these cases are designed to separate as high a proportion of active spermatozoa from the total ejaculate as is possible.

The effects of some of the procedures employed in such patients, in terms of the proportion of oocytes fertilised and the proportion of treatment cycles resulting in embryo replacement, are shown in Table 14.3. It can be seen that the standard centrifugation of semen culture medium (Purdy, 1982) resulted in 50 per cent of all oocytes being fertilised, with 54 per cent of these treatment cycles resulting in embryo replacement. These figures are increased to 56 and 75 per cent respectively when, after centrifugation,

Table 14.3 The effect of different methods of semen preparation on fertilisation rates in cases of male infertility (Cohen et al, 1985a)

	Proportion of oocytes fertilized (%)		Proportion of cycles resulting in embryo replacement (%)	
Centrifugation	52/104	(50)	21/39	(54)
Sedimentation after centrifugation	144/256	(56)	60/80	(75)
Layering before centrifugation	59/88	(67)	21/23	(91)

sedimentation of the suspension is allowed to occur for some hours; after which time the upper portion of the droplet is pipetted off and used for insemination. Good results were also obtained by another method of semen preparation termed 'layering', in which a quantity of culture medium is carefully pipetted onto liquefied semen and left to stand for up to 60 minutes at room temperature. Active spermatozoa swim upwards into the medium layer which is then removed, mixed with more culture medium as necessary and the resulting suspension centrifuged in order to produce the final insemination droplet. This procedure produces a final suspension which is relatively free of debris and cellular contaminants, whilst at the same time achieving a high concentration of motile spermatozoa. Using this technique, 67 per cent of all oocytes were successfully fertilised, with a remarkable 91 per cent of all treatment cycles resulting in embryo replacement. However, the latter method can only be employed in cases where the spermatozoa have sufficient progression to cross the semen–medium barrier and therefore for most cases of abnormal semen, sedimentation of non-motile spermatozoa, cells and debris following centrifugation is by far the superior method.

(e) Manipulation of oocytes

When pronuclei are not present 14–24 hours after insemination, the oocytes can be transferred to fresh culture medium and reinseminated using either an aliquot of the original sperm suspension or a freshly produced and prepared semen specimen, depending upon the situation. In cases where few active spermatozoa are available at insemination, because of low numbers in the semen and the inevitable wastage during preparation, parts of the cumulus mass surrounding the oocytes can be removed in order to create access to the zona pellucida.

WHY SHOULD IVF GIVE BETTER RESULTS THAN CONVENTIONAL TREATMENTS?

The fact that successful fertilisation of oocytes with subsequent pregnancy can be achieved in couples where the man has oligoasthenospermia of an extreme degree (in some cases $<0.5 \times 10^6$ motile spermatozoa/ml, Table

14.4), indicates that the poor chance of *in vivo* conception occurring in such cases is due to a simple mathematical problem; insufficient numbers of spermatozoa reaching the ampulla in time for fertilisation to be achieved. *In vitro* fertilisation enables an increase in the number of spermatozoal/oocyte contacts to occur, by by-passing sperm transport barriers. In the *in-vivo* situation huge numbers of spermatozoa need to be deposited in the vagina at intercourse in order to enable only a relatively small number to reach the mature oocyte in the fallopian tube. In the process, spermatozoa are 'lost' in the vagina, cervical mucus, uterotubal junction, the 'wrong' fallopian tube and the pouch of Douglas. This has been considered in the past to provide a form of selection process (Krzanowska, 1974; Ahlgren, 1975), enabling only 'good-quality' spermatozoa to be in a position to achieve fertilisation. However, good motility of spermatozoa does not necessarily correlate with good fertilising capacity or the absence of genetic abnormalities, and despite fears expressed previously (Shuber & Bain, 1982), none of the three centres who have published results of IVF using poor-quality semen have found any increase in the incidence of spontaneous abortion or fetal abnormality in these cases.

On the basis of these assumptions one could consider intra-uterine

Table 14.4 Seven couples in which the man had a motile sperm count of less than 0.5×10^6/ml and *in vitro* fertilisation was successful (Cohen et al, 1985a)

Cause of infertility	Age of female partner	Duration of infertility	Semen analysis			Proportion of oocytes fertilised and recovered	Outcome of treatment
			Concentration ($\times 10^6$/ml)	Percentage motility	Progressive activity		
Bilateral salpingectomy oligo-asthenospermia	29	8	2	20	Low	2/3 1/1	One child delivered
Bilateral occlusion oligo-asthenospermia	31	6	0.8	15	Low	1/2 1/1	One child delivered
Bilateral occlusion, asthenospermia	39	10	50	1	Low	1/1 2/2	One child delivered
Bilateral occlusion, oligo-asthenospermia	35	10	2	5	Moderate	1/1	One child delivered
Testicular teratoma, cryostorage of semen	31	6	21*	2	Low	7/12	Singleton pregnancy (aborted)
Oligo-asthenospermia	35	11	2	25	Moderate	1/4	One child delivered
Asthenospermia	33	6	31	1	Moderate	4/5	Triplet pregnancy (aborted)

*Post-thawing.

insemination but a recent comparison of IVF and intra-uterine AIH showed that IVF was the superior method (Hewitt et al, 1985). Intratubal insemination may be a more obvious method to choose, but results have not yet been published.

On a cautionary note it must be realised that the three groups who have published results on male infertility and IVF therapy to date, all have established IVF programmes with pregnancy rates in excess of 20 per cent per cycle for cases of tubal infertility with normal semen. Figure 14.1 shows how the proportion of cycles resulting in embryo replacement, in cases of male infertility, has risen over a 4-year period in one of these clinics as techniques improved. Clearly, as IVF therapy for male infertility requires specialised techniques, treatment should not be offered without first having established a viable and successful 'basic IVF' service, otherwise the results will almost certainly be disappointing.

Is it possible to predict which males will achieve fertilisation?

Since it is clear that pregnancies can be established from infertile men with extremely abnormal semen (Table 14.4), there are at present no established lower limits on which suitability for IVF treatment can be assessed. The

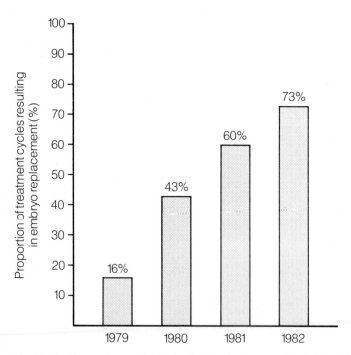

Figure 14.1   The incidence of successful *in vitro* fertilization in cases of male infertility in one clinic over a 4-year period (Trounson & Wood, Melbourne, Australia).

criteria for the various parameters of semen abnormality need to be re-evaluated in the light of IVF experience, and it may be that a separate set of definitions will be needed for IVF practice. In the meantime, one of the most important aspects, especially from the patient's point of view, is whether it is possible, in advance, to predict if fertilisation *in vitro* will be achieved. In order to answer this question, guidelines have been suggested based on observations made during previous IVF attempts when patients with differing semen problems have been treated and, in addition, various 'screening tests' have been proposed, based upon the ability of a given patient's spermatozoa to penetrate structures other than human oocytes.

PARAMETERS OF THE SEMEN ANALYSIS

(1) Sperm density

Low concentrations of spermatozoa have not been found to inhibit the fertilisation process, since 41 per cent of oocytes were fertilised by men with extreme oligospermia ($<5 \times 10^6$/ml) (Cohen et al, 1984b).

(2) Percentage motility

The percentage motility of spermatozoa does not correlate with the incidence of fertilisation; men with extreme asthenospermia (<5 per cent motility) fertilising human oocytes as often as men with moderate asthenospermia (16–20 per cent motility), the fertilisation rates being 63 and 60 per cent respectively (Cohen et al, 1984b).

(3) Motile sperm density

The motile sperm density can be calculated by multiplying the sperm density by the percentage motility, and one group have reported a significant reduction in fertilisation rates when severely oligospermic ($\leqslant 5 \times 10^6$ motile sperm per ml) samples were used compared with moderately oligospermic specimens (6–$11 \cdot 5 \times 10^6$ motile sperm per ml) (Yovich & Stanger, 1984).

Since the actual number of spermatozoa in each insemination droplet ($0 \cdot 5$–$2 \cdot 0 \times 10^5$ motile sperm per ml), was standardised in their practice, this would suggest a reduced capacity for fertilisation by spermatozoa from severely oligospermic men, yet despite this finding, some pregnancies were achieved in both groups. The importance of the motile sperm density has been questioned, however (Cohen et al, 1985a). The latter group only found a reduction in the incidence of fertilisation when the motile sperm density was $\leqslant 2 \times 10^6$ per ml, and even then seven pregnancies were achieved in 15 couples where the man had a motile sperm density of $<0 \cdot 5 \times 10^6$ per ml (Table 14.4), indicating that a low motile sperm density is by no means an absolute guide to the success or failure of IVF therapy.

(4) Forward progression of spermatozoa

It has been reported that *in vitro* fertilisation of oocytes does not occur regardless of the sperm density, if the initial semen sample contains spermatozoa with less than 20 per cent forward progression (Mahadevan & Trounson, 1984). However Cohen et al (1985a) found that in terms of both fertilisation and pregnancy rates, weak or abnormal progression of spermatozoa was not important.

(5) The presence of cells in the ejaculate

The fertilisation of oocytes *in vitro* is impaired by the presence of both phagocytic inflammatory cells and, to a lesser extent, by large numbers of cells of unknown type within the ejaculate, regardless of other semen parameters (Table 14.5). This may be due to inflammatory cells releasing cytotoxins reactive with the membranes of oocytes or spermatozoa, as demonstrated in the zona free hamster egg test (Berger et al, 1982). The detrimental effects of such cells may be minimised by the specialised semen preparation techniques outlined previously. Layering and sedimentation methods were particularly beneficial in these patients, with subsequent pregnancy rates ranging from 11 to 38 per cent per treatment cycle, despite the reduced fertilisation rates encountered (Table 14.5). It is therefore evident that predicting the outcome of IVF therapy by semen parameters alone is unreliable, and consequently more dynamic screening procedures have been proposed.

(6) *In vivo* cervical mucus penetration test

A poor postcoital test may be caused by a single detectable abnormality in the female or male partner, or by a combination of both subnormal cervical mucus and subnormal spermatozoa. *In vivo* and *in vitro* mucus penetration tests are useful tools in the general fertility assessment of a couple, but there are no clear guidelines in performing and interpreting the various assays (Blasco, 1984). Hull et al (1984) suggested that a low or poor postcoital test

Table 14.5 Fertilisation and pregnancy in cases with an abnormal semen analysis and the presence of cells in the specimen used for *in vitro* fertilisation (Cohen et al, 1985a)

Quantity and type of cells	No. of cycles (patients)		Oocytes fertilised/ recovered (%)		No. of replacements/ cycles		No. of pregnancies/ cycles	
Cells + +*	28	(22)	41/67	(61)	21/28	(75)	8/28	(29)
Cells + + +/+ + + +*	18	(15)	25/54	(46)	13/18	(72)	2/18	(11)
Phagocytic polymorphonuclear leukocytes	8	(7)	8/24	(33)	5/8	(63)	3/8	(38)

*Cell types unknown.

is correlated with a low incidence of *in vitro* fertilisation in couples with idiopathic infertility, provided that the test is performed under controlled conditions using constant time intervals and criteria for sperm survival. They therefore advised that the test be used as a criterion for such IVF couples. Results of the Bourn Hall group confirm that the incidence of fertilisation is reduced in couples with a poor postcoital test. However the incidence of implantation in such couples following embryo replacement is not affected, hence the policy of this IVF unit to treat patients with cervical mucus hostility.

Postcoital tests were performed in 15 out of 41 couples who received IVF therapy for exclusively male infertility (Cohen et al, 1984b). The *in vivo* mucus penetration of five patients was considered to be satisfactory and 65 per cent of oocytes were subsequently fertilised by spermatozoa from these men; however no pregnancies were induced following embryo replacement (Table 14.6). The postcoital test was poor in the 10 remaining cases and only 48 per cent of oocytes were fertilised in these cases, however four patients became pregnant following embryo replacement, demonstrating that the postcoital test has only a limited prognostic value for the prediction of IVF outcome in cases of male infertility.

Table 14.6   Limited prognostic value of postcoital tests for predicting the outcome of IVF in cases of male infertility (Cohen et al, 1984b)

Postcoital test result		Proportion of oocytes fertilised *in vitro* (%)		Proportion of patients with an embryo replacement	Proportion of patients achieving a pregnancy
Good	5	15/23	(65)	4/5	0/5
Poor	10	30/62	(48)	9/10	4/10

(7) The hamster egg penetration test

Species specificity of fertilisation in mammals is mainly caused by the zona pellucida, a glycoprotein layer surrounding the vitellus of the oocyte. Removal of the zona pellucida may reduce the specificity but interspecies fertilisation is rare. However the golden hamster oocyte forms an exception; its zona-free egg permits penetration by spermatozoa from other species, including that of the human (Yanagimachi et al, 1976). Zona-free hamster eggs have been used by many clinical centres worldwide for nearly 10 years, and it has been advocated as the best test available to date by which the fertilising ability of human spermatozoa can be assessed (Rogers et al, 1979; Aitken et al, 1982a; Hall et al, 1981; Karp et al, 1981). An elaborate review was recently written by the instigator of this controversial diagnostic test (Yanagimachi, 1984). Evaluation and follow-up of infertile men has demonstrated that the hamster egg test has little prognostic value as far as *in vivo* fertility is concerned (Overstreet et al, 1980; Cohen et al, 1982a; Rogers et al, 1982). This setback with regard to the diagnostic value of the test has, however, not reduced its application. On the contrary, more and more groups are employing the test, using their own patient selection criteria. In some instances, where the test has been restricted to idiopathic patients only, results seem to be promising (Aitken et al, 1982b). However follow-up studies have not yet been published. It has also been postulated that the hamster egg test has other uses, including the evaluation of male infertility treatments, chromosomal analysis of human sperm, and for the selection of couples before IVF is attempted (Yanagimachi, 1984).

Human spermatozoa that are able to penetrate zona-free hamster eggs may not necessarily be capable of fertilising a human oocyte *in vitro* with its intact zona pellucida (Overstreet et al, 1980). Occasionally non-motile, but living, spermatozoa in contact with zona-free hamster eggs may fuse with the vitellus membrane (Cohen et al, 1982b). Such phenomena have never been observed in human IVF, showing that motility is essential for zona pellucida penetration (Amelar et al, 1980). According to the findings of Overstreet et al (1980) and the assumptions of others (Yanagimachi, 1984; Aitken, 1984), spermatozoa from subfertile men should have less chance of penetrating the human zona pellucida than of fusing with the hamster egg membrane. However, in practice the opposite seems to be the case; the incidence of fertilisation of human oocytes being higher than that of zona-free hamster eggs using the same criteria for assessing and selecting infertile men (Cohen et al, 1982a, 1985a).

Spermatozoa from only one-quarter of infertile men investigated in the Netherlands in 1982 were capable of penetrating zona-free hamster eggs, which is in contrast to the results of human IVF, where more than three-quarters of infertile men, assessed at Bourn Hall, were able to fertilise at least one oocyte (Table 14.7). This suggests that the incidence of 'false negatives' will be high if the hamster egg test is used as a predictor of IVF outcome in cases of abnormal semen.

For any IVF screening test to be reliable it is necessary to determine the incidence of false positive and false negative predictions. In terms of the hamster egg test a false positive result means that penetration of the hamster eggs occurred but fertilisation of human oocytes did not; a false negative result implying that although hamster eggs were not penetrated, successful fertilisation of human oocytes occurred. Several studies have been published evaluating the hamster egg test as a screening procedure for patients seeking

Table 14.7   Relationship between human IVF and penetration of zona-free hamster eggs in cases of male infertility

	At least one hamster egg penetrated	At least one human egg fertilised
Male infertility	19/79 (24%)	84/102 (82%)
Asthenospermia only	3/42 (7%)	26/27 (97%)
Source	Cohen et al, 1982	Cohen et al, 1985a

Table 14.8 Limited value of hamster egg penetration tests for predicting IVF outcome in patients whose spermatozoa were unable to fertilise their wife's oocytes

Source	No. of investigated patients unable to fertilize human oocytes	Mean percentage of zona-free hamster eggs penetrated	Proportion of patients able to penetrate hamster eggs (incidence of false positives)
Margalioth et al (1983)	10	22	8/10
Wolf et al (1983)	6	82	6/6
Foreman et al (1984)	15	12	9/15
Ausmanas et al (1985)	6	34	6/6
Cohen et al (1985c)	9	4	3/9
Total	46	25	32/46

IVF therapy (Tables 14.8–14.10) and the results are especially interesting in those patients where human fertilisation failed for no discernible reason.

In general, spermatozoa that are capable of fertilising human oocytes, penetrate hamster eggs to a greater extent than spermatozoa that fail to fertilise human oocytes (41 per cent and 25 per cent respectively: Tables 14.8 and 14.9). However, spermatozoa from 32 out of 46 patients (71 per cent) who were unable to fertilise human oocytes, were able to penetrate at least one zona-free hamster egg, demonstrating a very high incidence of false positive tests (Table 14.8).

At the same time the incidence of false negative tests is also high. Spermatozoa from 14 out of 120 men (12 per cent) were unable to penetrate zona-free hamster eggs despite their ability to fertilise human oocytes (Table 14.9), false negative tests being reported by three of the five groups

Table 14.9 Limited value of hamster egg penetration tests for predicting IVF outcome in patients whose spermatozoa are able to fertilise their wife's oocytes

Source	No. of investigated patients able to fertilise human oocytes	Mean percentage of zona-free hamster eggs penetrated	Proportion of patients unable to penetrate hamster eggs (incidence of false negatives)
Margalioth et al (1983)	10	45	0/10
Wolf et al (1983)	20	58	2/20
Foreman et al (1984)	22	46	0/22
Ausmanas et al (1985)	49	39	6/49
Cohen et al (1985c)	19	18	6/19
Total	120	41	14/120

Table 14.10   Limited value of negative hamster egg penetration tests for the prediction of IVF

Source	No. of patients whose spermatozoa could not penetrate hamster eggs	Proportion of these patients able to fertilise human oocytes (incidence of false negatives)
Margalioth et al (1983)	2	0/2
Wolf et al (1983)	2	2/2
Foreman et al (1984)	6	0/6
Ausmanas et al (1985)	6	6/6
Cohen et al (1985c)	13	6/13
Total	29	14/29

investigating this test (Margalioth et al, 1983; Wolf et al, 1983; Foreman et al, 1984; Ausmanas et al, 1985; Cohen et al, 1985c).

The unreliability of negative hamster egg tests becomes even more apparent when men whose spermatozoa were unable to penetrate hamster eggs are evaluated (Table 14.10). Of the 29 such men investigated so far, fertilisation of the wife's oocytes was achieved by 14, demonstrating an incidence of false negative assays approaching 50 per cent.

These data demonstrate that considerable care must be taken when the hamster egg test is used as a tool for assessing a man's *in vitro* fertilising capacity. IVF specialists should not select infertile men solely on the basis of the interaction of spermatozoa with zona-free hamster eggs.

Recommendations for the treatment of male infertility

Many forms of male infertility will respond to IVF, and this enables new criteria to be recommended for the alleviation of such infertility. A comprehensive approach to the problem using conventional methods and IVF in combination is given in Table 14.11.

Further improvement in the results of treatment could arise through better methods of semen preparation and by pre-IVF medication of patients using the conventional treatments discussed earlier. Whilst many of these therapies have proved disappointing in terms of pregnancy rates when used alone, it should be remembered that they can often improve semen output, and this improvement may well be sufficient to allow concomitant IVF therapy to be successful.

Future prospects

The opportunity is now arising for the treatment of the infertile male to be completely revolutionised. By the micromanipulation of spermatozoa and oocytes it will shortly be possible to treat patients who are at present unsuitable for IVF, or in whom failure of fertilisation has previously occurred. Cumulus cells present a barrier to spermatozoa which may be removed, and the zona pellucida could be weakened enzymatically, thereby

Table 14.11 Recommendation for the treatment of male infertility

Forms of male infertility	Incidence	Conventional treatments used	Suitable for treatment by IVF*
I. Specific forms			
Varicocele	10–25%	Varicocelectomy/	Yes
Scrotal hyperthermia		hypothermia/AIH	
Immunity against spermatozoa	3–13%	Corticosteroids	Yes
Endocrine	1–3%	Gonadotrophins/GnRH	Yes
Azoospermia caused by			
Cryptorchism	4%	Orchidopexy/AID	
Epididymal or vasal obstruction	1–3%	Surgery/AID	
Congenital abnormality	4%	AID	
Other factors	10%	AID	
Retrograde ejaculation	Rare	Ejaculation with a full bladder/AIH	Yes
Physical deformity and impotence	Rare	—	
Seminal plasma deficiency	Rare	Vitamin C/AIH	Yes
Infections and venereal diseases	Unknown	Antibiotics	
II. Non-specific forms			
Oligospermia	25% ⎫		
Asthenospermia	12% ⎬ Split ejaculation/AIH?/	Yes
Teratozoospermia	5% ⎪ drugs?	
Combined zoospermia	10% ⎭		
Polyzoospermia	1%	—	Yes
Necrozoospermia	1%	—	Yes
Increased viscosity	Rare	Split ejaculation/ proteolytic enzymes, AIH	Yes
Variable sperm output	Unknown		Yes

* Provided 50 000/ml motile spermatozoa can be prepared with a minimum of 0·2 ml.

facilitating sperm penetration. The problem of zona pellucida penetration will be overcome in the near future by the use of microinjection, enabling non-motile spermatozoa to be placed in the perivitelline space or, in cases of fusion failure, even into the vitellus of the oocyte itself (Uehara & Yanagimachi, 1976). For patients with azoospermia of obstructive origin it may be possible to recover precursors of spermatozoa directly from the genital tract and, after *in vitro* maturation, these could also be used in the same manner.

REFERENCES

Aafjes J H, Van der Vijver J C M 1976 Men with reduced fertility. Dutch Journal of Medicine 120: 865

Aafjes J H, Van der Vijver J C, Schenck P E 1978 The duration of infertility: an important datum for the fertility prognosis of men with semen abnormalities. Fertility and Sterility 30: 423–425

Aafjes J H, Van der Vijver J C, Brugman F W, Schenck P E 1983 Double blind crossover treatment with mesterolone and placebo of subfertile oligozoospermic men; value of testicular biopsy. Andrologia 15: 531–535

Abdelmassih R, Fujisaki S, Fa'undes A 1982 Prognosis of varicocelectomy in the treatment of infertility, based on pre-surgery characteristics. International Journal of Andrology 5 : 452–460

Ahlgren M 1975 Sperm transport to and survival in the human fallopian tube. Gynaecologic Investigation 6 : 206–214

Aitken R J 1984 In vitro fertilisation for male infertility. European Journal of Fertility and Sterility 15 : 425–431

Aitken R J, Best F S M, Richardson D W, Djahanbakhkch O, Templeton A A, Lees M 1982a An analysis of semen quality and sperm function in cases of oligospermia. Fertility and Sterility 38 : 705–711

Aitken R J, Best F S, Richardson D W, Djahanbakhch O, Mortimer D, Templeton A A, Lees M 1982b An analysis of sperm function in cases of unexplained infertility : conventional criteria, movement characteristics and fertilising capacity. Fertility and Sterility 38 : 212–221

Amelar R D, Dubin L, Schoenfeld C 1980 Sperm motility. Fertility and Sterility 34 : 197–215

Ausmanas M, Tureck R W, Blasco L, Kopf G S, Ribas J, Mastroianni L 1985 The zona-free hamster egg penetration assay as a prognostic indicator in a human in vitro fertilisation program. Fertility and Sterility 43 : 433–437

Baker H W, Clarke G N, Hudson B, McBain J C, McGowan M P, Pepperall R J 1983 Treatment of sperm autoimmunity in men. Clinics in Reproduction and Fertility 2 : 55–71

Batterinck G J, Kremer J, Jager S 1983 The effect of oral Kallikrein treatment on sperm motility in asthenozoopermia. International Journal of Andrology 6 : 173–179

Berger R E, Karp L E, Williamson R A, Koehler J, Moore D E, Holmes K K 1982 The relationship of pyospermia and seminal fluid bacteriology to sperm function as reflected in the sperm penetration assay. Fertility and Sterility 37 : 557–564

Blasco L 1984 Clinical tests of sperm fertilizing ability. Fertility and Sterility 41 : 177–192

Buvat J, Ardaens K, Lemaire A, Gauthier A, Gosnault J P, Buvat-Herbaut M 1983 Increased sperm count in 25 cases of idiopathic normogonadotropic oligospermia following treatment with Tamoxifen. Fertility and Sterility 39 : 700–703

Carter J N, Tyson J E, Tolis G, Van Vliet S, Faiman C, Friesen H G 1978 Prolactin secreting tumors and hypogonadism in 22 men. New England Journal of Medicine 299 : 847–852

Charny C W 1979 Clomiphene therapy in male infertility : a negative report. Fertility and Sterility 32 : 551–555

Cohen J, Aafjes J H 1982 Proteolytic enzymes stimulate human spermatozoal motility and penetration ability into hamster ova. Life Sciences, 30 : 899–904

Cohen J, Weber R F A, Van der Vijver J C M, Zeilmaker G H 1982a In vitro fertilizing capacity of human spermatozoa with the use of zona free hamster ova : interassay variation and prognostic value. Fertility and Sterility 37 : 565–572

Cohen J, Mooyaart M, Vreeburg J T M, Zeilmaker G H 1982b Fertilization of hamster ova by human spermatozoa in relation to other semen parameters. International Journal of Andrology 5 : 210–224

Cohen J, Fehilly C B, Fishel S B, Edwards R G, Hewitt J, Rowland G F, Steptoe P C, Webster J 1984a Male infertility successfully treated by in vitro fertilization. Lancet 1 : 1239–1240

Cohen J, Edwards R G, Fehilly C B, Fishel S B, Hewitt J, Rowland G, Steptoe P C, Webster J 1984b Treatment of male infertility by in vitro fertilization : factors affecting fertilization and pregnancy. European Journal of Fertility and Sterility 15 : 455–465

Cohen J, Edwards R G, Fehilly C B, Fishel S, Hewitt J, Purdy J, Rowland G, Steptoe P C, Webster J 1985a In vitro fertilization : a treatment for male infertility. Fertility and Sterility 43 : 422–432

Cohen J, Edwards R G, Fehilly C B, Fishel S B, Hewitt J, Rowland G F, Steptoe P C, Walters D E, Webster J 1985b In vitro fertilization using cryopreserved donor semen in cases where both partners are infertile. Fertility and Sterility 43 : 570–574

Cohen J, Fehilly C B, Walters D E 1985c Prolonged storage of human spermatozoa at room temperature or in a refrigerator. Fertility and Sterility. (In press)

Comhaire F 1976 Treatment of oligospermia with tamoxifen. International Journal of Fertility 21 : 232–238

Comhaire F, Vermeulen L 1983 Effect of high dose oral Kallikrein treatment in men with idiopathic subfertility : evaluation by means of in vitro penetration test of zona free hamster ova. International Journal of Andrology 6 : 168–172 del Pozo E 1982 Hyperprolactinaemia in male infertility. Treatment with bromocryptine. In: Bain J et al (eds) Treatment of male infertility. Springer-Verlag, Berlin, pp 71–84

Dondero F, Isidori A, Lenzi A, Cerasaro M, Massilli F, Giorenco P, Conti C 1979 Treatment and follow-up of patients with infertility due to sperm agglutinins. Fertility and Sterility 31: 48–51

Dubin L, Amelar R D 1971 Etiological factors in 1294 consecutive cases of male infertility. Fertility and Sterility 22: 469–474

Dubin L, Amelar R D 1975 Varicolectomy as therapy in male infertility: a study of 504 cases. Fertility and Sterility 26: 217–220

Edwards R G, Steptoe P C 1980 A matter of life. William Morrow, New York

Edwards R G, Fishel S B, Cohen J, Fehilly C B, Purdy J M, Slater J M, Steptoe P C, Webster J 1984 Factors influencing the success of in vitro fertilization for alleviating human infertility. Journal of In Vitro Fertilization and Embryo Transfer 1: 3–23

Ferrie B G, Hart A J, Kyle K F 1982 Varicoceles: a ten year retrospective review. Scottish Medical Journal 27: 305–308

Fishel S B, Edwards R G 1982 Essentials of fertilization. In: Edwards R. G., Purdy J M Human conception in vitro. Academic Press, London, pp 157–179

Foreman R, Cohen J, Fehilly C B, Fishel S B, Edwards R G 1984 The application of the zona-free hamster egg test for the prognosis of human in vitro fertilization. Journal of in Vitro Fertilization and Embryo Transfer 1: 166–171

Franks S, Jacobs H S, Martin N, Nabarro J D N 1978 Hyperprolactinaemia and impotence. Clinical Endocrinology 8: 277–287

Getzoff P L 1955 Clinical evaluation of testicular biopsy and the rebound phenomenon. Fertility and Sterility 6: 465–474

Getzoff P L 1975 Surgical aspects of infertility. Clinical Endocrinology and Metabolism 4: 693–709

Gottesman I S, Bain J 1980 Subfertility and infertility in the male: a persistent dilemma. In Bain J, Hafez, E S E (eds), Diagnosis andrology. Martinus Nijhoff, Amsterdam, pp 79–86

Hall J L 1981 Relationship between semen quality and human sperm penetration of zona free hamster ova. Fertility and Sterility 35: 457–463

Hargreave T B, Elton R A 1982 Treatment with intermittent high dose methylprednisolone or intermittent betamethasone for antisperm antibodies: preliminary communication. Fertility and Sterility 38: 586–590

Hargreave T B, Haxdon M, Whitelas J, Elton R, Chisholm C O 1980 The significance of sperm agglutinating antibodies in men with infertile marriages. British Journal of Urology 52: 566

Hendry W F, Sommerville I F, Hall R R, Pugh C B 1973 Investigation and treatment of the subfertile male. British Journal of Urology 45: 670

Hendry W F, Stedronska J, Parslow J, Hughes L 1981 The results of intermittent high dose steroid therapy for male infertility due to antisperm antibodies. Fertility and Sterility 36: 351–355

Hewitt J, Cohen J, Krishnaswamy V, Fehilly C B, Steptoe P C, Walters D E 1985 Treatment of idiopathic infertility, cervical mucus hostility and male infertility: artificial insemination with husbands semen or in vitro fertilization? Fertility and Sterility 44: 350–355

Homonnai Z T, Peled M, Paz Q F 1978 Changes in semen quality and fertility in response to endocrine treatment of subfertile men. Gynaecologic and Obstetric Investigation 99: 244–255

Hovatta O, Koskimies A I, Ranta T, Stenman U H, Seppala M 1979 Bromocryptine treatment of oligospermia: a double blind study. Clinical Endocrinology 11: 377–382

Hull M G R, Joyce D M, McLeod F N, Ray B D, McDermott A 1984 Human in vitro fertilization, in vivo sperm penetration of cervical mucus and unexplained infertility. Lancet 2: 245–247

Johnsen S G 1978 Maintenance of spermatogenesis induced by hmG treatment by means of continuous hcg treatment in hypogonadotrophic men. Acta Endocrinologica 89: 763–769

Karpe L E, Williamson R A, Moore D E, Shy K K, Plymate R, Smith W D 1981 Sperm penetration assay: useful test in evaluation of male fertility. Obstetrics and Gynaecology 5: 620–623

Krzanowska H 1974 The passage of abnormal spermatozoa through the uterotubal junction of the mouse. Journal of Reproduction and Fertility 38: 81–90

Lamensdorf H, Compere D, Begley G 1975 Testosterone rebound therapy in the treatment of male infertility. Fertility and Sterility 26 : 469–472

Lome L G, Ross L 1977 Varicocelectomy and infertility. Urology 9 : 416–418

Lunenfield B, Mor A, Mani M 1967 Treatment of male infertility I. Human gonadotrophins. Fertility and Sterility 18 : 581–592

Margalioth E J, Navot D, Laufer N, Yosef S M, Rabinowitz R, Yarkoni S, Schenker J G 1983 Zona-free hamster ovum penetration assay as a screening procedure for in vitro fertilization. Fertility and Sterility 40 : 386–388

Mahadevan M M, Trounson A O 1984 The influence of seminal characteristics on the success rate of human in vitro fertilization. Fertility and Sterility 42 : 400–405

Mulcahy J J 1984 Scrotal hypothermia and the infertile man. Journal of Urology 132 : 469–470

Nilsson S, Edvinsson A, Nilsson B 1979 Improvement of semen and pregnancy rate after ligation and division of the internal spermatic vein : fact or fiction? British Journal of Urology 51 : 591–596

Overstreet J W, Yanagimachi R, Katz D F, Hayashi K, Hanson F W 1980 Penetration of human spermatozoa into human zona pellucida and the zona-free hamster egg : a study of fertile donors and infertile patients. Fertility and Sterility 33 : 534–542

Paulsen C A, Espeland D H, Michals E L 1970 Effects of hCG, hMG and hGH administration on testicular function. In : Rosenberg E, Paulsen C A (eds) The human testis. Plenum, New York, pp 547–562

Purdy J M 1982 Methods for fertilization and embryo culture in vitro. In : Edwards R G, Purdy J M (eds) Human conception in vitro. Academic Press, London, pp. 135–156

Rodriguez-Rigau L J, Smith K D, Steinberger E 1978 Relationship of varicocele to sperm output and fertility of male partners in infertile couples. Journal of Urology 120 : 691–694

Rogers B J, Van Campen H, Ueno M, Lambert H, Bronson R, Hale R 1979 Analysis of human spermatozoal fertilizing ability using zona-free ova. Fertility and Sterility 32 : 664–670

Rogers B J, McCarville C, Soderdahl D, Hale R 1982 Re-evaluation of the zona-free egg test with regard to its use in human fertility assessment. Fertility and Sterility 37a : 296

Ronnberg L 1980 The effect of clomiphene citrate on different sperm parameters and serum hormone levels in preselected infertile men : a controlled double blind crossover study. International Journal of Andrology 3 : 479–486

Rosemberg E 1976 Gonadotrophin therapy of male infertility. In : Hafez E S E (ed) Human semen and fertility regulation in men. Mosby, St Louis, pp. 464–475

Rowland G F, Forsey T, Moss T R, Steptoe P C, Hewitt J, Darougar S 1985 Failure of in vitro fertilization and embryo replacement following infection with chlamydia trachomatis. Journal of In Vitro Fertilization and Embryo Transfer 2(3) : 151–155

Russel J K 1960 Artificial insemination (husband) in the management of childlessness. Lancet 3 : 1223–1225

Schellen T C M 1970 Results with mesterolone in the treatment of disturbances of spermatogenesis. Andrologia 2 : 1–9

Schellen T M 1982 Clomiphene treatment in male infertility. International Journal of Fertility 27 : 136–145

Schill W B 1979 Treatment of idiopathic oligozoospermia by kallikrein : results of a double blind study. Archives of Andrology 2 : 163–170

Schill W B, Landthaler M 1981 Erfahrung mit dem antioestrogen Tamoxifen zur therapie des oligozoospermie. Hautartz 32 : 306–308

Schoenfield C Y, Amelar R D, Dubin L 1973 Stimulation of ejaculated human spermatozoa by caffeine : a preliminary report. Fertility and Sterility 24 : 772–775

Schrofner W G 1978 Restoration of male fertility five years after total hypophysectomy. Hawaii Medical Journal 37 : 331–334

Schulman J F, Schulman S 1982 Methylprednisolone treatment of immunological infertility in males. Fertility and Sterility 38 : 591–599

Shuber J, Bain J 1982 In vitro fertilization : future treatment for male infertility. In : Bain J et al (eds) Treatment of male infertility. Springer-Verlag, Berlin, pp 313–320

Trounson A, Wood C 1984 In vitro fertilization results 1979–1982 at Monash University, Queen Victoria and Epworth Centres. Journal of In Vitro Fertilization and Embryo Transfer 1(1) : 42–47

Uehara T, Yanagimachi R 1976 Microsurgical injection of spermatozoa into hamster eggs

with subsequent transformation of sperm nuclei into male pronuclei. Biology of
    Reproduction 15: 467–470

Vermeulen A, Vandeweghe M 1984 Improved fertility after varicocele correction: fact or
    fiction? Fertility and Sterility 42: 249–256

Verstoppen G R, Steeno O P 1977 Varicocele and the pathogenesis of the associated
    subfertility: a review of various theories II. Results of surgery. Andrologia 9: 293

Wolf D P, Sokoloski J E, Quigley M M 1983 Correlation of human in vitro fertilization with
    the hamster egg bioassay. Fertility and Sterility 40: 53–59

Yanagimachi R 1984 Zona-free hamster eggs: their use in assessing fertilizing capacity and
    examining chromosomes of human spermatozoa. Gamete Research 10: 187–232

Yanagimachi R, Yanagimachi H, Rogers B J 1976 The use of zona-free animal ova as a test-
    system for the assessment of the fertilizing capacity of human spermatozoa. Biology of
    Reproduction 15: 471–476

Yovich J L, Stanger J D 1984 The limitations of in vitro fertilization from males with severe
    oligospermia and abnormal sperm morphology. Journal of In Vitro Fertilization and
    Embryo Transfer 1: 172–179

Zorgniotti A W, Sealfon A I 1984 Scrotal hypothermia: new therapy for poor semen. Urology
    23: 439–441

Zorgniotti A W, Sealfon A I, Toth A 1982 Further clinical experience with testis hypothermia
    for infertility due to poor semen. Urology 19: 636–640

Timing of ovulation

Accurately determining the time of ovulation is of great importance to individuals interested either in the control or promotion of fertility. This is particularly true with reference to *in vitro* fertilisation (IVF). Success rates are markedly improved if oocytes which have resumed or completed the first meiotic division are used (Edwards, 1983). Conversely, prolonged delay will allow ovulation to occur with loss of the oocyte into the peritoneal cavity. Over the past decade many methods have been used to time ovulation including basal body temperature (BBT) charts, cervical mucus, breast skin temperature rhythms and salivary peroxidase levels (de Mouzon et al, 1984; Shah et al, 1984; Anderson et al, 1984). Because those methods rely on the hormonal events surrounding ovulation rather than ovulation *per se*, they can only provide a limited degree of precision. Similarly, although serial ultrasound scanning is an excellent method of following follicular growth and development, observing ovulation, or determining that ovulation has occurred, is of limited value in precisely timing ovulation (Seibel et al, 1981b; Marinho et al, 1982; Queenan et al, 1980). Ovulation has been shown to occur from a wide range of follicle diameters, and no acceptable reference point has been established to anticipate at what particular moment or follicle size ovulation will occur. This chapter will discuss the relationship of the luteinising hormone (LH) surge to two biological markers: (1) the stage of oocyte maturation if ovulation has not occurred; and (2) the presence of a fresh ovulatory stigma if ovulation has occurred. Background information will also be discussed.

Considerable information has accumulated over the past 25 years as to the time of ovulation in relation to the hormonal events of the normal menstrual cycle. Although 17β oestradiol (E_2), progesterone (P), follicle stimulating hormone (FSH) and LH have all been studied, the measurement of LH appears to be the most promising parameter of this event (WHO, 1980) (Table 15.1).

McArthur (1959) was the first to show a consistent midcycle LH surge by means of a rat ventral prostate assay. However, that study had no direct ovarian marker of ovulation. The only reference point was the BBT. A few months later, separately and independently, Taymor (1959) utilised the rat

Table 15.1   Summary of studies relating time of ovulation to onset of LH surge and LH peak

Reference	Hours from surge onset	Hours from LH peak
Taymor (1959)		26 (12–48)
Yussman & Taymor (1970)	32·8 (28–44)*	17·6 (16–24)*
Ferin et al (1973)	21–36	
Croxatto et al (1974)		15·5
Pauerstein et al (1978)		9 ± 2
WHO (1980)	32 (23·6–38·2)	16·5 (9·5–23·0)†
Garcia et al (1981)	27·3	17·5
Testart et al (1981)	36–38	
Seibel et al (1982b)	38	
Taymor et al (1983)	36–38	22–26

LH = Luteinizing hormone.   *Range.   †95 per cent confidence limits.

ventral prostate assay for LH together with corpus luteum biopsy as a marker of the time of ovulation. Six normally menstruating women collected 12 hour urine samples from the 11th to the 17th day of their cycles. Indicated surgery was performed, as well as an endometrial biopsy, between days 15 and 20. Peak levels of LH were found 24–48 hours before ovulation. Although the biological assays utilised were relatively insensitive, requiring pooling of urine samples, it was the first report describing the temporal relationship of LH to ovulation. It has since been found that plasma peaks precede urinary peaks, and may do so by as much as 48 hours (Roger et al, 1980).

The development of radioimmunoassay (RIA) in blood greatly simplified laboratory testing. It became possible to obtain more frequent sampling around the periovulatory period, and this made it possible to determine more precisely the patterns of LH discharge. Utilising a serum RIA for LH, blood was drawn at 8-hourly intervals and combined with corpus luteum biopsy. Despite the fact that dating of the corpora lutea by histological sections is imprecise, and may carry a 12-hour error, ovulation was found to occur 24–30 hours after the onset of the LH surge and 12–24 hours after the LH peak (Yussman & Taymor, 1970). Ferin et al (1973) studied two patients: one patient was observed to have an intact follicle 21 hours after the LH surge, and the second was found to have a corpus luteum at 36 hours. A slightly wider range of time was reported by Croxatto et al (1974). Using corpus luteum biopsy and LH assay these workers reported that ovulation occurred as early as 15·5 hours after the LH peak. A similar study by Pauerstein et al (1978), using a single a.m. sample for LH combined with corpus luteum biopsy, found ovulation to occur 9 hours after the LH peak.

The wide variation reported in the studies above probably reflects the relative infrequency of LH determinations, as well as the low number of patients. The World Health Organisation Task Force obtained serum samples at 8-hourly intervals around the time of ovulation from 107 patients, and evaluated the temporal relationship between the LH surge and the presence or absence of ovulation. Corpus luteum biopsy was employed. The

LH rise was found to occur 32 (23·6–38·2) hours prior to ovulation and the LH peak 16·5 (9·5–23) hours prior to ovulation (WHO, 1980). Their results were remarkably similar to those Taymor had obtained a decade before. Their report also determined that LH was a superior indirect parameter of impending ovulation than either progesterone (P), FSH, or oestradiol (E$_2$).

Similar information concerning the time of ovulation in relationship to LH, and which generally conforms to the observations noted above, comes from studies in which hCG was injected into human menopausal gonadotrophin (hMG) primed subjects, and the state of the follicle or ovary noted at laparoscopy. The majority of cases were examined less than 33 hours after hCG: 41 of 47 still had not ovulated. From 37 to 38·5 hours three of five had ovulated. From 40 to 42 hours two of three had ovulated. These studies indicated that ovulation occurs approximately 38 hours after the injection of hCG. Therefore the results of observations from induced ovulatory cycles appear to be quite similar to those events observed in a natural cycle.

Over the past few years, laparoscopy performed around the time of ovulation, combined with LH values obtained at more frequent intervals, has allowed further refinement of the timing of ovulation. Testart and associates (1981) performed follicle puncture for *in vitro* fertilisation at varying intervals after the onset of the LH surge. Blood samples were obtained four times daily. Ovulation was found to occur 36–38 hours after the onset of the LH surge, a finding consistent with previous reports. In order to further refine the time interval between the LH surge and ovulation we obtained blood samples at 3- or 4-hourly intervals and performed laparoscopy at or around the time of anticipated ovulation. All the corpora lutea were found 38 hours or more after the onset of the LH surge (Taymor et al, 1983). In one patient whose laparoscopy was performed exactly 38 hours after the onset of the LH surge, ovulation was noted to be in progress (Fig. 15.1). These recent reports suggest that the temporal relationship between the LH surge and ovulation is a consistent and precise event which requires approximately 38 hours.

A recent study which also used 4-hourly intervals for the LH assay and laparoscopic observation of the early corpus luteum set the mean time of ovulation from the onset of the LH surge at 27 hours and 20 minutes (Garcia et al, 1981). This significant departure from previous studies on the timing of ovulation probably reflects the difference in the manner of determining the onset of the LH surge. These authors arbitrarily selected an LH level of 60 mIU/ml as the onset of the LH surge. However, many times the LH surge begins well before 60 mIU/ml. It is therefore of extreme importance to examine carefully the methodology of each report, to determine the definition of the LH surge.

Because the LH surge is rather abrupt when blood samples are obtained at frequent intervals (Hoff et al, 1983), it is usually possible to detect the onset of the LH surge by plotting the LH values on graph paper. We have

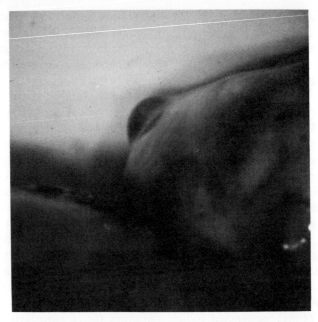

Fig. 15.1 Ovarian surface exactly 38 hours after onset of LH surge. Ovulation was observed to occur moments later

chosen to define the LH surge as the first point rising from baseline followed by a sustained rise. Other authors choose an LH value more than two standard deviations, or in some reports more than 180 per cent, greater than the mean of the preceding four LH values. In those instances where determining the onset of the LH surge was difficult we have employed a mathematical tool called cusum (Ransil et al, 1981).

The cusum of a group of serial measurements is a simple arithmetic calculation, as illustrated in Table 15.2 for luteinising hormone (LH) values. B is an appropriate baseline or reference value. It can be the initial value of a series of measurements, or the mean of the first few values. d_i is the difference between each LH value and the baseline. The cusum is the sum of these differences.

Table 15.2   Estimating the onset of the LH surge : Cumulative summation of sequential LH measurement

Hour	LH value	LH value-B*	Cusum
0	LH_1	$LH_1\text{-}B = d_1$	d_1
4	LH_2	$LH_2\text{-}B = d_2$	$d_1 + d_2$
8	LH_3	$LH_3\text{-}B = d_3$	$d_1 + d_2 + d_3$
$\vdots$	$\vdots$	$\vdots$	$\vdots$
n	LH_n	$LH_n\text{-}B = d_n$	$\sum_{i=1}^{n} d_i$

* Baseline value : LH_1 in the examples reported here.

If the serial values hover around the baseline value, the values of the d_i will oscillate between plus and minus. Their cumulative sum will remain close to, and oscillate about, 0. When the values begin to exceed the baseline value consistently, even by small amounts, the d_i will be consistently positive, as will their cumulative sum, which will increase markedly with each successive value. Conversely, for values consistently less than the reference value, the cusum will go increasingly negative. In this application we interpret the appearance of a sustained upswing from baseline as the onset of the LH surge.

Although LH is known to exhibit a pulsatile secretory pattern that varies in frequency and amplitude with the phase of the menstrual cycle, it has recently been established that the LH surge is governed by some kind of 24-hour neural clock (Fig. 15.2). Samples obtained from periovulatory women at 4-hourly intervals were assayed for LH. In all cases the onset of the LH surge was between 1 a.m. and 1 p.m. Seventeen of twenty subjects exhibited an LH surge between 5 a.m. and 9 a.m. These findings seem independent of whether or not the subjects received clomiphene citrate, and this implies that the LH surge is mediated by a central time-related mechanism located

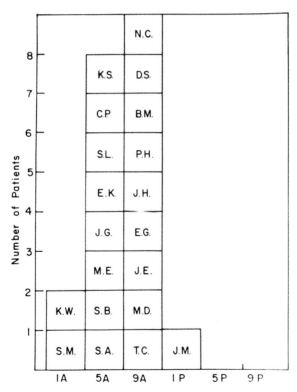

Fig. 15.2 Histogram showing the time of the onset of the LH surge. A 12 hour variation is noted, with the mean between 0500 and 0900 hours (Seibel et al 1982a)

higher than the hypothalamus. Although we did not demonstrate any seasonal variation, this has been demonstrated by others.

This does have a significant practical application. Patients undergoing *in vitro* fertilisation should be monitored for LH to detect an endogenous LH surge which could trigger ovulation to occur prior to oocyte retrieval. Because the LH surge occurs predominantly in the morning, a single a.m. sample for LH will alert the physician in most instances to impending ovulation. Obviously, much more frequent blood sampling would be necessary to anticipate exactly when ovulation might occur.

Emphasis has been placed on the accurate determination of the LH surge not only because of its predictive value in the timing of ovulation, but also because LH is at least associated with, if not responsible for, the resumption of oocyte maturation. There is also a temporal relationship between the LH surge and oocyte maturation. In order to better understand this relationship, a brief description of oocyte maturation follows.

Meiosis is a form of cell division which occurs only in gametes. It is a process which begins early in fetal life and is not completed until fertilisation occurs in the adult female almost two decades later. Its main purpose is to provide the means by which a diploid germ cell (2 n) which has four times the necessary chromatin (4 c) can exchange genetic material and ultimately result in a genetically distinct gamete which is haploid (1 n) and contains only the necessary amount of chromatin (1 c).

Three weeks after conception the primordial germ cells can be identified in the epithelium of the yolk sac near the developing allantois. These primordial germ cells progress by amoeboid action through the tissues of the yolk sac and the gut to the region of the developing kidneys (mesonephros) and finally into the adjacent genital ridge which will ultimately become the gonad. Beginning about 5 weeks gestation some of the primordial cells begin replication by mitosis and give rise to oogonia. Each of these oogonia are diploid (2 n) and each contains 46 chromosomes. By 5–6 months this process will result in six to seven million oogonia. During mitosis, two daughter cells genetically identical to the parent cell are produced. The oogonia undergoing mitosis pass through the four stages of cell life; G1 (the stage in which a cell carries out its primary function), S (synthesis of DNA), G2 (chromosome replication), and M (mitosis including prophase, metaphase, anaphase, and telophase). As a result of the DNA synthesis and chromosome replication, each oogonium still has 46 chromosomes, but has produced twice the amount of chromatin or DNA in anticipation of dividing into two genetically identical daughter cells during mitosis. However, beginning at 8–13 weeks, some of the oogonia with twice the amount of chromatin stop entering mitosis; instead they enter prophase of the first meiotic division. These oogonia are now called primary oocytes, and progress through the stages of meiotic prophase. During the leptotene stage of meiotic prophase, the 46 chromosomes containing twice the needed DNA are decondensed and *appear* as 46 single slender threads. During the next stage, zygotene, the homologous chromosomes align parallel to each other in synapses forming 23 bivalent pairs. However, each of the pairs has twice the needed DNA. Therefore each bivalent represents two times (2 n) the haploid number of chromosomes and four times (4 c) the needed amount of chromatin or DNA. At this point each chromosome splits longitudinally except at points of junction called centromeres. The four chromatids are now called tetrads. It is during the ensuing pachytene stage that the chromatids break and recombine, resulting in the exchange of genetic material. In the next stage of prophase, diplotene, the pairs of chromatids demonstrate mutual repulsion from each other except at the chaismata where 'crossing over' has occurred.

Due to atresia, the nearly seven million germ cells present at mid-term have declined to about two million. This phase is in general completed by or shortly after birth. At this point most of the oocytes have entered the first of two resting phases called the dictyate of dictyotene stage. This stage is exceedingly long and lasts from the time of birth until after puberty when ovulation occurs. Although apparently inert, oocytes in the dictyate stage do grow, and do show evidence of protein synthesis. Chromosomes decondense forming lateral projections which resemble lamp brushes and which replicate RNA.

During fetal life the follicle also develops. At approximately 8 weeks some of the primary oocytes become surrounded by a single layer of spindle-shaped cells which are the precursors of granulosa cells. These cells develop cytoplasmic processes which project to the plasma membrane of the oocyte. The oocyte and adjacent granulosa cells have become surrounded by a basal lamina which separates this complex, now called a primordial follicle, from the stroma. During the 5th–6th gestational month some of the spindle-shaped granulosa cells become cuboidal and begin to divide. This unit is called a primary follicle. Granulosa cell proliferation results in multiple layers of granulosa cells which contribute greatly to increasing follicle diameter. While up to four layers of granulosa cells are believed to be independent of hormonal control, hormones are definitely necessary to go beyond this point. These granulosa cells also synthesise and secrete a mucopolysaccharide substance, some of which becomes a translucent halo that surrounds the oocyte, called the zona pellucida. The cytoplasmic process from the granulosa cells traverses the zona pellucida and maintains close intimate association with plasma membrane of the oocyte. At about 7 months gestation some of the primary follicles form an antrum and thus become known as Graafian follicles. The oocyte is located eccentrically within the antrum surrounded by two or three layers of granulosa cells called the cumulus oophorus. Those granulosa cells comprising the cumulus which are contiguous with the wall of the follicle are known as the membranum granulosum. At the time of ovulation, cleavage occurs between the cumulus and the membranum granulosum, and the oocyte and its cumulus are extruded.

It is during the process of ovulation that resumption of meiosis occurs. At the onset of the LH surge the egg is still a primary oocyte. RNA synthesis ceases. The chromosomes become short and thick. This stage is called the germinal vesicle or diakinesis stage of meiosis, and the first meiotic prophase becomes complete. The nuclear membrane breaks down and the tetrads align themselves on the equator of the metaphase 1 plate. Tetrads rotate 90° and pull apart. One of the chromosomes still containing twice the necessary chromatin pinches off in a small blob of cytoplasm called the polar body. The polar body is located in the perivitelline space and contains one chromosome (1 n) and a double amount of chromatin (2 c). The oocyte is also now haploid (1 n) but contains twice the necessary chromatin (2 c). This stage is called metaphase II and the egg is called a secondary oocyte. This is the stage at the time of ovulation.

Metaphase II is the second resting phase of meiosis. The oocyte will remain in this stage unless fertilisation occurs. Should fertilisation occur, the remaining chromosome containing twice the chromatin (2 c) splits longitudinally and half the chromatin pinches off to the second polar body. The oocyte is now haploid and contains the proper amount of chromatin (1 n, 1 c). Therefore the process of meiosis, which begins in the early fetus, becomes complete only in the adult when fertilisation occurs.

Since LH is a reliable predictor of ovulation, we studied the temporal relationship between the LH surge and human oocyte maturation (Seibel et al, 1982b). Subjects consisted of infertile women undergoing routine diagnostic laparoscopy. They were admitted 2 days prior to anticipated ovulation. Blood was drawn initially at 4- and later at 3-hourly intervals by means of an intracath. Early each morning the bladder was filled by administering intravenous fluids and a pelvic ultrasound obtained. The previous day's blood samples were run each morning between 9 a.m. and 12 noon (Seibel et al, 1981a). Laparoscopy and oocyte retrieval was carried out at varying intervals after the LH surge. Follicular fluid was quickly examined for the presence of an oocyte and the stage of oocyte maturation assessed: germinal vesicle, diakinesis, metaphase I, and metaphase II (first polar body) (Vebele-Kallhardt, 1978). Between 4 and 8 hours after the LH surge the germinal vesicle stage was still present. Resumption of meiosis had occurred in all cases where oocytes were obtained more than 18 hours after the LH surge. Metaphase I oocytes were identified between 31 and 33 hours following the LH surge, whereas 28–38 hours following the LH surge oocytes in metaphase II were obtained. After 38 hours a corpus luteum was always obtained (Fig. 15.3).

These data are comparable with those observed with oocytes matured *in vitro* (Edwards, 1965). Most were in metaphase II 26–28 hours later, and in metaphase II after approximately 36 hours *in vitro*. Resumption of meiosis has also been studied *in vivo* following hCG injection (Jagiello et al, 1978).

Either germinal vesicle or metaphase I oocytes were identified in ovarian tissue removed 24–25 hours after hCG injection. Metaphase II occurred 25–

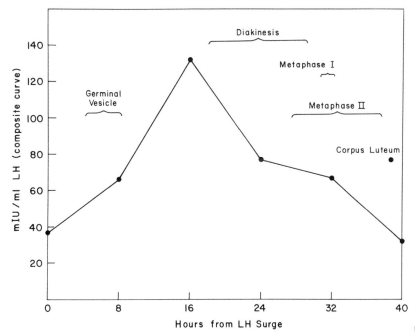

Fig. 15.3   The temporal relationship between the LH surge and oocyte maturation (Seibel et al 1982b)

29 hours after subsequent incubation *in vitro*. Similarly, Steptoe and Edwards (1970) reported *in vivo* maturation to either germinal vesicle, diakinesis or metaphase I, but rarely metaphase II in oocyte obtained 29–31 hours after hCG injection. A few of the metaphase I or earlier stage oocytes were transferred into culture media for 3–18 hours and were found subsequently to progress to metaphase II.

Of interest among the patients we studied was the fact that clomiphene citrate slightly delayed resumption of meiosis, and shortened the time interval of the oocyte maturing from metaphase I to metaphase II (Seibel et al, 1983). However, there was no difference between the temporal relationship of the LH surge and ovulation in either the clomiphene citrate-treated or non-treated patients. The impact and importance of delayed resumption of meiosis in clomiphene-treated patients, however, remains to be determined.

The ability to more accurately determine ovulation provides a potentially better method of natural family planning. The methods most commonly used have been changes in periovulatory cervical mucus and the biphasic changes which occur keeping a basal body temperature (BBT) chart. It is believed that the BBT nadir is usually located at the beginning of the LH surge, and the first high point on the BBT chart is 8 hours after ovulation (de Moupon et al, 1984). Large multinational studies which included a wide range of socioeconomic and cultural diversity have demonstrated that 93 per cent of women can be educated to recognise periovulatory cervical mucus changes. Only 5 per cent of previously fertile women became pregnant following proper instruction (WHO, 1981). However, it has also been demonstrated, by studies in which laparoscopies were performed on the first day of the BBT rise, that in one-third of cases, ovulation will have already occurred more than 24 hours earlier. Furthermore, in studies utilising AID in which insemination was delayed by more than 48 hours after the hyperthermic shift, no pregnancies occurred. Additional studies in which sexual intercourse was timed to alter sex preselection have demonstrated that there is no significant differences in sex ratio from varying intervals between the likely act leading to conception and the estimated day of ovulation (WHO, 1984). Studies such as these suggest that the vast majority of women are capable of detecting ovulation by changes in cervical mucus and hyperthermic shifts in the BBT. Subjects who fail to learn these techniques within three cycles have a high pregnancy rate. These methods of detecting ovulation allow patients to practice natural family planning with a significant degree of comfort, and allow physicians to schedule insemination treatments with a high degree of accuracy. However, these methods of timing ovulation are only rough parameters, and do not reflect precision in determining the exact moment of ovulation.

REFERENCES

Anderson W A, Ahluwalia B S, Westney L S, Burnett C C, Ruchel R 1984 Cervical mucus peroxidase is a reliable indicator for ovulation in humans. Fertility and Sterility 41 : 697
Croxatto H B, Carril I M, Cleviakoff S 1974 Time interval between LH peak and ovulation in women. In : Esling P J, Henderson R W (eds) Biological and clinical aspects of reproduction. Excerpta Medica, Amsterdam, p 282
deMoupon J, Testart J, LeFevre B, Pouly J-L, Frydman R 1984 Time relationships between basal body temperature and ovulation or plasma progestins. Fertility and Sterility 41 : 254
Edwards R G 1965 Maturation in vitro of human ovarian oocytes. Lancet 2 : 926
Edwards R G 1983 Studies on human conception. American Journal of Obstetrics and Gynecology 117 : 587
Ferin J, Thomas K, Johansson E D B 1973 Ovulation detection. In : Hafez E S E, Evans T N (eds), Human reproduction, conception and contraception. Harper & Row, New York, p 260
Garcia J E, Jones G S, Wright G L 1981 Prediction of the time of ovulation. Fertility and Sterility 36 : 308
Hoff J D, Quigley M E, Yen S S C 1983 Hormonal dynamics at mid cycle: a reevaluation. Journal of Clinical Endocrinology and Metabolism 57 : 792
Jagiello G, Karnicki J, Ryan R J 1978 Superovulation with pituitary gonadotropins: method for obtaining meiotic metaphase figures in human ova. Lancet 1 : 178
Marinho A O, Sallam H N, Goessens L K V, Collins W P, Rodeck C H, Campbell S 1982 Real time pelvic ultrasonography during the periovulatory period of patients attending an artificial insemination clinic. Fertility and Sterility 37 : 633
McArthur J W 1959 Midcycle changes in urinary gonadotropin excretion. In : Lloyd C W (ed) Recent progress in endocrinology of reproduction. Academic Press, New York, p 67
Pauerstein C J, Eddy C A, Croxatto H D, Hess R, Siler-Khodr T M, Croxatto H B 1978

Temporal relationships of estrogen, progesterone, and luteinizing hormone levels to ovulation in women and infrahuman primates. American Journal of Obstetrics and Gynecology 130: 876

Queenan J T, O'Brien G D, Bains L M, Simpson J, Collins W P, Campbell S 1980 Ultrasound scanning of ovaries to detect ovulation in women. Fertility and Sterility 34: 99

Ransil B J, Seibel M M, Taymor M L 1981 Estimating the onset of the LH surge by cumulative summation. Infertility 4: 295

Roger M, Grenier J, Houlbert C, Castanier M, Feinstein M C, Scholler R 1980 Rapid radioimmunoassays of plasma LH and estradiol $17-\beta$ for the prediction of ovulation. Journal of Steroid Biochemistry 12: 403

Seibel M M, Levesque L A, Taymor M L 1981a A rapid radioimmunoassay method for serum luteinizing hormone utilizing polyethylene glycol (PEG) and a double antibody method of separation. Fertility and Sterility 35: 36

Seibel M M, McCardle C R, Thompson E I, Berger M J, Taymor M L 1981b The role of ultrasound in ovulation induction: a critical appraisal. Fertility and Sterility 36: 573

Seibel M M, Shine W, Smith D M, Taymor M L 1982a Biological rhythm of the luteinizing hormone surge. Fertility and Sterility 37: 709

Seibel M M, Smith D M, Levesque L, Borten M, Taymor M L 1982b The temporal relationship between the luteinizing hormone surge and human oocyte maturation. American Journal of Obstetrics and Gynecology 142: 568

Seibel M M, Smith D M, Swartz S, Levesque L, Taymor M L 1983 Patterns of human preovulatory follicular fluid gonadotropin and postaglandin concentrations in vivo. Presented at the 30th Annual Meeting of the Society of Gynecologic Investigation, 17–20 March 1983, Washington, DC, p 108

Shah A, Rao K H S, Ruedi B, Magrini G 1984 Determination of fertility interval with ovulation time estimation using differential skin surface temperature (DST) measurement. Fertility and Sterility 41: 771

Steptoe P C, Edwards R G 1970 Laparoscopic recovery of preovulatory human oocytes after priming of ovaries with gonadotropins. Lancet 1: 638

Taymor M L 1959 Timing of ovulation by LH assay. Fertility and Sterility 10: 212

Taymor M L, Seibel M M, Smith D, Levesque L 1983 Ovulation timing by luteinizing hormone assay and follicle puncture. Obstetrics and Gynecology 62: 191

Testart J, Frydman R, Feinstein M C, Thebault A, Roger M, Schdler R 1981 Interpretation of plasma luteinizing hormone assay for the collection of mature oocytes from women: definition of a luteinizing hormone surge-initiating rise. Fertility and Sterility 36: 50

Uebele-Kallhardt B M 1978 Human oocytes and their chromosomes. Springer-Verlag, Berlin

World Health Organization Task Force 1980 Temporal relationship between ovulation and defined changes in the concentration of plasma estradiol-17β, luteinizing hormone, follicle-stimulating hormone, and progesterone. I. Probit analysis. American Journal of Obstetrics and Gynecology 15: 383

World Health Organization Task Force 1981 A prospective multicentre trial of the ovulation method of natural family planning. I. The teaching phase. Fertility and Sterility 36: 152

World Health Organization Task Force 1984 A prospective multicentre study of the ovulation method of natural family planning. IV. The outcome of pregnancy. Fertility and Sterility 41: 593

Yussman M A, Taymor M L 1970 Serum levels of follicle-stimulating hormone, and luteinizing hormone and of plasma progesterone related to ovulation by corpus luteum biopsy. Journal of Clinical Endocrinology and Metabolism 30: 396

Ultrasound in gynaecological practice

Gynaecological ultrasound was first used by Donald et al (1958) in the diagnoses of abdominal masses, and since then the changes and developments in ultrasound machines have resulted in widespread usage of this technique as a diagnostic and surgical tool in gynaecological practice.

Since its advent in the obstetric and gynaecological field in 1958, obstetricians have capitalised on this discovery and the use of ultrasound in obstetrics is routine in antenatal diagnosis and management (Campbell, 1966, 1974; Campbell & Thoms, 1977).

The evolution of ultrasound through A-scanning, bistable scanning and static B-scanning limited the use of gynaecological ultrasound. The incidence of false positive diagnoses, without real-time ultrasound, resulted in a large number of cystic pelvic lesions being diagnosed (O'Brien et al, 1984). Real-time ultrasound enabled visualisation of peristalsis in the bowel and thus cystic lesions previously diagnosed on static scans as ovarian cysts were now recognised as fluid-filled loops of intestine!

Large real-time linear ultrasound transducers prevent adequate visualisation of pelvic side walls and deep pelvic structures; hence it is only with the advent of real-time mechanical sector ultrasound that gynaecological ultrasound and ovarian scanning have become widely used in day-to-day practice.

Several workers have reported the use of gynaecological ultrasound in differentiating cystic from solid lesions when a clinical diagnosis is made (Reeves et al, 1980; Schlensker & Beckers, 1980; Minawi et al, 1984). The use of ultrasound as a preoperative investigation to differentiate an ovarian cyst from a fibroid needs no elaboration here, as it is well known that this diagnosis can now be made even by an inexperienced technician in a matter of seconds. I shall concentrate in this chapter on contemporary aspects of gynaecological ultrasound and will discuss two main features of gynaecological ultrasound.

The first part of this chapter is devoted to pelvic anatomy and ultrasound landmarks to enable gynaecologists to understand and use this technique as an adjunct to pelvic examination. This is followed by the progress made in screening for ovarian cancer and the use of gynaecological ultrasound in infertility management as well as the specialised use of ultrasound in *in vitro* fertilisation and embryo replacement (IVF) programmes.

PREREQUISITES OF GYNAECOLOGICAL ULTRASOUND EXAMINATION

It is important that a detailed menstrual and surgical history of the patient is taken so that ultrasound examination can be directed at appropriate organs in the pelvis.

The importance of a full bladder was first stressed by Donald (1963). A partially distended bladder can result in false negative diagnoses, when ovarian tumours are hidden by intestinal loops; and in false positive diagnoses, when fluid-filled intestinal loops or loculated adhesions are mistaken for ovarian cysts.

The patient should be in the supine position for all gynaecological ultrasound examinations except in cases where a vaginal probe may be used, in which case the semi-lithotomy position may be used.

PELVIC ANATOMY

A precise knowledge of pelvic anatomy and ultrasound landmarks is a prerequisite for any good gynaecological ultrasound examination.

Anatomically the pelvis may be divided into the greater or false pelvis and the lesser or true pelvis. The organs of reproduction lie within the true pelvis and therefore I shall confine myself to this region when discussing pelvic anatomy. The true pelvis is bound anteriorly by the pubic symphysis and the superior pubic rami, posteriorly by the pelvic surfaces of the sacrum and coccyx, and laterally by the ilium below the arcuate line and the inner surfaces of the body and superior ramus of the ischium (Gray, 1966). The anterior surface of these osseous structures can be visualised, but as they do not affect the reproductive tract I shall not discuss them further.

Muscles

The three principal muscles that are regularly visualised in gynaecological ultrasound examinations are the iliopsoas muscle, the obturator internus muscle and the levator ani. The two other muscles of the lesser pelvis, the coccygeus and piriformis, are located deep, posteriorly and cranially. They are not routinely visualised and, when imaged, cannot accurately be separated from the more inferiorly located levator ani muscle (Kurtz & Rifkin, 1983).

On ultrasound examination the iliopsoas muscle is relatively hypoechoic and discretely marginated. The interposed fascial sheath between the iliacus and psoas is easily noted by a bright linear echo. The bright reflector seen immediately posterior to the iliopsoas muscle is the anterior surface of the iliac bone.

The obturator internus muscle occupies a large part of the inner surface of the anterior and lateral pelvic walls. On ultrasound examination in the transverse plane, sections of this muscle are routinely imaged as an elongated and relatively hypoechoic muscle surrounded by the bright reflector of the obturator fascia (Sample, 1980).

The levator ani muscle lies caudad to the obturator internus muscle, and stretches across the pelvic floor to form the pelvic diaphragm. On ultrasound examination it lies at the level of the cervix and can be a helpful landmark, especially after hysterectomy, in judging the level below which the ovaries may not be seen. The hypoechoic nature of the muscle may be confused with normal ovarian echoes and care must be taken to differentiate between these two structures (Goswamy et al, 1983).

Blood vessels

In the author's opinion the pelvic blood vessels and the ureters are the most useful landmarks in localising the ovaries on ultrasound examination (Fig. 16.1).

The internal iliac vessels pass over the pelvic brim to descend to the true pelvis posteriorly and lateral to the ureter and ovary. The ovarian vessels enter the ovary from the lateral aspect.

Blood vessels are seen as tubular structures with bright walls and echofree lumina. Pulsations in the arteries are easily visualised using real-time

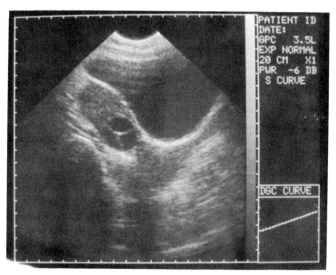

Fig 16.1 Anatomical landmarks. Longitudinal oblique scan through the pelvis showing the ovary containing three Graafian follicles. The internal iliac artery and ureter are seen as tubular structures posterolateral to the ovary

ultrasound and may be especially useful landmarks for assisting in ovarian identification when the normal anatomy is distorted either by disease or previous surgery.

Ureter

The ureter appears as a tubular structure with an echo-free lumen and lies anterior to the iliac vessels and posterior to the ovary. It does not pulsate and ureteric peristalsis can be seen as sparkling patterns of intermittent echos (Kurtz & Rifkin, 1983).

Reproductive organs

The vagina is imaged posterior to the full bladder and anterior to the rectum. It appears as a long reflector with the anterior and posterior walls being hypoechoic. A mid-line echo is seen as a thin bright line running parallel to the vaginal walls.

The uterus is pear-shaped and is pushed superiorly by a full bladder. Anteversion and retroversion are easily diagnosed and the ultrasound image is one of relatively low echoes. The normal uterine canal, corresponding to the apposed endometrial linings, usually thin and bright, is seen extending up to the mid-line of the uterus and surrounded by a relatively echo-free endometrium (Green, 1980). The thickness and brightness of the endometrial canal vary through the menstrual cycle, and in the secretory phase the endometrial echos are thicker and brighter than in the proliferative stage. The appearance of the endometrial cavity may be affected by the degree of bladder distension. A thick mid-line echo in a postmenopausal woman, not on hormone replacement therapy, should be regarded with suspicion, as this may be indicative of a hormone-secreting ovarian tumour.

Retroversion of the uterus may not only decrease echogenicity in the fundal region, the appearance mimicking those due to fibroids, but may also make the uterus appear globular (Fig. 16.2). Another problem experienced with uterine retroversion is that loops of intestine lying on the anterior surface of the fundus of the uterus interfere with adequate visualisation of the endometrial cavity and the ovaries. Head-down tilt or increased distension of the bladder are thus needed for adequate visualisation.

The fallopian tubes are not usually defined unless disease has caused distension and/or distortion.

The ovaries are usually seen lateral to the uterus; medial to the ovarian vessels and obturator internus muscle and fascia; superior to the levator ani muscle; and anterior to the internal iliac vessels and ureter. The methodology for ultrasound visualisation of the ovaries is described in detail elsewhere (Goswamy et al, 1983). The ovaries appear as ovoid structures with an echogenicity greater than that of the uterus and obturator internus muscles. During the ovulatory cycle the shape and appearance of the ovary may be

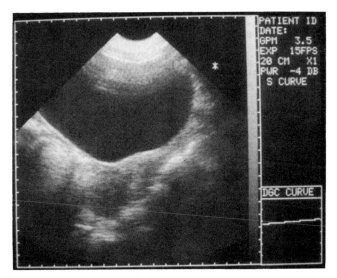

Fig. 16.2 Retroverted uterus. Longitudinal scan of a retroverted uterus. Note the globular shape of the fundus mimicking a fibroid, and the necessity of an extremely distended bladder to displace intestinal loops from the pelvis.

distorted by the presence of Graafian follicles or a corpus luteum. In the early post-menopause the ovaries contain low-level echoes and retain their ovoid shape, but change to linear or streak ovaries in the late menopause.

The ovaries are relatively mobile organs and their normal position described above may be altered by pelvic surgery, uterine enlargement or bladder or bowel distension. Thus the ovary may be visualised in the pouch of Douglas, at the pelvic brim, in the iliac fossa, just superior to the vaginal wall (especially in women who have undergone hysterectomy), or closely adherent to the pelvic side-wall, due to pelvic surgery or disease. A constant landmark, irrespective of ovarian position, is the pulsation noted at the point of entry of the ovarian vessels into the lateral aspect of the ovary, and this should always be observed, in addition to an absence of peristalsis, to ascertain correct visualisation of both ovaries.

SCREENING FOR OVARIAN CANCER

Ovarian cancer is the commonest cause of death from gynaecological malignancies, and kills more women than cervical and endometrial cancer combined (OPCS monitor, 1981). The overall 5-year survival rate has not changed over the past 20 years and remains at approximately 30–35 per cent (Doll et al, 1966, 1970; Jeffcoate, 1975; Ranney and Ahmad, 1979).

This poor survival is mainly attributable to late diagnosis. The failure to detect localised ovarian tumours (5-year survival rate: 85 per cent, equal to that of stage one endometrial or cervical cancer) is due to the insidious nature of the disease, to the unreliability of clinical examination, and to the lack of an ineffective early screening technique (Parker et al, 1970; Churches et al, 1974; Jones, 1975).

Several screening tests have been evaluated in the past; such as cervical cytology (Parker et al, 1971; Wagman & Brown, 1971), culdocentesis (Funkhouser et al, 1975; McGowan, 1975), ovarian cystadenocarcinoma-associated antigen (Bhattacharya & Barlow, 1975) and carcinoembryonic antigen (Samaan et al, 1976) and all of these have been found lacking in sensitivity, specificity or both.

Real-time mechanical sector ultrasonography has been used effectively to monitor follicular development (Hackeloer et al, 1979; Kerin et al, 1981; Sallam et al, 1982) in the ovarian cycle. When performed daily, follicular changes are observed so clearly that, in the author's experience, ovulation can be timed more accurately than with any other biophysical or biochemical technique currently available.

This methodology was successfully adapted to measure ovarian volume and determine morphology in climacteric women in an earlier pilot study (Campbell et al, 1982). Ovarian morphology and volume as assessed by ultrasound examination was compared to findings at laparotomy in 31 climacteric women. The correlation between ovarian volumes as determined by sonar with those observed at laparotomy was extremely encouraging ($r = 0.97$).

In March 1982 an Ovarian Scanning Clinic was set up at King's College Hospital, London to evaluate the use of real-time mechanical sector ultrasound in the detection of ovarian neoplasia in women over the age of 45 years. Any woman of appropriate age could request an ovarian scan, without the need for medical referral. Some women below the age of 45 years were also accepted if they were postmenopausal, as defined by cessation of menses for at least 1 year.

In total 5841 women were screeened. Subjects with normal ovaries were asked to return 1 year later for a repeat scan. Those with abnormal ovaries (see below) were rescanned 2–6 weeks later to determine whether the abnormality was still present, as it was indeterminate whether morphological changes occurred in postmenopausal ovaries. Patients with persistently 'abnormal' results were followed up by laparoscopy/laparotomy.

Because the ovary is relatively mobile, linear measurements change when ovarian position alters. Hence it is preferable to measure ovarian volume, a preference expressed by several authors (Campbell et al, 1982; Goswamy et al, 1983; Fleischer et al, 1983; Kurtz & Rifkin, 1983). Serial transverse scans allow the largest transverse (D1) and anteroposterior (D2) diameters to be determined and serial longitudinal scans allow the largest longitudinal diameter (D3) to be measured. The volume of an ovary, which approximates that of an ovoid is then calculated by the formula D1 × D2 × D3 × 0.523. The time taken to assess ovarian morphology and measure ovarian dimensions was 5 or 10 minutes.

Results

A total of 5841 new subjects were scanned up to March 1985. 5247 (89·8 per cent) women were noted to have normal ovaries and asked to return in a year for a repeat examination. 341 (5·8 per cent) women were found to have abnormal ovaries at the first scan but then noted to have normal ovaries at repeat scans 2–6 weeks later. 253 (4·3 per cent) women were found to have persistently abnormal ovaries and were referred to their local gynaecologist for laparoscopy/laparotomy.

Normal ovaries

Morphology—a morphologically normal ovary was defined as one that had a uniformly hypoechoic structure, an ovoid shape and a small echogenic outline. A total of 5588 women fulfilled these criteria in the study group.

The mean right ovarian volume in 1016 postmenopausal subjects reported in an earlier publication (Goswamy et al, 1983) was $3·71 \pm 1·42$ (S.D.)cm^3; the mean left ovarian volume in 1015 postmenopausal subjects in the same sample was $3·70 \pm 1·42$ (S.D.)cm^3. The percentage difference in volume between right and left ovaries in 990 subjects with normal morphology ranged between -68 per cent and $+92$ per cent, with a mean difference of $0·3 \pm 18·7$ (S.D.) per cent. The correlation between right and left ovarian volume was good ($r = 0·86$).

Abnormal ovaries

Morphological abnormalities could be classified into one of four categories:

1. Entirely cystic or unilocular ovary: this appears as a round or oval echogenic outline surrounding an echo-free centre.
2. Cystic ovary with multiple locules: the ovary has a dense echogenic outline which may be irregular. It contains multiple echo-free cystic spaces which vary in size and do not communicate with each other. The septa appear as thin or thick echogenic lines.
3. Cystic ovary with solid areas: the ultrasound appearance is of an enlarged ovary with echo-free cystic spaces and highly echogenic solid areas within the cyst.
4. Solid ovary with an irregular outine, with or without cystic spaces: the ovary may or may not be enlarged and has an irregular echogenic outline. The substance of the ovary may be seen as a hyperechoic or a hypoechoic area with cystic echo-free spaces (Fig. 16.3).

It is noted that, as in past publications (Goswamy et al, 1982, 1983) very similar ultrasound appearances were associated with widely differing histological diagnoses (Table 16.1).

This study is on-going at King's College Hospital to determine whether

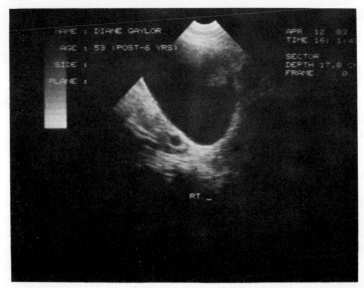

Fig. 16.3   Borderline malignancy serous cystadenocarcinoma. Longitudinal scan of the left ovary containing a cystic area surrounded by a thick echogenic outline. This echogenic outline differentiates this tumour from a Graafian follicle. Note the ureter and internal iliac artery lying posterior to the ovary

annual intervals for screening are adequate, and whether the incidence of malignancy is reduced in second or subsequent screens following removal of potentially malignant tumours in the population screened.

Discussion

The ideal screening test for ovarian cancer should be of high specificity and sensitivity, acceptable both to patients and medical staff, and cost-effective. It should be applied to a high-risk population. Apart from age, there are no high-risk factors for ovarian cancer. The age specific incidence is less than

Table 16.1   Comparison of sonar morphology and histological diagnoses in the first 3 years of the study at King's College Hospital

Ultrasound appearance	Histological diagnoses
1. Unilocular cystic ovary	Serous cysts, mucinous cystadenoma, stage I serous cystadenocarcinoma, serous cystadenomas
2. Multilocular cysts	Endometriomas, mucinous cystadenomas, metastatic sigmoid adenocarcinoma, metastatic adenocarcinoma of the breast
3. Cysts with solid areas	Benign cysts with adenofibromatous nodules, cystic teratomas, clear-cell carcinoma, serous cystadenocarcinoma stage I
4. Solid irregular ovary	Fibromas, metastatic adenocarcinoma of the breast

15/100 000 below the age of 40 years, but rises to 25/100 000 around 45 years and thereafter continues to rise, reaching 50/100 000 by the age of 70 years (OPCS Monitor, 1981). This would indicate that all women aged over 45 years, who possess one or both ovaries, should be screened for ovarian cancer.

It has been suggested that certain ultrasonographic features are associated with malignant changes, whereas others are associated with benign ovarian tumours. Morley & Barnett (1970) suggested that malignant change was indicated by the presence of more complex lesions with thick septa and solid areas, a view later supported by Koyabashi (1976). Morley & Barnett divided their results into 'correct' and 'helpful'. In their study ultrasound diagnosis of the nature of an ovarian neoplasm was 'correct' and confirmed by subsequent histological examination in 31 out of 59 patients (52 per cent); and was 'helpful' in 24 out of 49 patients (41 per cent). Koyabashi reported that ultrasound appearance permitted correct diagnosis in 69 per cent of benign cysts and 77 per cent of ovarian cancers. Therefore the failure rate reported by these authors was between 23 per cent and 48 per cent.

Meire et al (1978) described more complex criteria for differentiating between benign and malignant tumours. They reported that unilocular cysts with thin septa and locules were likely to be benign, whereas multilocular cysts with thin septa and nodules or multilocular cysts with thick septa (with or without nodules) were more likely to be malignant. However, the results from the study at King's do not agree with these conclusions, because in this series ultrasound appearance of abnormal ovaries bore little correlation to the histological diagnosis. For example the most benign ultrasound appearance, that of a unilocular cystic ovary, was associated with follicular or simple serous cysts and also found in association with a stage one serous cystadenocarcinoma. More sinister ultrasound appearances, of cysts with nodules, could be associated with benign neoplasms (such as simple cysts with adenofibromatous nodules, benign cystic teratomas and endometriomas) and could also be associated with premalignant tumours, such as papillary serous cystadenomas and even with frank malignancy, such as the clear-cell carcinoma and metastatic breast and sigmoid carcinomas. For these reasons I believe that ultrasound appearances are unreliable and that the only means by which a diagnosis can be made with certainty is by histological examination.

I believe that real-time mechanical sector ultrasound provides new hope for the early detection of ovarian cancer. It is quick, non-invasive, painless and provides results immediately.

However, the high incidence of benign tumours with no malignant potential that are removed may not be entirely satisfactory. One may argue that even benign unilocular cysts are prone to torsion and haemorrhage, and should therefore be removed electively to avoid emergency surgery.

On the other hand the incidence of torsion may be so low that it makes elective surgery a costly and unnecessary exercise. A control group of women, not being subjected to ultrasound screening, is urgently required.

The following questions remain unanswered:

1. What is the incidence of ovarian accidents in a control population?
2. What is the incidence of cancer deaths in a control population as compared to the screened group?
3. What is the incidence of cancer in repeat screens?
4. Is 1 year the right time interval (NB three cancers were detected at repeat annual scan, the first having been normal 1 year earlier)?
5. What is the cost-effectiveness of this as a screening procedure?

There is no doubt that real-time mechanical sector ultrasound can detect early ovarian cancer, which is not detected by clinical examination. None of the cancers diagnosed in the King's study were palpable even on examination under anaesthetic. There have been no reported false negatives in the screening programme as yet, and this is another encouraging feature.

The technique warrants further evaluation as an effective screening test for early ovarian cancer.

GYNAECOLOGICAL ULTRASOUND AS USED IN THE MANAGEMENT OF INFERTILITY

Follicular growth

Ultrasound monitoring of follicular growth in the ovarian cycle is now established practice in most fertility centres. It is an essential adjunct to diagnosis and treatment in all types of female infertility and in *in vitro* fertilisation programmes.

The possibility of visualising and monitoring follicular growth during the ovarian cycle was first postulated by Kratochwil et al (1972). Hackeloer et al (1977) used the technique for monitoring ovulation induction, and in a later publication (1979) reported good correlations between follicular diameters and plasma oestradiol levels in women in spontaneous menstrual cycles. Since then, several workers have reported successful use of real-time mechanical sector ultrasonography in the monitoring of follicular growth and rupture during the ovarian cycle (Queenan et al, 1980; O'Herlihy et al, 1980; Ylostalo et al 1981; Sallam et al, 1982).

Methodology

The patient is scanned in the supine position with a full bladder as for any other gynaecological ultrasound examination. Using the methodology previously cited in this chapter, the ovaries are located and the number of follicles present in each ovary is counted. The extent to which the bladder is filled will affect the shape of the Graafian follicles (Fig. 16.4). Hence measuring the maximum diameter in any one plan will not give reproducible

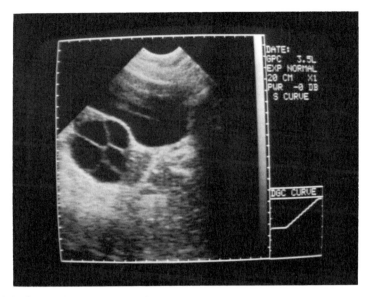

Fig. 16.4 Ovarian hyperstimulation. Scan photograph showing five Graafian follicles in an ovary stimulated by clomiphene citrate and human menopausal gonadotrophins. The odd shape of these follicles necessitates measuring four diameters before calculating the maximum mean follicular diameter for each follicle

results (Prins & Vogelzang, 1984). Therefore it is important to measure the mean follicular diameter for each follicle observed. On transverse scan the maximum transverse follicular diameter is measured, and on longitudinal scan the maximum longitudinal diameter and the maximum anteroposterior diameters are measured. The mean follicular diameter (MFD) may then be calculated for each follicle.

In cases of multiple follicular development in ovaries stimulated with clomiphene, with or without human menopausal gonadotrophins (HMG), the shape of the follicles may not be oval or round; thus the anteroposterior diameter may not be the same on longitudinal and transverse scans. In such cases the maximum transverse diameter and anteroposterior should be measured in the transverse plane and the maximum longitudinal and anteroposterior diameters should be measured in the longitudinal plane. A mean follicular diameter should then be calculated on these four diameters.

Ovarian changes during the follicular phase

Follicles may be seen in the ovaries as early as day 2 or 3 of the menstrual cycle, measuring 3–4 mm in size. Several workers have reported that the rate of growth of a follicle is between 1 and 2 mm per day (Hackeloer & Robinson, 1978; Smith et al, 1980; Queenan et al, 1980; Sallam et al, 1982) thus by day 12 the dominant follicle is 12–16 mm in size. Follicular rupture in a natural cycle occurs when the MFD is between 18 and 28 mm

(Hackeloer et al, 1979; Smith et al, 1980; Renaud et al, 1980; Sallam et al, 1982). In clomiphene cycles follicular rupture usually occurs between 18 and 24 mm (O'Herlihy et al, 1980; Vargyas et al, 1982), whereas the follicles seen in cycles stimulated by HMG are significantly smaller, between 16 and 20 mm (Ylostalo et al, 1979; Siebel et al, 1981; Marrs et al, 1983).

Signs of ovulation

It is essential that serial scans are performed during the ovarian cycle to ensure a correct diagnosis of ovulation being made. When follicular rupture has occurred the follicle may undergo one of the following:

1. Follicle collapses: on ultrasound examination this appears as an irregular echogenic line surrounding a compressed cystic area. This is attributed to partial emptying of follicular fluid from the follicle.
2. Follicle disappears: in this case the ovary attains its normal hypoechoic structure, ovoid shape and smooth echogenic outline. This is due to complete emptying of follicular fluid from the follicle.
3. Follicle enlarges and fills with internal echoes: in this case the follicle may or may not retain its smooth outline but the size increases and internal echoes of low-level density appear inside the follicle. These low-level echoes are attributed to blood clots in the follicle following follicular rupture.

The appearance of the corpus luteum may not be noted until 3 or 4 days after follicular rupture. When it is visualised it is seen as a unilocular cystic structure which may or may not contain low-density echoes inside it. A definitive diagnosis of a corpus luteum being present can only be made by laparoscopy, but a presumptive diagnosis may be made when it is seen to disappear in the early proliferative phase of a subsequent menstrual cycle. Hackeloer & Sallam (1983) state that the corpus luteum can be visualised in the mid-luteal phase as an oblong structure 30–35 mm in length and 20–25 mm in width. It consists of three concentric areas with different echocystic properties: a central echo-free area (possibly representing a blood clot), a surrounding mildly echogenic area (probably luteal tissue), and a peripheral strong echogenic outline of an ovarian stroma. This has not been confirmed by other workers. In the author's experience the only confirmation of a corpus luteum, on ultrasound examination, is a change in size and shape during the luteal phase accompanied by disappearance in the subsequent cycle. The echo-free area cannot always be seen in the luteal phase; thus a single scan of the ovary at this stage may not show evidence of a corpus luteum.

When postovulation endometrial changes (see below) are seen in the luteal phase one may presume more definitely that ovulation has taken place at some time preceding the scan.

Uterine changes in the menstrual cycle

Cyclic changes in uterine size and endometrial echoes are noted in the menstrual cycle.

Size

The uterus grows gradually during the proliferative stage, and this can be measured on ultrasound examination. It has been claimed that an increase in size in the luteal phase is seen in conception cycles and a decrease in size is noted in non-conception cycles (Mason & Adams, 1983). This has not been confirmed by others, and needs further investigation.

Endometrium

Changes in the endometrium have been noted during the menstrual cycle, and correlate well with plasma oestradiol and progesterone levels (Hackeloer & Sallam, 1983). In the early proliferative phase the endometrium is seen as translucent and thin (Kurtz & Rifkin, 1983) on either side of the mid-line echo. In the late proliferative phase the endometrium increases in thickness and cells of the superficial layer may be separated by oedema fluid which is ultrasonically demonstrated by a hyporeflective area (Fig. 16.5). Following ovulation the endometrium shrinks in thickness as the oedema of the superficialis is lost; thus dense echogenic echoes appear on either side of the ultrasound mid-line echo.

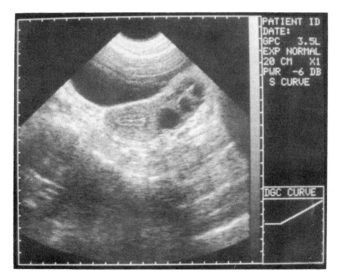

Fig. 16.5 Endometrial ring. Transverse scan showing the uterus and one ovary. The endometrial ring with a midline echo is present in the follicular phase. Three Graafian follicles can be seen in the ovary

Hackeloer (1984) studied the endometrium in the luteal phase in 62 cases and suggests that the thickness of the secretory endometrium correlates with the hormone profile and pregnancy rates following ovulation induction and insemination. No pregnancy was seen with an endometrial diameter lower than 30 mm at days 18–21. These results have not been confirmed by other workers.

APPLICATION OF ULTRASOUND IN THE MANAGEMENT OF INFERTILITY

(1) Timing of intercourse and artificial insemination

Monitoring follicular growth during the ovarian cycle can be a useful aid to timing of intercourse and artificial insemination, instead of relying on inaccurate methods such as basal body temperature (BBT) charts and average cycle lengths. In a study done at King's College Hospital (1981, unpublished data) it was noted that ultrasound evidence of ovulation occurred on the day of drop in BBT in four out of 19 cycles monitored, in patients who failed to conceive after six AID cycles.

Kerin (1979) reported the use of ultrasound monitoring for timing of insemination in an AID programme. Insemination was carried out daily after a mean follicular diameter of 15 mm was achieved, and continued until ultrasound signs of ovulation were observed. The fecundibility rate increased to 14 per cent, when ultrasound monitoring was used, as compared to 7 per cent when only BBT charts were used. Marinho et al (1982) reported a similar increase from 6 to 12 per cent when ultrasound was used instead of BBT charts.

(2) Monitoring clomiphene citrate (CC) therapy

Ultrasound scanning has been used to monitor patients on CC therapy, and a good correlation has been reported by Vargyas et al (1982) between plasma oestradiol concentrations and follicular diameters. The number of follicles, the size of the follicles and the occurrence of multiple ovulation can be observed.

Luteinised unruptured follicle syndrome (LUF) occurs in up to 34 per cent of CC cycles or spontaneous cycles, and can be accurately diagnosed using ultrasound monitoring (Liukkonen et al, 1984). The leading follicle is noted to achieve a maximum size between 20 and 24 mm, and then seen to regress (1–2 mm per day) during the luteal phase. When this change in mean follicular diameter is noted in the presence of endometrial thickening a diagnosis of LUF can be made with sufficient confidence. Treatment with an injection of hCG, appropriately timed, may be implemented as recommended by O'Herlihy et al (1982).

(3) Human menopausal gonadotrophin therapy

Ultrasound may be used in conjunction with hormonal monitoring, or may be used on its own. When ultrasound is used in conjunction with 24-hour urinary oestrogens it has resulted in diminishing the incidence of multiple pregnancy as well as the severity of hyperstimulation syndrome (Hackeloer et al, 1977; Siebel et al, 1981; Fink et al, 1982).

When ultrasound is used as the sole method of monitoring, hCG is administered when one or two follicles achieve a mean follicular diameter of 20 mm. If more than two follicles are noted at 20 mm or above (mean follicular diameter), hCG is withheld and the cycle abandoned (Sallam et al, 1982). It has been shown that ultrasound used as the sole method of monitoring has proved to be as successful as hormone monitoring on its own in preventing multiple pregnancy and diminishing the severity of incidence of hyperstimulation syndrome (Sallam et al, 1983). The cumulative pregnancy rate after 9 months of the study done by Sallam et al (1983) was higher in the ultrasound-monitored group than the oestradiol-monitored group.

In a study by Fink et al (1982), where patients were monitored using ultrasound as well as using 24-hour urinary oestrogen monitoring, it was noted that ultrasound was a poor predictor of multiple pregnancy. Out of five women with multiple pregnancy from 17 women who conceived during this study, three showed only one mature follicle at the time of hCG injection. This would indicate that smaller follicles may yield mature oocytes and result in multiple pregnancy. The evidence from IVF programmes confirms that small follicles in hMG-stimulated cycles do yield mature oocytes resulting in pregnancies, and therefore ultrasound should be used in conjunction with oestrogen monitoring to prevent multiple pregnancies occurring. Haning et al (1983) have shown that plasma oestradiol is superior to ultrasound and urinary oestrogens as a predictor of ovarian hyperstimulation during ovulation induction with hMG.

(4) *In vitro* fertilisation

(a) Monitoring response to ovulation induction

Ultrasound is used to monitor ovarian response in IVF treatment cycles following drug therapy using CC with or without hMG and other ovulation induction agents.

The information gained by ultrasound as regards the site, the number and size of follicles is an invaluable adjunct to endocrine monitoring.

Follicular size correlates well with optimal maturation since follicles with an MFD of 18–25 mm were found to have a normal complement of granulosa cells in a study by McNatty et al (1979). In the normal cycle the correlation between follicular size and plasma oestradiol concentrations shows a linear correlation ($r = 2.0968$) (Hackeloer et al, 1979). However, in induced cycles the combined use of ultrasound and serum oestradiol levels for the prediction of impending ovulation has given conflicting results. This is attributed to the recruitment of various cohorts of follicles which are at different stages of function and maturation. Mantzavinos et al (1983) found no correlation between serum oestradiol levels and the size of the largest follicles, and only a moderate correlation with the number of follicles. Tarlatzis et al (1984) found that serum oestradiol levels on the day of hCG administration were similar in women developing one large follicle (greater than 15 mm MFD) and those developing three large follicles. The mean follicular volumes in the patients did not differ.

It would therefore be reasonable to assume that the individual follicle in monofollicular cycles contributes more to peripheral oestradiol levels than the individual follicle in multifollicular cycles. The maturity of follicles in stimulated cycles is not necessarily reflected by the size of the follicles.

In the author's experience, ultrasound should be used in conjunction with endocrine monitoring for IVF cycles as the two methods complement each other and aid in accurate timing of oocyte recovery.

Ultrasound assessment of the endometrium in stimulated cycles in an IVF programme may help in timing of oocyte recovery. In a study by Smith et al (1984) the reflectivity and thickness of endometrium was assessed as an additional ultrasound parameter to monitor patients. A change in reflectivity of the endometrium from darker than the myometrium to equal to and brighter than the myometrium, during the proliferative phase, was graded from D to A: D, being early proliferative, then through C and B to A, being late proliferative.

Endometrial thickness was measured as the distance between the reflective surface of the endometrium on the anterior wall of the uterus and the opposite surface on the posterior wall of the uterus. In patients where follicular size was the sole indicator for hCG injection, as compared to patients who had follicular size plus endometrial changes monitored, the oocyte retrieval rates were similar (2·9 and 3·0 per patient). However, the fertilisation rate was better in the second group (82·5 per cent) as compared to 59·2 per cent of the first group. The pregnancy rates in the two groups did not differ. They infer that endometrial changes should be considered when monitoring IVF cycles. This needs further evaluation because the grading system used is open to question, and the pregnancy rate was no different in the two groups.

Ultrasound-guided oocyte recovery

Trans-vesical ultrasound-directed oocyte recovery was first described by Susan Lenz and co-workers (1981) as a simple technique that could be performed successfully under local anaesthetic. It is superior to laparoscopy in cases where the ovaries are buried under bowel adhesions, but can also be used for laparoscopically accessible ovaries.

The technique was evaluated further by others (Goswamy et al, 1984; Feichtinger & Kemeter, 1984; Wikland and Hamberger, 1984) and shown to be a successful method for recovering oocytes in IVF programmes. However, follicles in the pouch of Douglas were difficult to aspirate and in cases where endometriosis resulted in both ovaries being bound down by adhesions in the pouch of Douglas another route was sought to make oocyte recovery possible. Dellenbach et al (1984) described the transvaginal route using abdominal ultrasound guidance; thus ovaries in the pouch of Douglas were now accessible for ultrasound-directed oocyte recovery.

In cases where adhesions result in only part of the ovary being visible through a distended bladder the transurethral route is used. This was described by Parsons et al (1985) as an alternative route to transabdominal oocyte recovery.

In the author's opinion, from experience with more than 200 such surgical procedures, the route for ultrasound-directed oocyte recovery should be dependent on ovarian position. The choice of route is as follows:

1. ovary lateral to uterus and adjacent to bladder: transabdomino-vesical;
2. high ovary just deep to abdominal wall and not adjacent to bladder: transabdominal;
3. high ovary lateral to uterus and partially adjacent to bladder: transurethral.
4. low ovary in the pouch of Douglas: transvaginal.

Complications of ultrasound-directed oocyte recovery

1. *Pain* When ultrasound oocyte recovery is done using local infiltration anaesthesia to the abdominal wall, a premedication is required as entry of the needle into the ovary can be painful. The pain following different routes has not been assessed and some workers claim that the vaginal route is less painful than the abdominal route (Dellenbach et al, 1984). This has not been confirmed by other workers.
2. *Infection* The incidence of urinary tract infection or exacerbation of pelvic inflammatory disease is minor. However, because sterility in the vagina is difficult to achieve, this needs to be taken into account when attempting the vaginal route.
3. *Haematuria* This tends to be minor and transient, rarely persisting beyond 24 hours postoperatively. A case requiring 8 units of blood transfusion, where endometriosis in the uterovesical pouch was not previously diagnosed, has occurred in the author's experience. A preliminary laparoscopy, as work-up prior to IVF treatment, may have prevented this complication.
4. *Puncture of internal iliac vessels* This has occurred on three occasions in the author's experience and has not required any surgical interference. It is self-limiting and should not cause problems unless the vessels have been torn or lacerated.

5. *Bowel injury*   This has never occurred in the author's experience because a full bladder displaces intervening bowel loops between the bladder and the ovary.

Results. At Bourn Hall the practice has been to use ultrasound-directed oocyte recovery for patients with inaccessible ovaries.

Between 1 March 1985 and 15 August 1985 a total of 61 patients underwent ultrasound directed oocyte recovery. The results are shown in Table 16.2. The oocyte recovery rate, the fertilisation rate, and pregnancy rates were the same as those with laparoscopic oocyte recovery during the same period of time. The rate of ectopic pregnancies has been higher than with laparoscopic oocyte recovery, and this needs further evaluation, as does the risk of miscarriage.

SAFETY OF ULTRASOUND

Epidemiological studies do not indicate any hazard associated with perinatal ultrasound imaging.

The American Institute of Ultrasound in Medicine (AIUM) made the following statement in October 1983.

> Diagnostic ultrasound has been in use for over 25 years. Given its known benefits and recognised efficacy for medical diagnosis, including use during human pregnancy, the American Institute of Ultrasound in Medicine addresses the clinical safety of such use. No confirmed biological effects on patients or instrument operators caused by exposure at intensities typical of present diagnostic instruments have ever been reported.
>
> Although the possibility exists that such biological effects may be identified in the future, current data indicate that the benefit to patients of prudent use of diagnostic ultrasound outweighs the risk, if any, that may be present.

It is difficult to make firm statements about the clinical safety of diagnostic ultrasound. The experimental and epidemiological bases for risk assessment

Table 16.2   Results of ultrasound-directed oocyte recovery on 61 patients with laparoscopically inaccessible ovaries at Bourn Hall clinic (1 March–15 August 1985)

	No.	Comments
Oocyte recoveries (OR)	61	
Oocytes obtained	322	5·3 oocytes/patient
Failed oocyte recoveries	Nil	
Embryo replacements (ER)	56	91·8% of OR
3 embryos replaced	37	60·7% of OR
		66·1% of ER
Pregnancies	14	1 ectopic (7·1%)
		2 miscarriages (14·2%)
		11 ongoing
Pregnancy rate		23% per OR
		25% per ER

are far from complete. However, much work has been done with no evidence of harm in the clinical setting. The AIUM clinical safety statement forms an excellent basis for formulating a response to patients' questions and concerns.

THE FUTURE OF GYNAECOLOGICAL ULTRASOUND

As machines get better and imaging improves, the possibilities of ultrasound imaging are limitless.

Blood flow studies are providing encouraging information in obstetrics (Griffin et al, 1983). With the advent of Doppler and the possibility of offset mechanical sector systems it should be possible to measure uterine and ovarian blood flow. The changes in blood flow associated with tumour development, or with changes in the ovarian cycle, will provide more information and surely aid better diagnosis and treatment of the cancer patient as well as helping to reduce the misery of infertile patients. Ultrasound is just starting to show its potential in gynaecology and there is still a lot of research to be done in using this diagnostic tool to its full potential.

REFERENCES

AIUM Safety Statements 1983 Journal of Ultrasound in Medicine 2: R10
Bhattacharya M, Barlow J J 1975 Tumour associated antigen for cystadenocarcinoma of the ovary. National Cancer Institute Monograph 42: 25–33
Campbell S 1968 An improved method of fetal cephalometry by ultrasound. British Journal of Obstetrics and Gynaecology 75: 568–571
Campbell S 1974 The assessment of fetal development by diagnostic ultrasound. Clinics in Perinatology. 1: 507–519
Campbell S, Thoms A 1977 Ultrasound measurement of the fetal head to abdominal circumference ratio in the assessment of growth retardation. British Journal of Obstetrics and Gynaecology 84: 165–174
Campbell S, Goessens L, Goswamy R, Whitehead M I 1982 Real-time ultrasonography for determination of ovarian morphology and volume. A possible early screening test for ovarian cancer? Lancet 1: 425–426
Churches C K, Kurrle G R, Johnson B 1974 Treatment of carcinoma of the cervix by combination of irradiation and operation. American Journal of Obstetrics and Gynaecology 118: 1033–1040
Dellenbach P, Nisand I, Moreau L, Feger B, Plumere C, Gerlinger P et al 1984 Transvaginal sonographically controlled ovarian follicle puncture for egg retrieval. Lancet 1: 1467
Doll R, Payne P, Waterhouse J 1966 Cancer incidence in five continents. International Union Against Cancer/Springer, New York
Doll R, Muir C, Waterhouse J 1970 Cancer incidence in five continents, vol. II. International Union Against Cancer/Springer, New York
Donald I 1963 Use of ultrasonics in diagnosis of abdominal swellings. British Medical Journal ii: 1154–1155
Donald I, McVicar J, Brown T G 1958 Investigation of abdominal masses by pulsed ultrasound. Lancet 1: 1188–1195
Feichtinger W, Kemeter P 1984 Laparoscopic or ultrasonically guided follicle aspiration for in vitro fertilization? Journal of In Vitro Fertilization and Embryo Transfer 1(4): 244–249
Fink R S, Bowes L P, Mackintosh C E, Smith W I, Georgiades E, Ginsburg J 1982 The value of ultrasound for monitoring ovarian responses to gonadotrophin stimulant therapy. British Journal of Obstetrics and Gynaecology 89(10): 856–861

Fleischer A C, Wentz A C, Jones H W III, Everett-James Jr A 1983 Ultrasound evaluation of the ovary. In: Hobbins J C, Winsberg F, Berkowitz R L (eds) Ultrasonography in Obstetrics and Gynaecology, 2nd edn. Williams & Wilkins, London, pp 209–225

Funkhouser J W, Hunter H K, Thompson N J 1975 Diagnostic value of cul-de-sac aspiration in detection of ovarian carcinoma. Acta Cytologica 19: 538–541

Goswamy R K, Campbell S, Whitehead M I 1982 Establishment of normal ranges for ovarian volumes and identification of enlarged ovaries by real-time mechanical sector sonar in postmenopausal women. In: Lenski R A, Morley P (eds) Ultrasound 1982. Pergamon Press Oxford, pp 615–619

Goswamy R, Campbell S, Whitehead M I 1983 Screening for ovarian cancer. Clinics in Obstetrics and Gynaecology 10(3): 621–643

Goswamy R, Vaid P, Parsons J, Matson P, Whitehead M I 1984 IVF and embryo transfer—an outpatient procedure. Journal of In Vitro Fertilization and Embryo Transfer 1: 111

Gray H 1966 Osteology. The bones of the lower limb (ossa membri inferioris). In: Goss C M (ed) Anatomy of the human body, 28th edn. Lea & Febiger, Philadelphia, pp 236–245

Green B 1980 Pelvic ultrasonography. In: Sarti D A, Sample W F (eds) Diagnostic ultrasound text and cases. G K Hall, Boston, pp 502–589

Griffin D, Cohen-Overbeek T, Campbell S 1983 Fetal and utero-placental blood flow. Clinics in Obstetrics and Gynaecology 10(3): 565–602

Hackeloer B J 1984 Ultrasound scanning of the ovarian cycle. Journal of In Vitro Fertilization and Embryo Transfer 1(4): 217–220

Hackeloer B J, Robinson H P 1978 Ultrasound examination of the growing ovarian follicles. Geburtshilfe und Frauenheilkunde 38: 163–168

Hackeloer B J, Sallam H N 1983 Ultrasound scanning of ovarian follicles. Clinics in Obstetrics and Gynaecology 10(3): 603–619

Hackeloer B J, Nitshke S, Daume E 1977 Ultrasonics of ovarian changes under gonadotrophin stimulation. Geburtshilfe und Frauenheilkunde 37: 185–190

Hackeloer B J, Fleming R, Robinson H P, Adam A H, Coutts J R T 1979 Correlation of ultrasonic and endocrinologic assessment of human follicular development. American Journal of Obstetrics and Gynecology 135: 122–128

Haning R V, Austin C W, Carlson I H, Kuzma D L, Shapiro S S, Zweibel W J 1983 Plasma estradiol is superior to ultrasound and urinary oestriol glucoronide as a predictor of ovarian hyperstimulation during induction of ovulation with menotropins. Fertility and Sterility 40: 31–36

Jeffcoate N 1975 Tumours of the Ovary. In: Principles of gynaecology, 4th edn. Butterworth, London–Boston, pp 447–484

Jones H W III 1975 Treatment of adenocarcinoma of the endometrium. Obstetrical and Gynaecological Survey 30: 147–169

Kerin J F P 1979 Determination of the optimal timing of insemination in women. In: Richardson D, Joyce D, Symonds M (eds) Frozen human semen. Royal College of Obstetricians and Gynaecologists, London, pp 105–132

Kerin J F, Edmonds D K, Warnes G M, Cox L W, Seamark R F, Matthews C D et al 1981 Morphological and functional relations of Graafian follicle growth to ovulation in women using ultrasonic, laparoscopic and biochemical measurements. British Journal of Obstetrics and Gynaecology 88: 81–89

Koyabashi M 1976 Use of diagnostic ultrasound in trophoblastic neoplasms and ovarian tumors. Cancer 38: 441–452

Kratochwil A, Urban G, Friedrich F 1972 Ultrasonic tomography of the ovaries. Annales Chirurgiae et Gynaecologiae Fenniae 61: 211–214

Kurtz A B, Rifkin M D 1983 Normal anatomy of the female pelvis. In: Hobbins J C, Winsberg F, Berkowitz R (eds) Ultrasonography in obstetrics and gynaecology. Williams & Williams, London, pp 193–208

Lenz S, Lauritsen J G, Kjellow M 1981 Collection of human oocytes for in vitro fertilization by ultrasonically guided follicular puncture. Lancet 1: 1163–1164

Liukkonen S, Koskimies A I, Tenhunen A, Ylostalo P 1984 Diagnosis of luteinized unruptured follicle (LUF) syndrome by ultrasound. Fertility and Sterility 41(1): 26–30

Mantzavinos T, Garcia J E, Jones H W 1983 Ultrasound measurement of ovarian follicles stimulated by human gonadotrophins for oocyte recovery and in-vitro fertilization. Fertility and Sterility 40: 461–465

Marinho A O, Sallam H N, Goessens L, Whitehead M I, Collins W P, Campbell S 1982 Pelvic ultrasonography during the periovulatory period of patients attending an AID clinic. Fertility and Sterility 37: 633–638

Marrs R P, Vargyas J M, March C M 1983 Correlation of ultrasonic and endocrinologic measurements in human menopausal gonadotrophin therapy. American Journal of Obstetrics and Gynaecology 145: 417–421

Mason W P, Adams J 1983 Clinical aspects of LH releasing hormone treatment. Journal of Obstetrics and Gynaecology 4: 70

McGowan L 1975 Peritoneal fluid profiles. National Cancer Institute Monographs 42: 75–79

McNatty K P, Moore Smith D, Makris A, Osathanondh R, Ryan K J 1979 The microenvironment of the human antral follicle: Interrelationships among the steroid levels in antral fluid, the population of granulosa cells, and the status of the oocyte in vivo and in vitro. Journal of Clinical Endocrinology and Metabolism 49: 851–860

Meire H B, Farrant P, Guha T 1978 Distinction of benign from malignant ovarian cysts by ultrasound. British Journal of Obstetrics and Gynaecology 85: 893–899

Minawi M F, El-Halafawy A A, Hadi M A, Hamid E A, Derballa S, Wahby O 1984 Laparoscopic gynaecographic and ultrasonographic vs clinical evaluation of a pelvic mass. Journal of Reproductive Medicine 29(3): 197–199

Morley P, Barnett E 1970 The use of ultrasound in the diagnosis of pelvis masses. British Journal of Radiology 43: 602–616

O'Brien W F, Buck D R, Nash J D 1984 Evaluation of sonography in the initial assessment of the gynaecologic patient. American Journal of Obstetrics and Gynecology 149: 598–602

O'Herlihy C, de Crespigny L J, Robinson H P 1980 Monitoring ovarian follicular development with real time ultrasound. British Journal of Obstetrics and Gynaecology 87: 613–618

O'Herlihy C, Pepperell R J, Robinson H P 1982 Ultrasound timing of human chorionic gonadotrophin administration in clomiphene stimulated cycles. Obstetrics and Gynaecology 59: 40–45

OPCS (Office of Population Census Survey) Monitor 1981 Deaths by Cause D.H.2 81/1

Parker R T, Parker C H, Wilbanks G D 1970 Cancer of the ovary. Survival studies based upon operative therapy, chemotherapy, and radiotherapy. American Journal of Obstetrics and Gynecology 108: 878–888

Parsons J, Riddle A, Booker M, Sharma V, Goswamy R, Wilson L et al 1985 Oocyte retrieval for IVF by ultrasonically guided needle aspiration via the urethra. Lancet 1: 1076–1077

Prins G S, Vogelzang R L 1984 Inherent sources of ultrasound variability in relation to follicular measurements. Journal of In Vitro Fertilization and Embryo Transfer 1(4): 221–225

Queenan J T, O'Brien G D, Bains L M, Simpson J, Collins W P, Campbell S 1980 Ultrasound scanning of ovaries to detect ovulation in women. Fertility and Sterility 34: 99–105

Ranney B, Ahmad M I 1979 Early identification, differentiation and treatment of ovarian neoplasia. International Journal of Gynecology and Obstetrics 17: 209–218

Reeves R D, Drake T S, O'Brien W F 1980 Ultrasonographic versus clinical evaluation of a pelvic mass. Obstetrics and Gynaecology 55(5): 551–554

Renaud R L, Macler J, Dervain I, Ehret M C, Avon C, Plas-Roser S et al 1980 Echographic study of follicular maturation and ovulation during the normal menstrual cycle. Fertility and Sterility 33: 272–276

Sallam H N, Marinho A O, Collins W P, Whitehead M I, Campbell S 1982 Monitoring gonadotrophin therapy by real-time ultrasonic scanning of ovarian follicles. British Journal of Obstetrics and Gynaecology 89: 155–159

Sallam H N, Whitehead M I, Collins W P, Campbell S 1983 A retrospective analysis of two methods of monitoring gonadotrophin therapy. Paper presented at the IXth World Congress on Fertility and Sterility, Dublin, June 1983

Samaan A N, Smith J P, Rutledge F N, Schultz P S 1976 The significance of measurement of human placental lactogen, human chorionic gonadotrophin, and carcinoembryonic antigen in patients with ovarian cancer. American Journal of Obstetrics and Gynecology 126(2): 186–189

Sample W F 1980 Gray-scale ultrasonography of the normal female pelvis. In: Sanders R C, James A E (eds) The principles and practice of ultrasonography in obstetrics and gynaecology. Appleton-Century-Crofts, New York, pp 75–89

Schlensker K H, Beckers H 1980 The use of ultrasound in the Diagnosis of Pelvic Pathology. Archiv für Gynaecologie 229: 91–105

Siebel M M, McArdle C R, Thompson I E, Berger M J, Taymor M L 1981 The role of ultrasound in ovulation induction: a critical appraisal. Fertility and Sterility 36: 573–577

Smith D H, Picker R H, Sinosich M, Saunders D M 1980 Assessment of ovulation by ultrasound and estradiol levels during spontaneous and induced cycles. Fertility and Sterility 33: 387–395

Smith B, Porter R, Ahuja K, Craft I 1984 Ultrasonic assessment of endometrial changes in stimulated cycles in an in vitro fertilization and embryo transfer program. Journal of In Vitro Fertilization and Embryo Transfer 1(4): 233–238

Tarlatzis B C, Laufer N, De Cherney A H 1984 The use of ovarian ultrasonography in monitoring ovulation induction. Journal of In Vitro Fertilization and Embryo Transfer 1(4): 226–232

Vargyas J M, Marrs R P, Kletzky O A, Mishell D R 1982 Correlation of ultrasound measurement of ovarian follicle size and serum estradiol levels in ovulatory patients following clomiphene citrate for in vitro fertilization. American Journal of Obstetrics and Gynaecology 144: 569–573

Wagman H, Brown C L 1971 Ovarian cytology. An application of cytology in an attempt at the early detection of ovarian carcinoma. British Journal of Cancer 25(1): 81–84

Wikland M, Hamberger L 1984 Ultrasound as a diagnostic and operative tool for in vitro fertilization and embryo replacement (IVF/ER) programs. Journal of in Vitro Fertilization and Embryo Transfer 1(4): 213–216

Ylostalo P, Ronnberg L, Jouppila P 1979 Measurement of the ovarian follicle by ultrasound in ovulation induction. Fertility and Sterility 3: 651–655

Ylostalo P, Lindgren P G, Nillius S J 1981 Ultrasonic measurement of ovarian follicles, ovarian and uterine size during induction of ovulation with human gonadotrophins. Acta Endocrinologica 98: 592–598

Nuclear magnetic resonance imaging in obstetrics and gynaecology

INTRODUCTION

Magnetic resonance imaging (MRI) is a new technique for viewing the internal anatomy of the body. It is based on the phenomenon of nuclear magnetic resonance (NMR) which was discovered simultaneously in 1946 by Bloch et al and Purcell et al, and for which they were jointly awarded the 1952 Nobel Prize for physics. They showed that when certain atomic nuclei are placed within a magnetic field and then stimulated by radio waves of a particular frequency, they will re-emit some of the absorbed energy in the form of radio signals; this is known as nuclear magnetic resonance. NMR spectroscopy became the province of physicists and chemists as a powerful tool for the elucidation of the structure of matter at the molecular level. Some 30 years later, in a letter to *Nature*, Lauterbur (1973) published the first magnetic resonance image of two tubes of water. It is now clear from the large volume of published work that this method represents a significant advance in medical imaging.

The Department of Physics at Nottingham University, in conjunction with the University Hospital, made a substantial contribution to research into harnessing magnetic resonance as an imaging technique (Mansfield and Maudsley, 1976; Mansfield et al, 1978; Hinshaw et al, 1978, 1979; Hawkes et al, 1980). Prototype clinical imaging systems were first set up early in 1980 in Nottingham, London and Aberdeen. Subsequent progress has been rapid; its value in the assessment of pathology in the nervous system and musculoskeletal system has been clearly demonstrated (Worthington, 1983). Johnson et al (1984) were the first to image the fetus and indicate the potential value of MRI in obstetrics.

The pelvis is suitable for examination by MRI because of the minimal effect of respiratory motion on the pelvic organs. In gynaecology MRI has potential in both assessment and staging of malignant disease. Fetal movement in the first and second trimesters of pregnancy limits the resolution that can be obtained, but maternal anatomy is particularly well defined.

311

PHYSICAL PROPERTIES

There are several bands of radiation within the electromagnetic spectrum which can penetrate human tissues and so be harnessed for imaging. The recently developed MRI uses radiofrequency radiation (RF) in the presence of a carefully structured magnetic field to generate high-quality cross-sectional images of the body. These images portray the distribution density of hydrogen nuclei and parameters relating to their motion, the so-called T_1 and T_2 relaxation times, in the tissue water and lipids. When used properly the method appears to be unassociated with any significant hazards (Budinger, 1981; Wolffe et al, 1982). Although there is no evidence to suggest that the developing embryo would be harmed by the exposure conditions during NMR imaging, the guidelines of the National Radiological Protection Board (1983) recommend the exclusion of pregnant patients during the first trimester when organ development is taking place, except where the pregnancy is to be electively terminated.

Production of the NMR signal

Most of the images to date have been based on the hydrogen nucleus or proton, which is favourable from the NMR standpoint because it gives a relatively high signal and is abundant in biological tissues. Because protons have both an associated magnetic field and a spin they can be regarded as tiny bar magnets spinning about an axis. When a group of such protons is exposed to a magnetic field, a majority of these nuclear magnets will align in the direction of the field. In addition, their axes will be both tilted and caused to rotate like a small gyroscope. The frequency of this so-called precessional movement is directly proportional to the strength of the applied field. If now a pulse of radiowaves from a coil is imposed on the protons a strong interaction or resonance will occur when their frequency coincides with the precessional frequency of the protons. The energy absorbed by the protons is re-emitted after a short interval as a tiny nuclear signal, and this can be detected in a coil surrounding the sample. This signal has an initial size which is proportional to the density of protons. It then dies away exponentially as the disturbed protons, which were all initially moving in phase, return or relax back to their original state. As they do so they exchange energy both with their surroundings and between themselves. The so-called T_1 relaxation time is the time that it takes for the protons to return to their original state, and the T_2 time is related to the time that it takes for the precessing nuclei to get out of step with one another. Different sequences of radiowaves have been devised so that the resulting nuclear signal is weighted to different degrees by the proton density and the T_1 and T_2 relaxation times. The nuclear signal is also influenced by bulk flow of protons, and MRI therefore offers the potential to gain useful insights into blood flow by a non-invasive technique. As with computed tomography (CT), the display of soft tissue detail is at a premium, and there is with NMR imaging the additional advantage of being able to manipulate the contrast between tumours in order to highlight pathological changes by altering the pattern of radiowaves which is applied. This is done by changing the time constants associated with the different sequences of radiowaves.

Localisation of the NMR signal

Since the resonant frequency is proportional to the strength of the main magnetic field, if this varies in a known fashion then the resonant frequency in different regions will be different. This is achieved by the use of so-called field gradient coils contained within the main magnet. By separating out the different frequency components in the complex nuclear signal each can be ascribed to a particular location in a given cross-section. Each area element or pixel is therefore labelled by being associated with a different resonant frequency.

Selection of the position and thickness of the imaging plane

Because the radiowaves from the transmitter coil cannot be collimated into a narrow beam, as can X-rays, on account of their much greater wavelength; there is a fundamental difference in the method of selecting the body plane to be imaged. Both the position and thickness of this plane are selected by confining the collection of signals to the desired region. This is achieved by tailoring the frequency content of the radiowaves so that within the field conditions only a selected strip of protons is excited. This is the basis of the so-called method of selective excitation. This means that the position of the imaging plane is selected without moving the patient, and that the additional perspectives of direct sagittal and coronal views are available in addition to the more conventional transverse axial sections.

Components of an NMR imaging system

All NMR scanners have the same basic components: a magnet, which may be resistive or superconducting, within which are gradient coils to produce variations in the main field. Surrounding the part to be imaged is an appropriately sized radio transmitter and receiver coil (Fig. 17.1). Ancillary equipment is required to generate and analyse the NMR signals from which the final image is constructed. This is presented as an analogue grey scale display of the signal in each picture element within a given anatomical cross-section and a typical matrix size is 128×128 with a slice thickness of 1 cm. By appropriate manipulation of the NMR signals abstraction of numerical values of the proton density and relaxation times can be made. One of the few drawbacks to NMR imaging is that its low inherent sensitivity requires long imaging times of typically 2–20 minutes. Methods have now been

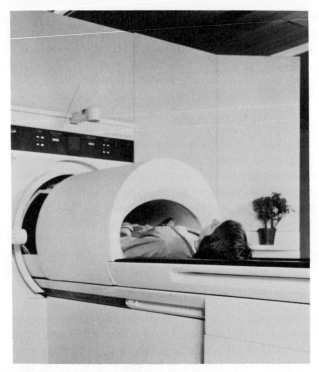

Fig. 17.1   Picker 0·15 Tesla resistive system.

developed which allow multiple slices to be acquired during a single exposure, thus effectively reducing the data acquisition time for each section. The interpretation of images requires a knowledge of the conditons under which the data were collected. The signal values of NMR can vary widely for a given tissue and the grey scale ordering of tissues is not constant as with CT.

THE NORMAL FEMALE PELVIS

The unique abilities that magnetic resonance is capable of providing is perhaps best demonstrated initially by looking at the anatomy of the normal female pelvis. Pulse sequences giving T_2 weighted images have been found to provide the best anatomical delineation. Figure 17.2a is a sagittal MRI scan taken in the mid-line of a normal femal volunteer. Subcutaneous fat, due to the high number of mobile protons, has a high-intensity signal with this sequence. The uterus and cervix have an intermediate-intensity signal of uniform density. Urine within the bladder has both a long T_1 and T_2 relaxation time and has a low-density signal. Cortical bone with a lack of mobile protons is represented as a black line. Muscles and viscera fall within an intermediate range. If the T_2 weighting is increased the uterus has a

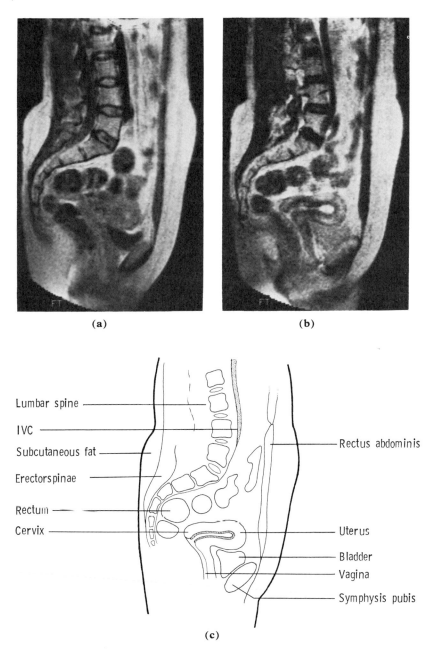

(a)   (b)

Lumbar spine

IVC

Subcutaneous fat

Erectorspinae

Rectum

Cervix

Rectus abdominis

Uterus

Bladder

Vagina

Symphysis pubis

(c)

Fig. 17.2   The normal female pelvis: (a) T_2 weighted sagittal image; (b) longer T_2 weighted image; (c) Diagrammatic section of the female pelvis.

distinctive appearance (Fig. 17.2b). There is now differentiation of the uterus into its respective constituents. The myometrium has an intermediate-intensity signal in contrast to the endometrium which has a signal of high intensity. Encircling the endometrium is a low-intensity band within the myometrium. An annotated illustration is shown in Figure 17.2c for comparative purposes. The nature of this layer is uncertain and has been ascribed to the stratum basalis (Hricak et al, 1983). Our preliminary studies have indicated that this is more likely to be a compacted muscle layer at the myometrial–endometrial junction. This is important with regard to assessing the depth of myometrial invasion in early endometrial carcinomas. Continuation of this layer is seen into the cervix; although less evident it is nevertheless distinct. With this particular sequence the nucleus pulposus of the intervertebral discs has a high-intensity signal, which is reduced and eventually lost in progressive degenerative diseases of the spine (Chaftez et al 1983).

The normal ovary is more difficult to visualise, having an intermediate-intensity signal with most T_2 weighted sequences. Follicular cysts within the ovary often highlight its position, and are shown particularly well on a transverse axial image slice (Fig. 17.3). Image slices in the transverse plane are comparable to that provided by computerised tomography; although fat, with its high signal intensity, facilitates easier identification of muscle planes. Understanding the unique qualities of multiplanar imaging, tissue characterisation and increased resolution that MRI is able to provide is an important prerequisite before its application to pathology.

GYNAECOLOGICAL PATHOLOGY

The uterus

As indicated above the uterus has already been shown to have a distinctive appearance when certain T_2 weighted pulse sequences are used. This is of

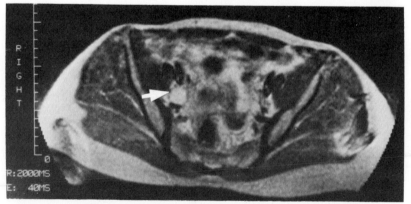

Fig. 17.3 T_2 weighted: transverse axial view through the mid-pelvis demonstrating follicular cyst in left ovary (arrow).

particular interest with regard to the staging of early endometrial adenocarcinoma. Adenocarcinoma of the endometrium has a signal of similar high intensity to normal endometrium when using a T_2 weighted pulse sequence. Therefore it is possible in stage I tumours to demonstrate invasion into the myometrium and to measure the depth from the serosa. This has important prognostic significance. We have imaged 15 cases of stage I tumours, 12 of which have shown an excellent correlation with pathological findings following hysterectomy (Powell et al, 1986b). In two cases foci of adenomyosis were indistinguishable from tumour, and in one the scan was unsatisfactory. The low-intensity band previously described is of particular value in assessing superficial invasion. Figure 17.4 is a parasagittal image using a T_2 weighted pulse sequence of an endometrial adenocarcinoma. The tumour is sited at the fundus of the uterus and has breached the low-intensity band. In those patients with deeply invasive disease it is absent. Both ultrasound and CT examination fail to give this sort of information. At present it is not possible to differentiate atypical hyperplastic endometrium from an early non-invasive tumour. Endometriotic deposits in the pelvis also possess a high-intensity signal when T_2 weighted sequences are used. We have regularly identified endometriotic deposits down to 5 mm size. Endometriotic ovarian cysts also have a characteristic high-intensity signal on both T_1 and T_2 weighted sequences.

The intermediate signal seen from the myometrium in T_2 weighted

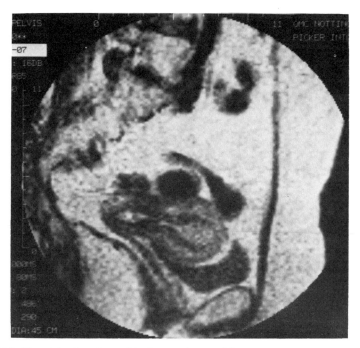

Fig. 17.4 T_2 weighted: endometrial adenocarcinoma of the uterus.

sequences is reflected in leiomyomata (Fig. 17.5). This is a greatly enlarged uterus with multiple leiomyomata. Calcified areas within are shown as low-intensity areas. Leiomyomata can be easily recognised as they present a characteristic appearance distinguishing themselves from other common tumours in the pelvis.

The cervix

Advanced carcinoma of the cervix has an intermediate signal intensity with both T_1 and T_2 weighted sequences. This means its appearances are less distinctive. Nevertheless, magnetic resonance still has several advantages over CT. The high-intensity signal from fat within the pelvis acts as an excellent contrast to the edge of an advancing cervical tumour. Two transverse axial images, just above, and at the level of the heads of femur are shown through a large carcinoma of the cervix (Figs 17.6a and 17.6b). Both ureters are dilated and the tumour is invading into the rectum. The pelvic side walls are not involved. No potentially hazardous intravenous contrast agents are used—unlike CT. Metastatic disease to the lymph nodes is difficult to assess, and MRI relies on similar criteria to that of CT, i.e. an alteration in size and morphology. Magnetic resonance's multiplanar imaging facility allows early FIGO stage I and II cervical tumours to be seen in the sagittal perspective (Fig. 17.7). This allows assessment of

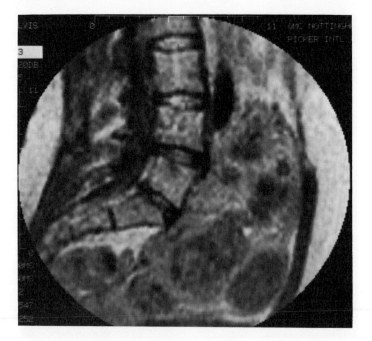

Fig. 17.5 T_2 weighted : large uterine fibroid.

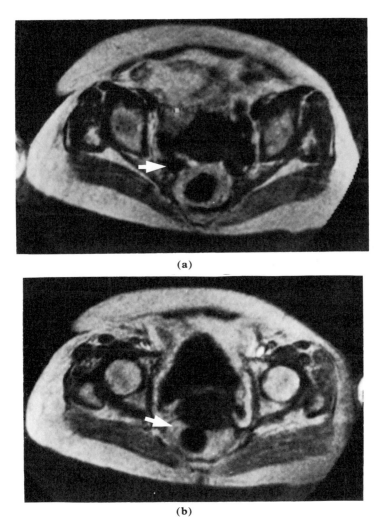

(a)

(b)

Fig. 17.6   T₂ weighted: Advanced cervical carcinoma: (a) transverse axial image at level of femur head: tumour invading into rectum (arrow); (b) mid-pelvis view; tumour involving ureters (arrow).

extension both upwards into the body of the uterus and downwards into the vaginal vault.

Figure 17.7 demonstrates a tumour which has completely replaced the cervix and is invading into the uterine body. A careful comparison between MRI and CT is necessary before conclusions are drawn as to which is the more appropriate technique for imaging of this disease.

The ovary

MRI is a suitable imaging modality for the investigation of ovarian pathology. Both ultrasound and CT have limitations in this respect and

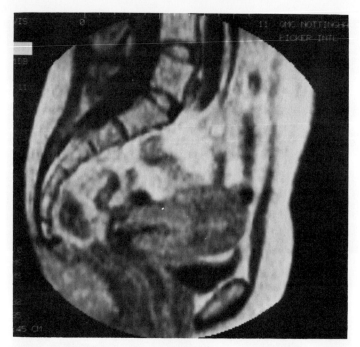

Fig. 17.7   T$_2$ weighted : early carcinoma of the cervix.

MRI's ability for tissue characterisation, as well as providing morphological information, is well demonstrated. Johnson et al (1984) were the first to demonstrate the potential value of MRI in assessment of benign and malignant ovarian disease. Although the normal ovary may be on occasions difficult to identify, pathology of the ovary changes its appearance. Figure 17.8a is a transverse section through an ovarian cyst in a 34-year-old woman. Using a T$_2$ weighted pulse sequence the cyst contents have a very high signal intensity which is of uniform density, surrounded by the low-intensity signal from the cyst wall. Behind the cyst is a transverse section across the uterine body. Using a T$_1$ weighted pulse sequence, this time in the sagittal plane, the cyst contents have a similar signal to that of urine within the bladder, implying a fluid component (Fig. 17.8b). The pathological diagnosis was of a benign cystadenoma. Areas of malignant change within ovarian cysts of this nature may be seen and early invasion through the wall demonstrated. Figure 17.9a is a sagittal image of a cyst lying superior to the bladder. A T$_2$ weighted pulse sequence appears to demonstrate a benign cyst of uniform intensity, when the T$_2$ weighting is altered the true nature of this lesion is apparent (Fig. 17.9b). An area of different intensity at the cyst base is seen, corresponding to a malignant solid area within. The cyst wall is seen to be breached at this site by the invading tumour. The pathology specimen is demonstrated for correlation (Fig. 17.9c). Magnetic resonance therefore has the potential for staging primary ovarian cancer and in the

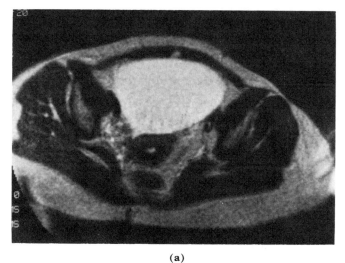

(a)

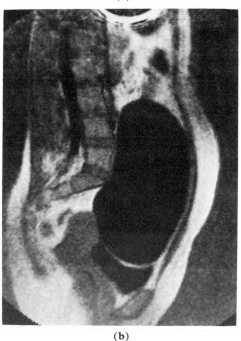

(b)

Fig. 17.8   Benign cystadenoma: (a) T_2 weighted: transverse axial image; (b) T_1 weighted: sagittal image.

detection of early recurrence because of the distinctive appearance of malignant ovarian disease with MRI. A trial is in progress comparing CT, ultrasound, immunoscintigraphy and MRI in the detection of recurrent disease. Early results have so far been encouraging; MRI appears to have

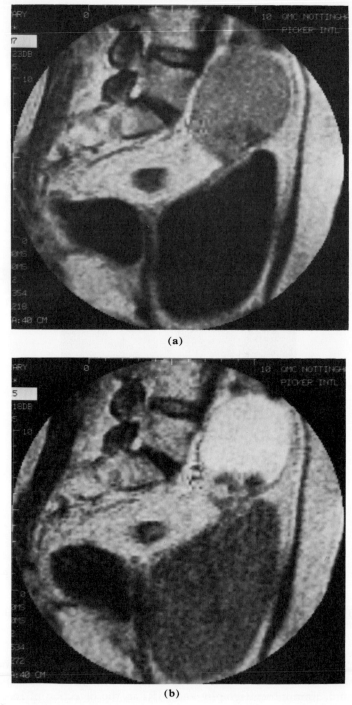

Fig. 17.9 Malignant ovarian cyst: (a) T_2 weighted; (b) longer T_2 weighting.

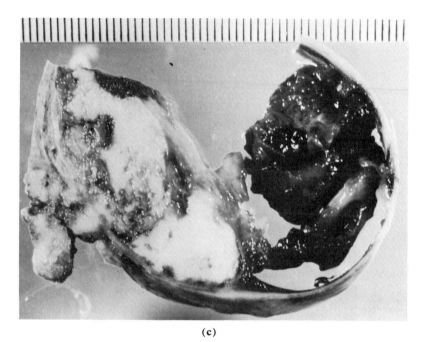

(c)

Fig. 17.9   (c) Malignant ovarian cyst: the pathological specimen.

distinct advantages over other imaging modalities and may reduce the need for unnecessary surgery.

OBSTETRICS

Maternal anatomy

Ultrasound, it is generally accepted, has a certain limitations in imaging maternal anatomy, particularly with the uterine lower segment. The internal os of the cervix may be difficult to locate and the internal structure of the cervix is not visible. This may be due to a combination of problems, such as incomplete filling of the bladder, acoustic shadowing from the presenting part, and inexperience on the part of the ultrasonographer (Goldberg, 1978). MRI avoids these drawbacks and is not operator-dependent. Excellent images of the maternal anatomy can be produced with particular view to the cervix. We have found motion artefact due to maternal respiration to be insignificant.

In all obstetric cases we have examined by MRI the bony pelvis has been well defined. The landmarks of the true pelvis are depicted as low- or no-signal areas due to the cortical bone around the symphysis pubis and sacrum (Figs 17.10a–c). Although the vogue for X-ray pelvimetry is now passing, most obstetricians still require pelvimetric measurements for their management of the breech presentation (Barton et al, 1982). Measurement of

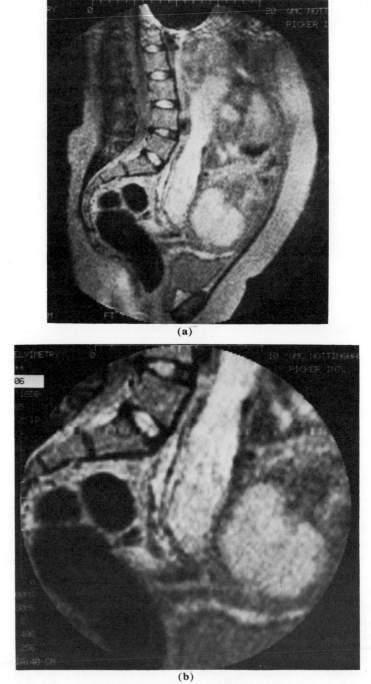

Fig. 17.10   Thirty-four-week pregnancy : (a) T_2 weighted : sagittal view ; (b) T_2 weighted : the cervix.

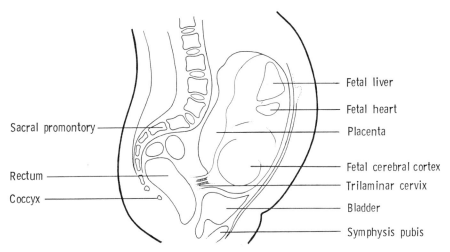

Fig. 17.10   (c) The pregnant female pelvis.

anteroposterior inlet and outlet diameters can be calculated, using the computer cursor from the MR image. A small correction factor is needed to correct for field inhomogeneities. The bispinous measurement is taken from a transverse image, the ischial spines presenting a characteristic appearance in this plane (Fig. 17.11). No correction factor was found to be needed in the transverse plane. Twenty-five women requiring X-ray pelvimetry also had the measurements taken by MRI (Powell et al, 1985). We have found an excellent concordance with the conventional X-ray pelvimetry but without the inherent hazards of exposing the fetus to ionising radiation. A pulse sequence with T_2 weighting can produce good anatomical definition. Imaging time totals 15 minutes to complete the examination.

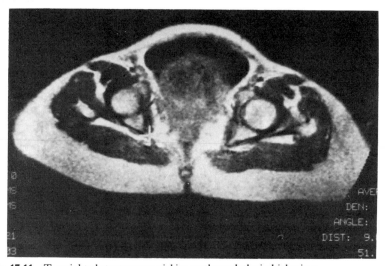

Fig. 17.11 T_2 weighted : transverse axial image through the ischial spines.

The characteristic appearance of the cervix with MRI has been noted. In pregnancy the cervix has a distinctive trilaminar structure (Figs. 17.10a and 17.10b). This is again best seen using a T_2 weighted pulse sequence. The highest signal in the centre of the cervix is from the mucous plug within the cervical canal. On either side is a prominent band, the true nature of which has not yet been determined. Both internal and external os are easily located. The placenta with a T_2 weighted pulse sequence also has a high signal intensity, which means the location of the placental site is straightforward. Therefore the relationship between the internal os and the lower edge of the placenta is well seen (Fig. 17.10). Thirty women having had a diagnosis of placenta praevia by ultrasound, underwent an MRI examination (Powell et al, 1986a). In six of these the ultrasound findings were incorrect in the degree of praevia. Accurate localisation by MRI will lead to a reduction in false positivities seen with ultrasound, particularly when the placenta has a posterior situation (Edelstone, 1977). This will therefore reduce unnecessary hospitalisation and surgery.

The distinctive appearance of the cervix offers an unparallel technique for the study of the physiological changes occurring during pregnancy. This may help towards our understanding of cervical incompetence, failure of ripening, and the response of the cervix to such drugs as prostaglandins.

The prominent signal from the nucleus pulposus has been noted earlier. We have observed a significant number who have a reduction in signal in the discs (see Fig. 17.14). In 60 women so far examined by MRI, 15 have some degree of disc degeneration. Back pain is increased during pregnancy and there is an associated increased incidence of disc herniation (Bishop et al, 1983). Whether our observations are of a temporary nature related to the relaxation of ligaments known to occur in pregnancy, or permanent, is being investigated.

Ultrasonographic examination is the main diagnostic technique in the detection of trophoblastic disease. Recent reports have documented the non-specificity of ultrasound in first-trimester molar pregnancies and invasive trophoblastic disease (Fleischer et al, 1978). Molar tissue has a characteristic appearance with MRI (Powell et al, 1986c). Figure 17.12 shows a sagittal scan of a hydatidiform mole using a T_2 weighted pulse sequence. The vesicular pattern within the molar tissue can be seen The myometrium is also clearly shown as a separate structure, and may allow for accurate assessment of invasion. The high specificity for trophoblastic disease using MRI leads us to believe that this will be a very useful technique for the early detection of recurrent trophoblastic disease associated with a rising hCG titre. Due to the high signal associated with molar tissue local metastasis in the vagina and pelvis, as well as distant disease, should be detected.

The fetus

Magnetic resonance imaging for the present is not a real-time technique; therefore any movement of the fetus during imaging will impair the

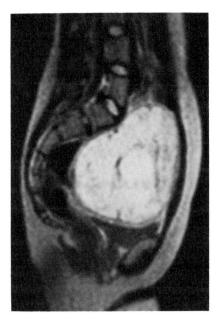

Fig. 17.12 T_2 weighted : hydatidiform mole.

resolution. This will be most apparent during the first and second trimesters of pregnancy. Imaging of fetal anomalies during this period will therefore remain, at least for the time being, the province of ultrasound. Figure 17.13 is a parasagittal scan of a 16-week fetus with a large cystic hygroma. This is trapped between an anterior and posterior wall fibroid. The ultrasonographic examination was superior and also demonstrated oedema of the fetal trunk, suggestive of Turner's syndrome, which was subsequently confirmed. The fetus in the third trimester presents a different picture. Figure 17.14 is a coronal section through the cerebral cortex of the fetus at 36 weeks' gestation. A T_2 weighted pulse sequence is best for differentiating the anatomy of the fetal brain. The lateral ventricles are seen with the tentorium cerebelli, and the cerebellum CSF gives a low-intensity signal. The high-intensity signal area around the head is due to subcutaneous fat in the scalp. The low signal intensity area immediately below this is the calvarium. The spinal cord is seen arising from the brain stem on this particular image slice. Inversion recovery sequences for fetal brain imaging have not been found to be of value. The fetal brain is featureless, indicating a long T_1 relaxation time (Fig. 17.15). This would agree with other studies on the preterm newborn infant (Johnson et al, 1983), since at this stage of brain development myelination is just commencing. T_1 weighted pulse sequences do highlight subcutaneous fat in the fetus (Fig. 17.15). Measurement of this layer has been proposed as a potential indicator of fetal well-being (Stark et al, 1985). In the severely growth-retarded fetus it is absent or severely thinned. It

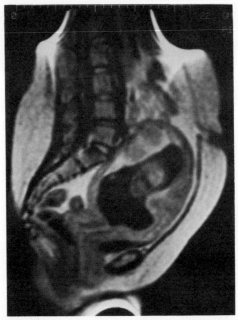

Fig. 17.13 T₂ weighted : parasagittal view of a 16-week fetus with a cyst hygroma.

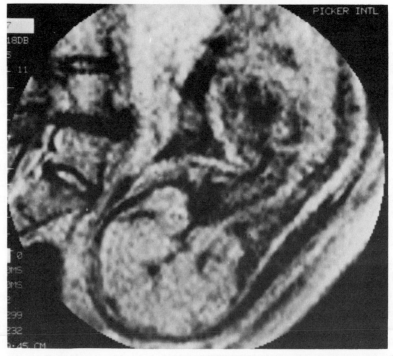

Fig. 17.14 T₂ weighted : coronal section fetal brain at 36 weeks gestation. Loss of signal seen at disc space L4/5.

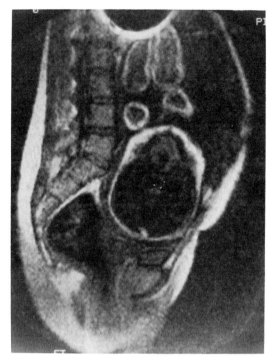

Fig. 17.15   T₁ weighted: 34-week-pregnancy.

remains to be seen whether this will rival or complement the ultrasound diagnosis.

Fetal lungs have a characteristic appearance with MRI having a moderately long T_2 relaxation time due to fluid within (Fig. 17.16a). Using a T_2 weighted pulse sequence, the fetal lungs have a high signal intensity. In stark contrast is the fetal heart which, due to rapid blood flow, is black and has little signal (Fig. 17.16b). Measurement of the relaxation times of fetal lung may provide a non-invasive technique for the assessment of fetal lung maturity. The fetal liver occupies a large proportion of the fetal abdomen and is of medium intensity (Fig. 17.10).

CONCLUSIONS

Magnetic resonance imaging is the latest technological advance in imaging technique. The main advantage over other imaging systems is its capability of tissue differentiation, as well as providing excellent morphological information. The method is still capable of further development and experiments to improve image resolution and reduce scanning time are in progress. Real-time echo-planar magnetic resonance imaging is being researched and developed in the Department of Physics at Nottingham University by Professor P Mansfield. *In vivo* spectroscopy using high field

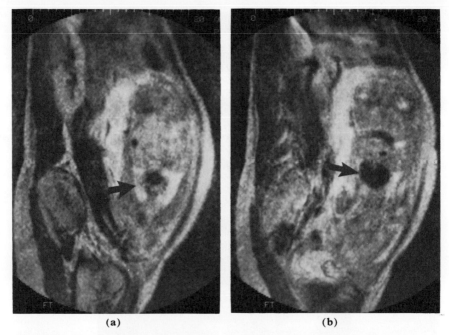

(a)   (b)

Fig. 17.16   T$_2$ weighted: 36-week pregnancy: (a) fetal lungs (arrow); (b) fetal heart (arrow).

magnet systems is also being investigated (Bottomley et al, 1983), and this will provide insight into metabolic activity in the tissues.

Our experience with MRI leads us to the conclusion that it can already materially assist in the clinical assessment of patients where other techniques have limitations or fail to disclose any abnormality. In research the opportunities are many and inviting, and it remains to be seen how many of these enquiries can be translated into clinical benefit.

ACKNOWLEDGEMENTS

We would like to thank Mr Stephen Chipperfield, Superintendent Radiographer in the Department of MRI at the University Hospital; also Mr John Williams and Dr Gordon Higson of the Department of Health and Social Security for their continued advice and encouragement.

REFERENCES

Barton J J, Garbaciak J A, Ryan G M 1982 The efficacy of x-ray pelvimetry. American Journal of Obstetrics and Gynecology 143: 304–311
Bishop E, Cefalo R 1983 Signs and symptoms of pregnancy, J B Lipincott, Philadelphia, pp 78–81
Bloch F, Hansen W W, Packard M E 1946 Nuclear induction. Physiological Reviews 69: 127–136

Bottomley P A, Hart H R, Edelstein W A 1983 NMR imaging/spectroscopy system to study both anatomy and metabolism. Lancet ii: 273–274

Budinger T F 1981 Nuclear magnetic resonance (NMR) in vivo studies: know thresholds for health effects. Journal of Computer Assisted Tomography 5: 800–811

Chaftez N I, Genant H K, Moon K L, Hilms C A, Morris J M 1983 Recognition of lumbar disc herniation with NMR. American Journal of Radiology 141: 1153–1156

Edlestone D I 1977 Placental localisation by ultrasound. Clinical Obstetrics and Gynecology 20: 285–296

Fleischer A C, James A E, Krause D A, Mills J B 1978 Sonographic patterns in trophoblastic disease. Radiology 126: 215–220

Goldberg B B 1978 The identification of placenta praevia. Radiology 128: 255–256

Hawkes R C, Holland G N, Moore W S, Worthington B S 1980 Nuclear magnetic resonance tomography of the brain: a preliminary clinical assessment with demonstration of pathology. Journal of Computer Assisted Tomography 4: 577–586

Hinshaw W S, Andrew E R, Bottomley P A, Holland G N, Moore W S, Worthington B S 1978 Display of cross-sectional anatomy by nuclear magnetic resonance imaging. British Journal of Radiology 51: 273–280

Hinshaw W S, Andrew E R, Bottomley P A, Holland G M, Moore W S, Worthington B S 1979 An in-vivo study of the forearm and hand by thin section NMR imaging. British Journal of Radiology 52: 36–43

Hricak H, Alpers C, Crooks L E, Sheldon P E 1983 Magnetic resonance imaging of the female pelvis—initial experience. American Journal of Radiology 141: 1119–1128

Johnson I R, Symonds E M, Kean D M et al 1984 Imaging the pregnant human uterus with nuclear magnetic resonance. American Journal of Obstetrics and Gynecology 148: 1136–1139

Johnson M A, Pennock J M, Bydder G M et al 1983 Clinical NMR imaging of the brain in children: normal and neurologic disease. American Journal of Radiology 141: 1005–1018

Johnson I R, Symonds E M, Worthington E S, Johnson J, Gyngell M, Hawkes R C 1984 Imaging ovarian tumours by nuclear magnetic resonance. British Journal of Obstetrics and Gynaecology 91: 260–264

Lauterbur P C 1973 Image formation by induced local interactions: examples employing nuclear magnetic resonance. Nature 242: 190–191

Mansfield P, Maudsly A A 1976 Planar and line-scan spin imaging by NMR. Proc. XIXth Congress Ampere, Heidelberg, pp 247–252

Mansfield P, Pykett I L, Morris P G, Coupland R E 1978 Human whole body line-scan imaging by NMR. British Journal of Radiology, 51: 921–922

Mansfield P 1984 Real-time echo-planar imaging by NMR. British Medical Bulletin, 40(2): 187–190

McCarthy S M, Stark D D, Filly R A, Callen R W, Hricak H, Higgins C B 1985 Obstetrical magnetic resonance imaging: maternal anatomy. Radiology, 154: 421–425

National (British) Radiological Protection Board 1983 Revised guidance on acceptable limits of exposure during nuclear magnetic clinical imaging. British Journal of Radiology 56: 974–977

Powell M C, Buckley J, Symonds E M, Worthington B S 1985 Magnetic resonance imaging and pelvimetry. Radiology 157(P): 190

Powell M C, Buckley J, Price H, Symonds E M, Worthington B S 1986a Magnetic Resonance and placenta praevia. American Journal of Obstetrics and Gynecology 154: 565–569

Powell M C, Womack C, Buckley J, Worthington B S, Symonds E M 1986b Magnetic resonance imaging and Stage 1 endometrial adenocarcinoma. British Journal of Obstetrics and Gynaecology 93: 353–360

Powell M C, Buckley J, Symonds E M, Worthington B S 1986c Magnetic resonance imaging and hydatidiform mole. British Journal of Radiology 59: 561–564

Purcell M, Torrey H C, Pound R V 1946 Resonance absorption by nuclear magnetic resonance moments in a solid. Physiological Reviews 69: 37–38

Stark D D, McCarthy S M, Filly R A, Callen P W, Hricak H, Parer J T 1985 Intra-uterine growth retardation: evaluation by magnetic resonance. Radiology 155: 425–427

Wolff S, Crooks L E, Brown P 1982 Tests for DNA and chromosomal damage by nuclear magnetic resonance imaging. Radiology 136: 707–710

Worthington B S 1983 Clinical prospects for nuclear magnetic resonance. Clinical Radiology 34: 3–12

Surgical pelviscopy: review of 12 060 pelviscopies, 1970–85

Until recently intra-abdominal endoscopic procedures in gynaecology were used mainly for diagnostic indications. However technical developments during the past decade, pioneered at the University Department of Obstetrics and Gynaecology in Kiel, have transformed this diagnostic procedure into a broad spectrum of intra-abdominal endoscopic surgery which could replace approximately 80 per cent of laparotomies previously performed for ovarian and tubal surgery and, indeed, 50 per cent of all laparotomies in gynaecological practice. Prerequisities for this, however, are a considerable skill in pelviscopy (laparoscopy) and the availability of a full set of appropriate, and for the most part newly designed, instruments.

It is evident that with the conventional diagnostic instruments and apparatus for laparoscopy an easy application to endoscopic surgery cannot be made without additional instruments.

APPARATUS FOR ENDOSCOPIC INTRA-ABDOMINAL SURGERY

The endoscopic optic Wisap with a 30° viewing angle of 5 and 10 mm diameter and fluid crystal cables (e.g. Semm surgical pelviscopes, allowing full frame slides and colour prints without flash) are necessary for good intra-abdominal diagnosis and surgery. For extended endoscopic surgery, however, the electronically controlled OP-PNEU-Electronic must replace the old CO_2-PNEU which was developed about 20 years ago. This apparatus measures the static intra-abdominal pressure electronically and continuously, and allows any necessary replacement of gas up to a flow of 5 litres per minute to be automatically monitored. Even in cases requiring repeated instrument changes, where there is considerable gas loss, surgery is possible under the same constant conditions which exist at laparotomy. But without the use of the electronically controlled insufflator lengthy endoscopic surgical intervention is virtually impossible.

Of vital importance to the surgeon is the possibility of quick and secure haemostasis. Ovarian and tubal surgery during laparotomy may be associated with profuse bleeding, whereas endoscopic surgical intervention should be performed with a minimum of blood loss. A possible explanation for the bleeding at laparotomy may be that blood vessel paralysis is provoked during the open procedure but not during pelviscopy. The same may be true of postoperative bowel ileus.

In general surgery there are two systems for haemostasis:

1. haemostasis by suture and ligation,
2. haemostasis by high-frequency current coagulation.

After a long period of development all suture and ligation techniques used for laparotomy are now available for intra-abdominal endoscopic surgery.

Haemostasis can easily be achieved with the Roeder loop (Ethi-ligator) for bleeding vessels which can be grasped and pulled through (Figs 18.1 and 18.2). This is recommended for arterial bleeding, especially in the area of the mesosalpinx or in the utero-ovarian ligament, and also for occluding extensive ovarian wounds after large cyst wall resection or for the ligation of bleeding vessels after extended adhesiolysis of the omentum with or without partial resection. This catgut-loop ligature can be placed with an applicator through a 5 mm cannula. After 20 years of experience and a few thousand applications of the Ethi-ligator, we have never observed any secondary haemorrhage due to faulty application of the loop knot.

Bleeding tissue which can not be pulled through this loop, such as ovarian incisions or other intraperitoneal wounds, can be more effectively closed by

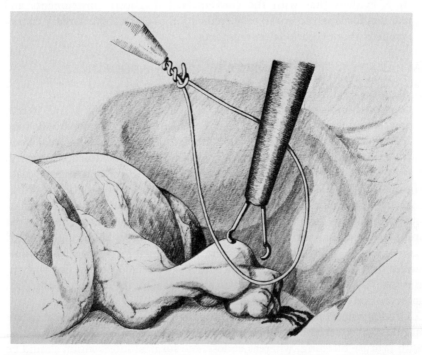

Fig. 18.1   Bloody adhesiolysis: the bleeding adhesion is grasped with the atraumatic forceps through a Roeder loop.

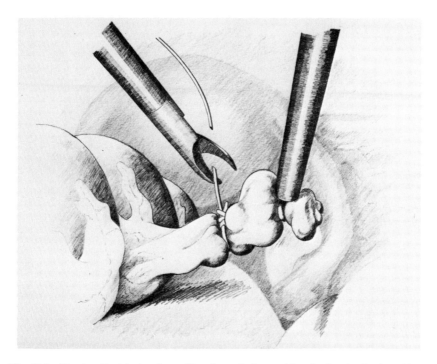

Fig. 18.2   Bloody adhesiolysis: after pulling down the knot with a plastic tube the thread is cut.

sutures using the endosuture set (Ethicon) with an extracorporeal knot. When the wound edges are pierced with a needle, with the help of a 5 mm and a 3 mm needle-holder, the needle and suture are brought out through the suture applicator. The Roeder gliding knot is performed extracorporeally, and after pulling it down with a plastic tube into the abdomen the knot is fixed and the excess suture material is cut. We distinguish between 'bloody adhesiolysis' when the adhesions are at first separated (Fig. 18.3) and afterwards ligated with the Roeder-loop (see Fig. 18.2), and non-bloody adhesiolysis for stronger vascularised adhesions when it is better to ligate them before cutting. For this manoeuvre we use an endosuture set. It is necessary first to ligate the vascularised tissue by surrounding the adhesions with the endoligation thread. After performing an extracorporeal knot it is pulled down across the adhesion, which then can be separated bloodlessly with the hook scissors. An additional Roeder loop guarantees safe ligation.

For very fine sutures—for example, those used for fixation of the everted ampullary end of the tube, or for performing the purse-string suture after endoscopic appendectomy, we recommend this suture technique with intra-abdominal knotting with a 6/0 resorbable material of polydioxan (Ethicon).

This broad range of loop ligation, endoligation and endosuture, with extracorporeal and intracorporeal loop knotting, gives the endoscopic surgeon the ability to stop nearly all provoked bleeding and to join distended

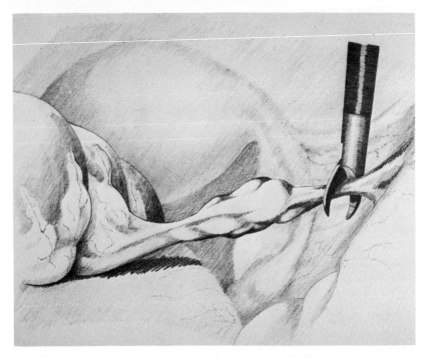

Fig. 18.3   Bloody adhesiolysis: vascularised adhesions are sharply dissected with the hook-formed scissors.

layers of the peritoneum in the area of the visceral as well as the parietal peritoneum.

During pelviscopy it is not possible to spend much time ligating all bleeding. High-frequency current is unacceptable for intra-abdominal endoscopic haemostasis procedures; therefore we have replaced that method by our 'endocoagulation system', in which the human body has no contact with the electric current. We use destructive heat only at a temperature of 100°C to coagulate protein for performing optimal haemostasis.

High-frequency current (monopolar or bipolar) is absolutely contraindicated for ovarian haemostasis as it follows the path of lowest resistance and flows mainly through the vessels and nerves of the ovary. These structures are therefore excessively heated. The destruction of thermolabile enzymes starts at 57°C and brings about destruction of the ovarian vessels and nerve supply. As it is desirable not to damage the highly sensitive ovarian tissue during diagnostic and therapeutic procedures, use of high-frequency current should be rejected as the means of maintaining haemostasis.

The use of high-frequency current into closed spaces, as in the abdominal cavity, is also contraindicated because the surgeon is unable to watch the path of the current and identify the areas which are being heated and possibly destroyed. The best method for using heat to achieve haemostasis is by endocoagulation at 100°C. At this temperature protein coagulates, as in the boiling of an egg, and is visible. The coagulated tissue is later not sequestered, as happens after high-frequency burning with resultant carbonisation. The little-coagulated tissue will be repaired by migration of histiocytes and fibroblasts from below, and therefore the formation of adhesions is less likely to occur.

The Wisap Endocoagulator especially developed for this purpose can be used with a 12 volt or 110/220 volt source, and electronically monitors excessive heat of the crocodile forceps, or the myoma enucleator or the point coagulator.

Instruments for endoscopic intra-abdominal surgery

The instrumentation for endoscopic surgery which has been developed during the past two decades comprises modifications of commonly used instruments in general surgery, such as forceps, scissors, needle-holders and suction devices. Every instrument should be available before starting endoscopic intra-abdominal surgery, as one missing instrument may result in failed procedures, necessitating laparotomy.

Some instruments have to be mentioned specifically: The set of instruments for dilation of the entry wound is extremely helpful. It permits a nearly atraumatic dilatation of the 5 mm trocar sheath incision to one of a diameter of 11 mm which would accommodate large endoscopes, larger forceps and the tissue-puncher. Some instruments must be available in 5 and 11 mm diameters, such as the grasping or big-mouth forceps. The tissue-puncher is necessary for morcellation of larger tumours, e.g. myomas, and larger fibroids or pieces of ovarian tissue. For the uncontaminated removal of the appendix after resection a special appendix extractor is available. Special applicators and needle-holders facilitate intra-abdominal suturing.

Apparatus for lavage of the lower pelvis

It is important to wash the operation field during pelviscopy, and the Wisap Aquapurator has been designed for this purpose. This has a bivalent washing tube which allows accurate flushing of the lower pelvis with saline solution during and after surgical intervention. The lavage with 1 to 3 litres of sterile 37°C saline solution is necessary during pelviscopic surgery to provide a clean operative field. At the end of this surgical intervention the original cleanliness of the lower pelvis is re-established. In our opinion this lavage also prevents postoperative adhesions. Every time endoscopic surgery is performed, particularly in the management of a partially ruptured ectopic pregnancy, the Aquapurator is considered an item of basic apparatus without which conservative or radical management of a tubal pregnancy cannot be commenced. The ampullary end of the Fallopian tube can then be flushed out with the washing tube and a clear view obtained for pelvic surgery.

TYPICAL PELVISCOPIC PROCEDURES

Each patient has to be prepared and instructed as for a laparotomy. The bowels should be properly purged. In a 15° Trendelenburg position the bowel slips into the upper abdomen, allowing the surgeon to obtain a better view into the pelvis than during a laparotomy. Endoscopic surgery should be performed under general endotracheal anaesthesia. An extensive review of the establishment of a pneumoperitoneum and the basi instrument handling is to be found in my *Atlas of Pelviscopy and Hysteroscopy* (1976/77), and the *Atlas of Endoscopic Intra-abdominal Surgery* (1983a & b).

The seven security steps must be kept in mind: needle-test; aorta–palpation test; followed by Snape test; Hiss-phenomenon; aspiration test; manometer test; volume-test (Semm, 1976, 1983b).

The intra-abdominal gas pressure is preselected on the OP-PNEU-electronic and regulated automatically.

The Veress needle should only be inserted when the aorta and the big common iliac vessels are palpated. The distance between skin (e.g. the umbilicus) and these vessels is often very small, and therefore the vessels may be situated only 1 or 2 cm behind the umbilicus. The pelviscopic trocar should always be inserted by using the Z-incision technique. All other surgical instruments needed are placed 1 cm below the pubic hairline. Two trocar sheaths for instrumentation are required as a minimum. Two or three puncture sites, and the use of a magnifying glass, may be necessary to diagnose extragenital endometriosis. It should be remembered that 20 per cent of endometriotic spots are retro-ovarian and not visible without elevation of the ovaries.

If the umbilical view is insufficient the endoscope can be introduced through a trocar introduced into the lower abdomen. From this perspective adhesions or other pathological findings in the upper abdomen can easily be diagnosed and manipulated.

For tubo-ovarian surgery and bowel separation the use of a magnifying glass fitted over the eyepiece of the pelviscope is essential. This gives a 2–6-fold magnification; therefore it is possible to perform endoscopic operations under micro-surgical conditions.

An old maxim of endoscopists is 'The endoscopist will see only the things he knows, and he will not see the things he does not know.' The endoscopic surgeon may add: 'The endoscopist should do nothing other than what is routine during a normal laparotomy. There are no exceptions in endoscopic surgery.'

General adhesiolysis

Lysis of adhesions after a previous laparotomy represents a special field of surgical pelviscopy.

Omental adhesiolysis and partial resection can easily be performed with complete haemostasis, either by sharp division and haemostasis later using the loop applicator (bloody adhesiolysis), or by using the endoligation technique prior to sharp division (bloodless separation). The latter method is essentially the same as that during a laparotomy, and should be the preferred method in the middle and upper abdomen.

Ovariolysis and salpingolysis

For division of peri-ovarian peri-tubal adhesions two secondary puncture sites with 5 mm trocar in the pubic area are usually necessary. After the haemostatis has been carried out with the crocodile forceps the ovary should be freed from adhesions by sharp and blunt dissection with a hook scissors. Sometimes the fallopian tube and the ovaries can be delivered from the adhesions, by using the myoma enucleator. We believe that this technique prevents later adhesions.

Fimbrioplasty and salpingostomy

Endoscopic intra-abdominal surgery is useful for fimbriolysis, using two atraumatic forceps in combination with chromosalpingoscopy (dye insufflation) under an automatically controlled pressure of 100–250 mmHg (manual insufflation is absolutely inadequate). If the dye insufflation demonstrates a hydrosalpinx, the distal tube can be opened during pelviscopy as long as the insufflation pressure is kept constantly by the use of the Universal Insufflator (Fikentscher and Semm) at a pressure of 200–300 mmHg. For this procedure a coagulation strip 2 cm in length and 4 mm wide is produced with the point coagulator for haemostasis before the incision with special microscissors, or a knife eversion of the old ampullary and fimbriae occur. Fimbriae are fixed with the endosuture, using 4 to 6/0 resorbable suture (polydioxan) material with intracorporeal knotting technique. Our pregnancy rate (632 cases) is 37 per cent, as shown in Table 18.1.

Table 18.1 Pregnancy rates in 632 infertility patients following operative pelviscopy and chromotubation for correction of peripheral tubal lesions over a period of 10 years

	n	Resulting intra-uterine pregnancies		Live births	
		n	%	n	%
Pelvic endometriosis*(3-step therapy)	255	122	48	114	44
Ovariolysis*	60	13	22	13	22
Salpingolysis*	75	26	35	22	29
Fimbrioplasty*	150	48	32	40	27
Salpingostomy*	92	27	29	25	27
Total	632	236	37	214	34

* In cases of multiple treatment the predominant one is indicated.

Myomectomy

Subserous myomas can be removed by pelviscopy nearly bloodlessly, using a specially developed heated myoma enucleator in combination with infiltration of octapressin (1 : 100). Any haemostasis necessary following the enucleation of the myoma should be performed at 110–120°C with constant rotation of the point coagulator, e.g. myoma enucleator. If the wound edges are too separated, one or two endosutures with extracorporeal knotting will join them together. We now have 186 cases with no postoperative evidence of subsequent adhesions of bowels to the myomectomy scars (proved by re-pelviscopy). This is a common occurrence following myomectomy and laparotomy, and we believe that the difference can be explained as follows: the 100°C coagulated protein covers the wound for many days: no migration of fibrin, fibroblasts or histiocytes occurs, and as the coagulated protein will be replaced from the interior no adhesions should occur. After enucleation of the myoma the tissue can be easily morcellated with the tissue-puncher.

Conservative endoscopic treatment of tubal pregnancy

The conservative treatment of tubal pregnancy is facilitated by pelviscopy because of the reduced bleeding associated with this technique. The lower abdomen is cleaned of blood and clots with the help of the Aquapurator under the assistance of the electronic CO_2 insufflator. After infiltration of the mesosalpinx with octapressin (20–30 ml, 1 : 100 diluted) the involved part of the tube is coagulated for haemostasis at its antemesenteric aspect with a point coagulator and is opened in a longitudinal direction. The conception is usually extruded spontaneously from the tube by traction, or if necessary can be removed with the biopsy or spoon forceps. The edges of the linear salpingotomy incision are closed with endosuture using the extracorporeal or intracorporeal knotting technique. In more than 80 per cent of cases the tube and potential fertility is saved. Postsurgical adhesions are rare. The tubal patency remains in more than 80 per cent of patients.

Radical operation for tubal pregnancy

If the age of the patient does not dictate conservative management, or if the extent of the damage is too great, the fallopian tube can be grasped, ligated and cut with the 'three knot technique' in a manner similar to that used for oophorectomy (see later). Such treatment is easier to perform than tubal conservation.

Ovarian biopsy

The excision of a cylindrical portion of tissue for ovarian biopsy is performed by pushing down and rotating the trocar sheath after the ovary has been fixed by the two catch-hooks of the biopsy forceps. Any necessary haemostasis is performed with the point coagulator.

Ovarian-cyst puncture and ovarian-cyst enucleation

Ovarian retention cysts, theca-luteal cysts or cystoma ovarii simplex—if clearly identified as such—should be aspirated with the puncture needle. Small cysts can be aspirated by connection to a syringe, and the larger ones with the Aquapurator. If the benign nature of a cyst can be presumed after endoscopic magnification removal of chocolate cysts or dermoid cysts can be performed as effectively as during a laparotomy.

The low incidence of bleeding during endoscopic ovarian surgery is an advantage when enucleating ovarian cysts. The ovarian wound area edges are closed with the endosuture technique using extracorporal knots. It is remarkable that hardly any adhesions were observed at hundreds of re-pelviscopies after endoscopic ovarian surgery.

Ovariectomy

By using the 'three knot technique' ovariectomy can be carried out in an optimal manner by pelviscopy (Fig. 18.4). After ligation with the 'three ligator techniques' the ovary is removed by sharp dissection using the hooked scissors (Fig. 18.5) and—if necessary—morcellation (Fig. 18.6) of

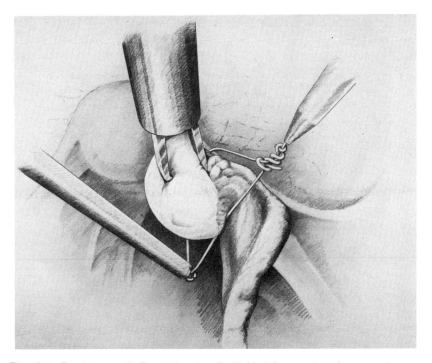

Fig. 18.4 Ovariectomy: the Roeder loop is pulled behind the ovary into the mesovarium with the help of the atraumatic forceps.

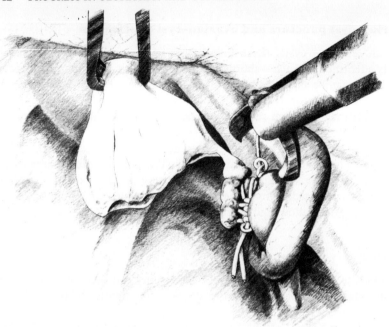

Fig. 18.5 Ovariectomy : after fixing the Roeder loop the ovary is pulled to the left and then disconnected with the hook-formed scissors. The three-times ligated stump of the ovary is coagulated at 90°C in order to avoid later formation of adhesions.

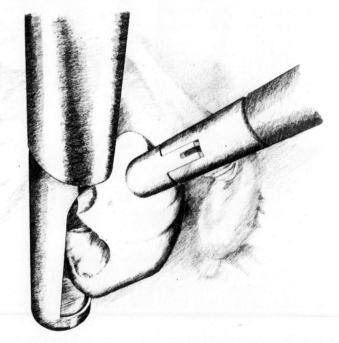

Fig. 18.6 Ovariectomy : the ovary is morcellated and collected into the 11 mm diameter tube of the morcellator.

the tissue using a specially developed tissue-puncher called 'Automorz'. The tissue stump is coagulated with the point coagulator to provide postoperative adhesions.

Adnexectomy

If the indications are appropriate it is simpler to perform an adnexectomy rather than oophrectomy. During adnexectomy a part of the fallopian tube is ligated simultaneously in the stump of the vessels of the mesovaricum, which prevents the tissue stump from slipping out of the ligature. Should the infundibulopelvic ligament or the utero-ovarian ligament slip because of insufficient suturing, the vessel pedicles must be ligated with separate Ethi-loop ligatures. Emergency laparotomy for bleeding has not been necessary in several hundred endoscopic adnexectomies.

Typical procedure in cases of endometriosis

Modern endocoagulation techniques allows the coagulation of endometriotic implants even on the dome of the bladder. A simple colour test (thermocolour test) to identify areas of endometriosis can be made by using this endocoagulation technique. Endometriotic implants coagulated with 100°C in this manner turn brown, while the coagulated healthy peritoneum changes to a whitish colour. For widespread pelvic endometriosis we perform a three-phase therapeutic regime.

Phase 1: *Endocoagulation* by *pelviscopy* of all endometriotic implants, adhesiolysis, salpingolysis, ovariolysis, and removal of endometriomas as described above.
Phase 2: Three to six months of hormonal suppression of the endometriosis by progestogens or antigonadotrophics.
Phase 3: Second-look pelviscopy for evaluation of the previous treatment and for final correction of any fimbrial disease, e.g. salpingostomy.

Tubal sterilisation

The endocoagulation technique for tubal sterilisation is in my opinion the safest method for the patient, and also in order to preserve full endocrinological function of the ovary. After coagulation of the Fallopian tubes the tube is cut with a hook scissors without involving the adjacent vessels, which are vital for ovarian function. The tubal stump is peritonealised in order to prevent later fistula formation. If desired such divided tubes can easily be reanastomosed under microsurgical conditions because only 1 cm is lost at the time of sterilisation.

Omentum adhesiolysis

For lysis of the most strongly vascularised postoperative omental adhesions, only the endoligation technique can be recommended.

Bowel adhesiolysis

After previous abdominal surgery bowel adhesions may provoke gastrointestinal symptoms or chronic abdominal discomfort, which might require a relaparotomy. After a routine preoperative bowel preparation we always commence with a diagnostic laparoscopy and in more than 90 per cent the bowel adhesions may be simply divided by pelviscopy under magnifying-glass control. Any resulting serosa defects can be closed using the endosuture technique with an extracorporeal knot. If the lumen of the bowel is opened the wound must be closed with endosuture and intra-abdominal knotting, using 4/0 suture material as in laparotomy.

SUMMARY

New developments in apparatus and instruments for endoscopy have allowed us to transform diagnostic laparoscopy into surgical pelviscopy (endoscopic intra-abdominal surgery). We are able to perform haemostasis by endocoagulation, loop ligation, endoligation and endosutures with extracorporeal or intracorporeal knots. This gives us the possibility of performing a broad spectrum of endoscopic intra-abdominal surgery. These techniques include general adhesiolysis in the abdomen with partial omental resection, salpingolysis, ovariolysis, fimbrioplasty or salpingotomy with suture fixation of the ampulla under microsurgical conditions, conservation or radical treatment of ectopic pregnancy, ovarian biopsy, ovarian cyst puncture and/or cyst removal with consecutive ovarian suture, ovariectomy or adnectomy, or myomectomy.

The patients have to be prepared without exception as if for normal laparotomy, in order that endoscopic intervention may be turned into a laparotomy with no additional risk from the initial endoscopic management.

BIBLIOGRAPHY

Acosta A, Buttram V C, Besch P K et al 1973 A proposed classification of pelvic endometriosis. Obstetrics and Gynecology 42 : 19
Bruhat M A 1980 Treatment of ectopic pregnancy by means of laparoscopy. Fertility and Sterility 33 : 411
Cohen M R 1975 Surgical laparoscopy in infertility. Journal of Reproductive Medicine 15 : 51
Diamond E 1977 Lysis of postoperative pelvic adhesions in infertility. Fertility and Sterility 28 : 1203
Dubuisson J B 1979 Early control laparoscopy after tubal microsurgery. Journal de Gynécologie Obstétrique et Biologie de la Reproduction (Paris) 8 : 655
Fragenheim H 1980 Diagnostische und operative Laparoskiopie in der Gynäkologie Marsaille Verlag, Wien

Gaisford W D 1975 Peritoneoscopy: a valuable technique for surgeons. American Journal of
    Surgery 130: 671
Gayan P 1978 Extraction of an ectopic intrauterine device by laparoscopy. Revista Chilena de
    Obstetricia y Ginecologia 43: 305
Gomel V 1977 Salpingostomy by laparoscopy. Journal of Reproductive Medicine 18: 265
Hasson H M 1980 Window for open laparoscopy. American Journal of Obstetrics and
    Gynecology 137: 869
Kleppinger R K 1978 Ovarian cyst fenestration via laparoscopy. Journal of Reproductive
    Medicine 21: 16
Kolmorgen K, Hauβwald H R, Havemann O, Wergien G 1978 Ergebnisse nach
    Ovarialzystenpunktion unter laparoskopischer Sicht. Zentralblatt für Gynäkologie 100: 289
Ladipo O A 1980 Laparoscopic removal of extra uterine Lippes-loop. Journal of the
    International Medical Association 72: 701
Mintz M 1977 Risks and prophylaxis in laparoscopy—a survey of 100 000 cases. Journal of
    Reproductive Medicine 18: 269
Palmer R 1974 Safety in laparoscopy. Journal of Reproductive Medicine 13: 1
Semm K 1976/77 Pelviskopie und Hysteroskopie—Farbatlas und Lehrbuch, F. K. Schattauer,
    Stuttgart, 1976 (W. B. Saunders, Philadelphia, 1977; French. edn. Masson, Paris, 1977;
    Spain edn. Toray-Masson SA, Barcelona, 1977, Portuguese edn. Editora Manole LTDA,
    Sao Paulo, 1977)
Semm K 1980 Technical progress in pelviscopic surgery by operative laparoscopy. American
    Journal of Obstetrics and Gynecology 138: 121
Semm K 1982 Pelviscopic ovarian surgery. In: Fioretti P, Martini L, Melis G B, Yen S S C
    (eds) The menopause: clinical, endocrinological and pathophysiological aspects. Serono
    Symposium No. 39. Academic Press, London, pp 235–243
Semm K 1983a Pelviscopy—Hysteroscopy and fetoscopy. Series of 240 slides and textbook.
    Edited by K. Semm, Kiel, 1980 (English edn., French edn., Kiel 1981; Spanish edn., Kiel,
    1983)
Semm K 1983b Advances in pelviscopic surgery. Current problems in obstetrics and
    gynecology, vol. V, no. 10. Year Book Medical, Chicago.
Semm K 1983c Die operative Pelviskopie. In: Schwalm, H., Döderlein C, Wulf K.-H. Klinik
    der Frauenheilkunde und Geburtshilfe. Urban & Schwarzenberg, München Wien
    Baltimore; 1st series 1970; 2nd series 1978; 3rd series 1983
Semm K 1983d Advances in pelviscopic surgery. Current problems in obstetrics and
    gynecology, vol. V, no. 10. Year Book Medical, Chicago
Semm K 1983e Endoscopic appendectomy. Endoscopy 15: 59
Semm K 1984 Operationslehre für endoskopische Abdominal-Chirurgie operative
    Pelviskopie—operative Laparoskopie F. K. Schattauer, Stuttgart
Semm K 1986a Operative manual for endoscopic abdominal surgery—operative pelviscopy—
    operative laparscopy. Year Book Medical, Chicago
Semm K 1986b Tecnica operativa per la chirurgia abdominale endoscopica. Martinucci
    Publicazioni Mediche, Naples, Italy
Semm K 1986c Operative pelviscopy. British Medical Bulletin 42: 284–295
Swolin K 1977 Laparoscopy as an operative tool in female sterility. Journal of Reproductive
    Medicine 19: 167
Sulewski J M 1980 The treatment of endometriosis at laparoscopy for infertility. American
    Journal of Obstetrics and Gynecology 138: 128

A gender identity crisis in males and females

Transsexualism is believed to have existed since antiquity (Green, 1969). Only few isolated studies were reported in the medical literature during the early 1900s and little had appeared in the lay press.

Public interest in transsexualism and sex reassignment surgery was first aroused by the sensationalism of Christine Jorgenson's case (Hamburger, 1953; Jorgenson, 1967). It was Jorgenson who popularised the notion that a man who felt like a woman could 'change' sex. Since then, several names of alleged successes have made the headlines from time to time, for example, those of Roberta Cowell, Jan Morris and a relatively recent addition to the list, Tula.

After several decades of experience with hormone therapy, coupled with advances in the techniques of plastic surgery, sex reassignment surgery is now available to both male and female transsexuals. Although the first sex reassignment surgery was performed more than half a century ago (Abraham, 1931), the controversy and emotion stirred by the use of this procedure in the management of transsexualism are unmatched by most other psychiatric issues.

With an increasing number of patients seeking sex reassignment surgery (Tsoi et al, 1977; Berger et al, 1977; Volkin, 1979), brought about in part by the availability of the surgery, media exposure, and the establishment of gender identity clinics all over the world, it has become imperative and beneficial that clinicians (general practitioners, internists, gynaecologists and others) have a better understanding of the syndrome and its management. This is because the chance of encountering a transsexual among their patients is high.

TRANSSEXUALISM

The process of developing sexual awareness and gender identity can be a painful business. It is common to find girls who are 'tomboyish' or boys who are 'girlish'. Furthermore, adolescents often have 'crushes' on friends or adults of the same sex. For most people these experiences represent only fleeting moments of their lives, and they soon outgrow these early childhood pains. However, there are others who are acutely aware of their abnormal sexuality and realise that their gender identity seems somewhat disoriented. They can neither be described as completely heterosexual nor homosexual. The pains generated by such a dilemma during early childhood continue into adulthood and torment them until help is obtained. Comparing the pains she experienced during her sex reassignment surgery, Tula said 'but it was worse living with the pain of being a woman in a man's body' (Campbell, 1983). Individuals with such a predicament are known as transsexuals. Males who want to be females are often referred to as male transsexuals; conversely females desiring to be males are known as female transsexuals.

Transsexualism is defined as a disturbance of gender identity in which persons anatomically of one sex have an intense and persistent desire for medical, surgical and legal 'change' of sex so that they may live as members of the opposite gender (Friedman et al, 1976). April Ashley, born as George Jamieson, said of herself, 'I was taunted for being like a girl, and yes, I wanted to be one, . . . I was convinced a monstrous mistake had been made, and only my being a woman would correct it' (Fallowell & Ashley, 1982).

Male transsexuals are often not diagnosed as such. Macroanalyses of these patients may reveal traits resembling other psychosexual patients, chiefly transvestites, who obtain some degree of sexual arousal from cross-dressing, or homosexuals, who know themselves to be men but obtain gratification mainly or exclusively from other men. To the undiscerning clinician, transsexuals are frequently considered as psychotic with delusional confusion in their gender identity. Although overlaps with the other two conditions mentioned are not denied, transsexuals are currently accepted as a distinct subgroup of psychosexual patients.

One of the more recent advancements in the management of transsexualism is the emphasis on purity of definition. This is brought about by advances in psychological investigative techniques. The advent of these techniques has led to the detection of patients presenting as homosexuals or fetishistic transvestites who later develop into transsexuals (Ball, 1981).

Transsexualism is generally accepted to vary independently of other mental disorders and to occur in individuals of varying personality types (Friedman et al, 1976). True transsexuals are distinct from those either known as secondary or 'wish-to-be' transsexuals whose gender dysphoria is a consequence of other psychosis (Laub & Fisk, 1974; Friedman et al, 1976). They are identified with, and behave like, members of the opposite sex from their earliest childhood. Their childhood behaviour may include cross-dressing and role-playing as members of the opposite sex. During adolescence and later, they do not find cross-dressing to be sexually arousing. Overtly they may appear to be homosexual, a label which they vehemently deny, although their sexual attentions from the time of puberty have been directed to members of the same sex. They consider their genitals as foreign, and their one obsession in life is to get rid of them. For these patients, surgery is the finishing touch rather than a sudden leap into either femaleness for the male transsexual, or maleness for the female transsexual.

Incidence

Reported incidence of transsexualism showed wide variation, ranging from 1 : 42 000 to 1 : 100 000 (Walinder, 1968; Pauly, 1968; Hoenig & Kenna, 1974; Ross et al, 1981). Hoenig & Kenna (1974) commented that the overall prevalence of transsexualism is difficult to establish as most of the usual epidemiological parameters for an accurate estimation are not available. Furthermore, studies in the 1960s and early 1970s were found to be plagued with methodological problems, chief among them being the lack of universally accepted criteria to diagnose true transsexualism (Lothstein, 1982). The rapprochement of psychoanalysis in studies of transsexualism in the mid-1970s and early 1980s had indicated that many patients at gender identity clinics are actually secondary transsexuals (Laub & Fisk, 1974; Friedman et al, 1976). These are patients who under stress, and a variety of unconscious motivations, identify themselves as transsexuals and express a regressive wish for the sex reassignment surgery. The existence of such patients among the true transsexuals raises problems not only to the estimation of prevalence, but also to the central issue of how these patients should be managed.

There is general agreement that transsexualism occurs two to four times more frequently in males than in females (Walinder, 1968; Pauly, 1968; Hoenig & Kenna, 1974). The reasons for deviation from this ratio in some of the more recent reports are not clear (Walinder, 1971; Ross et al, 1981). One possible reason is the demographic changes that occur over the years. New gender identity clinics recently established tended to attract more of the male than the female transsexuals, because of the relatively simpler procedures for sex reassignment of male to female. Generally female transsexuals prefer to go to more established gender clinics. The proposed reason for the decline in the male to female ratio is reflected in our experience in Singapore. Our unit remains the only experienced centre for the management of both male and female transsexuals. The numerous new centres that were established in Singapore only offer male to female sex reassignment surgery. Patients who are impatient with the long wait for their sex change surgery, and the bother of more elaborate pre-surgical work-up, are attracted to these clinics. This has resulted in the apparent reduction in male to female ratio in our centre over the past couple of years.

Preponderance of male over female transsexuals

Several reasons for the preponderance of male transsexuals have been outlined by Green (1974):

1. All children identify first with the most significant other person in their life—the mother. While the male must discontinue his identification with a female figure on the road to his male identity, the female skips this first hurdle towards her femaleness.
2. Contemporary society affords females more latitude for cross-sex expression. Although this status is changing in several countries, in most others the conservative view still prevails. Females can dress in men's clothes, live together, and engage in intimate relationships without the same degree of stigmatisation encountered by males. Thus the pressure to reduce social alienation by bringing anatomy into conformity with socially accepted patterns of behaviour is greater for males.
3. The basic mammalian state is anatomically female and may be behaviourally feminine. While androgen, the masculinising hormone, is required to produce maleness in the fetus, no sex hormones produced by the fetus appear to be necessary for femaleness. Sex-dimorphic behaviour is regulated by the differentiated brain. The differentiation of the brain, which occurs at specific time periods during the early development, appears to be influenced by the presence and the extent of androgen effects. This conclusion is largely derived from works in lower mammals, some data from primate studies and scanty information from the human (Dorner & Staudt, 1972; Forest et al, 1980; MacLusky & Naftolin, 1981). If masculinity is dependent on the presence of adequate amounts of androgen effect at critical time periods, it is therefore more vulnerable to an unfinished or 'imperfect' outcome.
4. The construction of a cosmetically acceptable and functional vagina is a more practical goal than the construction of an artificial penis.

Aetiology

The term transsexuals was first coined by Benjamin (1966) to identify a group of psychosexually disturbed patients who resemble, but are distinct from, the better-known and more intensely studied homosexuals and transvestites. Many of the controversies in the early 1960s revolved around the debate on the existence of transsexualism as a distinct psychosexual syndrome, the criteria for their diagnosis, and the use of sex reassignment surgery as a viable treatment modality for them (Brady & Brodie, 1978). Disagreements in these areas had made the management of transsexualism a difficult task, a difficulty compounded by the complexity and controversy of the diagnostic procedures and the involvement of emotionally highly charged value judgement.

Many theories were proposed to explain the aetiology of transsexualism. They can be classified into two broad categories—the psychodynamic and the organic theories. Which of these theories is correct is currently a matter of intense debate. Many clinical behavioural scientists, psychologists and endocrinologists have a great interest in the outcome of the debate. The controversy concerns not only the aetiology of transsexualism but also the more embracing issue of the effects of endocrine versus socio-environmental factors in gender identity differentiation and gender orientation in humans.

The psychodynamic theory

Experience with the management of hermaphroditism has helped to conceptualize the 'assignment theory' which is most commonly quoted to explain the development of gender identity (Money et al, 1955). Typically the best 'prognosticator' of gender identity is the sex of assignment followed by consistent and unambiguous rearing (Money et al, 1955). The underlining assumption of this theory is the premise that gender identity can develop independently of, and in contrast to, gonadal histology, karyotype, internal genitals, and even external genitals and secondary sexual characteristics, singly or in combination. Work with pseudohermaphrodites has demonstrated an early emergence of gender identity in the first 2–3 years of a child's life. The development of gender identity and gender role behaviour is similar to imprinting (and can be compared to early language acquisition) which begins at 12 months, reaching a critical period at 18 months, and being relatively well established by $2\frac{1}{2}$ years (Money et al, 1955). Although these authors asserted that 'gender role may not be changed' at a later age, they presented data showing increasing risk of ambiguity of gender with increasing age at the time of assignment (Money et al, 1956).

Evidence for the powerful effects of early social environmental conditioning on gender identification came largely from successful gender identity of hermaphroditic children whose sex had been assigned at birth. Furthermore children with both ambiguity of their sex organs at birth and subsequent exposure to confusing changes brought about by the onset of puberty, usually identify firmly with their assigned gender. This occurred in spite of the presence of secondary sexual characteristics which are discordant with their sex of rearing (Ehrhardt, 1979). Additional support for this theory came from the observation that the most common factors amongst transsexuals are parental deprivation, unsatisfactory parental behaviour patterns, and poor father–son and mother–daughter relationships (Walinder, 1967; Newman, 1970; Stoller & Baker, 1973; Hore et al, 1973).

There was, however, opposition to the assignment theory. Gender role behaviour of patients with prenatal endocrine syndromes or a history of maternal exposure to hormones during pregnancy was found to be affected (Money & Ehrhardt, 1972; Ehrhardt & Meyer-Bahlburg, 1979). Girls exposed to high levels of androgen during fetal life, as a result of either maternal drug treatment or of congenital adrenal hyperplasia, were found to show markedly increased rough-and-tumble play, decreased parenting rehearsal, etc. Proponents of the assignment theory, however, suggested that such a shift in the sex-dimorphic behaviours normally falls within the wide range of behaviours accepted for a given gender. Since males and females show wide variations and much overlap in gender-role behaviour, gender identity usually agrees with the sex of assignment. They affirmed that gender identity can develop and be maintained even in contrast to what are presumably direct effects of hormones on the brain. They further suggest that if confusion about a child's sex of rearing persists beyond infancy in the mind of parents and other family members, there is a risk of ambiguity in the child's gender identity formation. Transsexualism is therefore thought to be caused by either conscious or unconscious rearing of the child in opposition to his or her anatomical gender.

Neuroendocrine theories

There are numerous organic theories formulated to explain the development of gender dysphoria. A genetic cause had been ruled out when the karyotypes of children with gender identity disorders were found to be normal (Green, 1976; Rekers et al, 1979). More recently, Eicher and co-workers from Munich found that most male and female transsexuals had an H-Y antigen status which was concordant with their desired sex rather than with their anatomical sex (Eicher et al, 1979; Spoljar et al, 1981). However, their findings were not reproducible in their more recent study involving double-blind matched controls (Eicher et al, 1981). The technique for detection and quantitation of H-Y antigen is known to be complex and quite often the kind of result obtained is dependent on the skill of the analysts. The current consensus is that the development of transsexuality cannot be explained by specific deviation in H-Y antigen.

The neuroendocrine theory is by far the most well-studied hypothesis. The basic premise is that 'the extent of androgen (testosterone) exposure of the brain in utero and during the early postnatal period and at puberty has more effect in determining male-gender identity than does the sex of rearing. Androgens are presumed to act as inducers in utero and neonatally and as activators at puberty' (Imperato-McGinley et al, 1979).

Prenatal abnormality of sex hormone production and of hormone utilisation by the central nervous system should be reflected in aberration of sex hormone production after puberty, according to this theory. Therefore the search for endocrine indicators for homosexuality and transsexuality has concentrated on the sex hormones, starting with urinary hormone extraction earlier in this century, and focusing on plasma hormone levels during the past decade. For males, this search has been largely negative (Wilson & Fulford, 1977; Goh et al, 1979; Meyer-Bahlhurg, 1980; Futterweit, 1980). Relatively fewer reports were available for females. Raised levels of testosterone were shown in females with gender-identity disorders, including transsexuality (Gartrell et al, 1977). However, the results could represent artefacts in sampling by the inclusion of other pathological cases in the control group.

In more recent years the major focus of psychoendocrine research on sexual orientation has shifted from the hormone situation in adulthood to the role of prenatal hormones. Dorner, the most forceful proponent of this theory, suggested that two mating centres exist in rats. The medial preoptic/ anterior hypothalamic region is mainly involved in the regulation of male sexual behaviour (mounting, intromission, ejaculation) and the ventrome-dial nuclear region is for the regulation of female behaviour (lordosis) (Dorner & Staudt, 1968, 1969; Staudt & Dorner, 1976). The differentiation of these centres is under the control of perinatal hormones. If perinatal androgens are high they will lead to the predominant organisation of the 'male centre'; if androgens are low the 'female centre' will predominate. Predominance of the male or female centre predisposes an individual for a specific sexual orientation. Dorner proposed that an error in this process of differentiation would lead to disorder in gender identity. He categorises homosexuality as a 'central nervous pseudohermaphroditism' (Dorner, 1976). This view currently has wide acceptance (Bell et al, 1981; MacCulloch & Waddington, 1981; McConaghy, 1982).

In contrast to Dorner's works on lower mammals, Karsch et al (1973) found little influence of prenatal hormones on gonadotrophin regulation in non-human primates. Studies of girls with congenital adrenal hyperplasia reveal that exposure to high levels of testosterone prenatally, may 'masculinise' but not 'defeminise' them; that is, the male behaviour pattern is superimposed on a female one (Kolata, 1979).

Further, Dorner's rat model suffered from several major difficulties. The rat model and theory predict that prenatal androgen deficiency in males will lead to feminine sexual behaviour, interpreted as male homosexuality. In practice, he found predominant 'homosexuality' in prenatally androgenised female rats only after gonadectomy and testosterone administration in adulthood. If left intact, the rats showed just a slight increase in mounting behaviour but a very clear predominance of female sexual behaviour. Furthermore the rat model does not predict preferential homosexuality in gonadally intact females, which is the typical condition of human female homosexuals.

A second problem is that most systemic manipulation of sex hormones in the pre- or perinatal stage of development results not only in shifts of sex-dimorphic behaviour and in structural changes of the underlying brain systems, but also in corresponding alterations of the genitalia. By contrast, typical human homosexuals or transsexuals have normal gender-appropriate genitalia.

Failing to detect differences in static hormone levels between patients with gender-identity disorders and normal subjects, the emphasis then turns to the detection of dynamic or functional characteristics that could indicate the existence of a prenatal hormone abnormality. The positive oestrogen feedback on LH has been suggested as such an indicator.

In the physiological state oestrogen positive feedback mechanism exists only in the female. The LH surge at mid-cycle has been implicated to be responsible for triggering off ovulation. Dorner showed that, in transsexual and homosexual men, the positive feedback on LH elicited by oestrogen is stronger than in heterosexual men. Corresponding results were demonstrated in female transsexuals (Dorner et al, 1975; Seyler et al, 1978; Dorner, 1981). The reports of a somewhat feminised pattern of LH response in male transsexuals and a somewhat defeminised, masculinised pattern in female transsexuals, if replicable by other laboratories, may have potentially great significance for a neuroendocrine theory of sexual orientation. The interpretation of Dorner and co-workers' data, however, is not simple. Short (1979) cautioned the acceptance of the apparent positive feedback effects seen in Dorner's works, since a rebound of LH levels (slight elevation above baseline levels) in men can follow the release of oestrogen-induced suppression. He further suggested that the phenomenon should not be confused with the pronounced LH elevation seen in the positive feedback in women. To fit in the mechanism of positive feedback, there are two essential criteria that should be met.

First, the enhanced LH secretion, and to a lesser extent FSH, should occur in the presence of high levels of oestrogen. This criterion is probably not met in Dorner's investigation as it is not known what the oestrogen levels were in Dorner's subjects when the apparent 'positive feedback' effect occurred (Dorner et al, 1975). Given a half-life of about 20 minutes, it is unlikely that, 72–96 hours after the intravenous dose of oestrogens, the levels of oestradiol would be significantly higher than basal concentration.

Second, oestrogen positive feedback in normal women often results in a several-fold increase in LH levels. The average increase of LH over baseline levels in Dorner's study was only about 20 per cent. It is, therefore, likely that his observation represents a LH rebound rather than a positive feedback effect. We had demonstrated this phenomenon of LH rebound following releases from suppression caused by oestrogen administered either acutely (Goh, 1980) or chronically (Goh et al, 1981).

In a more recent study, male transsexuals who had no previous history of hormone therapy, and had no surgical intervention to their problem of gender dysphoria, responded to an acute high dose of oestradiol (depot preparation) with a classical male-type response (Goh et al, 1984). Basal LH concentrations and the pituitary responsiveness to LHRH were significantly suppressed. On the other hand, in transsexuals who had been primed previously with oestrogens, an acute high dose of oestradiol was able to elicit a positive feedback response (Goh et al, 1984). Plasma gonadotrophin levels and the pituitary responsiveness to LHRH were shown to increase several-fold over the baseline levels. Furthermore this phenomenon occurred in the presence of high levels of oestradiol. This result indicates that there is no feminisation of the hypothalamic–pituitary axis of male transsexuals. The result also provides additional information for our understanding of the oestrogen positive feedback in humans. It emphasises the importance of excluding patients with previous history of steroid hormone therapy in studies that are designed to search for endocrine correlates to the problem of gender dysphoria.

The neuroendocrine theory was given a boost recently by the case reports on gender-reversal in a group of male pseudohermaphrodites in the Dominican Republic (Imperato-McGinley et al, 1979). Because of 5α-reductase deficiency, testosterone in these subjects is not metabolised to dihydrotestosterone, resulting in severe ambiguity of the external genitalia. These individuals were reared as females from birth. However, at puberty virilisation took place, their voices deepened, penile growth took place, the testes descended, and they experienced erection. Most of the patients who were reported to be raised unambiguously as females changed to male identity and orientation. The authors inferred that testosterone exposure during the prenatal, perinatal, and especially pubertal, states of development is the most significant factor in the normal differentiation of male identity. This is in contrast to the more widely held contemporary assignment theory (Money & Ehrhardt, 1972; Money, 1977).

Serious doubts were cast on Imperato-McGinley's basic premise that the Dominican male pseudohermaphrodites were unambiguously raised as girls (Rubin et al, 1981; Meyer-Bahlburg, 1982). Several other cases of male pseudohermaphrodites due to 5α-reductase deficiency were reported in other countries (Opitz et al, 1971; Walsh et al, 1974; Saenger et al, 1978). Subjects were claimed to be similarly raised as girls, as with the Dominican kindreds. Among them, some experienced testosterone-induced activation of puberty prior to medical intervention, while others were treated before puberty. However, unlike the Dominican kindreds, most of these subjects did not experience gender-reversal. Therefore it may be possible that the majority of the Dominican subjects, due to the widespread knowledge of their family history, their not-so-ambiguous genitalia, the lack of privacy in their community living and the traditional society they were in, were not raised unambiguously as girls. They could have experienced gender-identity confusion during childhood which fostered their masculine gender emergence at puberty (Kolata, 1979). Imperato-McGinley recently stated that in fact the Dominican children knew that something was odd by 6–7 years of age (Ehrhardt & Meyer-Bahlburg, 1979).

Another line of evidence in support of a neuroendocrine theory for sexual differentiation of gender identity comes from studies of neuron distribution and its influence by steroid hormones. In 1973 Raisman & Field found sex-related differences in the distribution of synaptic connections of nerve cells in the preoptic area of rat brains, which is adjacent to the hypothalamus. They showed that when newborn rats are castrated during the critical period, but not later, they develop a female pattern of synaptic connections. And when newborn females are given testosterone during the critical period, they develop a male pattern of synaptic connections. Such sex differences in brain areas were noted by others too (Gorski et al, 1978, 1980; Goy & McEwen, 1980).

In rats, sex differences in the brain are brought about by oestrogen. Oestrogen receptors are found to increase rapidly in number about 2 days before birth, and continue to about 4–5 days after birth (the end of the critical period). McEwen (1981) found that there is a high concentration of oestrogen receptors in the cerebral cortex during the critical period, but that these receptors start to disappear after 14 days. This finding is especially intriguing because of the function of the cerebral cortex; it is the highest neural centre—the area where speech, hearing, thinking, and consciousness are controlled. Could this also be the seat of the sex dimorphic differentiation of the brain, which leads to the development of the male and female gender identity and gender orientation? A clear picture is now beginning to emerge of how the sex-related differences in rat brains occur. Whether these exact mechanisms have counterparts in human brain development is still unclear.

Most investigators now regard the factors contributing to the development of gender identity to be neither 'nature' nor 'nurture' alone, but rather an interaction of hormonal and psychosocial influences. The data from the Dominican kindred and others (Gajdusek, 1977; Imperato-McGinley et al, 1979; Meyer-Bahlburg, 1982) contribute to the growing body of evidence that prenatal and pubertal hormone exposure interacts with environmental factors to influence behavioural development in humans. What arose from these more recent studies is that expression of sex-dimorphic behaviour is the result of a complex interaction between hormonal influences on brain function and psychosocial and environmental forces. What is more important for future research is to delineate the relative contributions of both sets of influences on each specific behaviour. Such an understanding would have tremendous implication in the management of transsexualism and other psychosexual disorders.

MANAGEMENT OF TRANSSEXUALISM

In spite of the many clinical studies of transsexualism, very little is actually known about the social–psychological and medical–surgical effects of sex reassignment surgery on patients. Follow-up studies in the 1960s concentrated mainly on gross social psychological effects of the surgery. In spite of several instances of negative results (Benjamin, 1966; Money & Primrose, 1968; Randell, 1969), these studies claimed that the success or 'cure' rates were between 68 and 86 per cent. The reason for the post-operation improvement in socioeconomic functioning of transsexuals was attributed to the sex reassignment surgery. As a result of these studies the consensus in the 1960s and early 1970s was that sex reassignment surgery is the treatment of choice for transsexualism.

The early claim that sex reassignment surgery is the only viable treatment modality for transsexualism had proven to be counterproductive. Claims of successes led to its widespread use and, in many countries, the surgery is available on a fee-for-service basis. Consequently many self-proclaimed transsexuals were receiving this mode of surgical treatment secretly. This factor, together with the high mobility of transsexuals after their sex change operation, resulted in few cases being available for follow-up studies. The early claims of high success rates which were based on evaluation of small numbers of patients are questionable (Lothstein, 1982; Ball, 1981).

The monopoly of the use of the sex reassignment surgery in the management of transsexuals had also resulted in the exclusion of traditional psychiatric intervention from the treatment. Too few patients were available for studies which might lead to a better understanding of the nature of their psychological stress. A lack of such an understanding rendered many psychiatrists unprepared to respond adequately to the transsexual phenomenon. However, more studies using improved psychoanalytical methods were carried out in the mid-70s and early 1980s. Evidence from these studies provided support to the early claim that the sex reassignment surgery led to a better social and economic status for the patients. This is only true for a highly select group of gender-dysphoric patients. These studies also revealed that most patients, who would otherwise undergo the surgery, were not true transsexuals, and could adjust to a non-surgical solution through psychotherapy (Lothstein, 1982; Ball, 1981); they need psychotherapy not surgery (Newman & Stoller, 1974). What is more disturbing is the finding that many of the gender-dysphoric patients were characterised as having severe psychopathology which was unaltered by the sex reassignment surgery (Sturup, 1976; Meyer & Reter, 1979; Hunt & Hampson, 1980; Lothstein, 1980; Rollin, 1982). Surgery and hormones are not effective treatment for major instability, and certainly not for sociopathic personality characteristics.

Transsexualism is an emotionally crippling disease that impinges on all developmental stages (Edgerton et al, 1982). While sex reassignment surgery has definite medical–surgical and psychological limitations, there is evidence suggesting that some gender-dysphoric patients benefit primarily from it (Hunt & Hampson, 1980). The problem is how to identify these patients. Conservatively, and in the light of conclusions of more recent studies, thorough screening—rather than ruthless exclusion of doubtful cases, and prolonged pre-surgery observation—leads to successful results with excellent individual, social and sexual adjustment.

The lack of a simple litmus test to predict which patients will benefit from sex reassignment surgery has created a tremendous ethical unease among professionals managing transsexuals. To provide guidance for this particularly difficult area of patient management, the Harry Benjamin International Gender Dysphoria Association has developed 'standards' that set minimal requirements of care. A team approach is recommended. The 'standards' require that a patient should have the gender disorder for at least 2 years, and that a person with this condition be known to a clinical behavioural scientist, and be his or her patient, for at least 3 months. Hormone therapy should be initiated only upon the recommendation of the clinical behavioural scientist. The endocrinologist of the team should be aware of the risk factors or side-effects of the hormone therapy. He needs to appraise the patient in the light of those risks. Regular monitoring of relevant blood chemistries and routine physical examinations must be included.

Hormone therapy

Hormone therapy serves two functions. Before irreversible surgical intervention is considered, hormone therapy will result in reversible (chemical) castration; testicular and penile atrophy in the male and cessation of menstruation in the female. These serve to diminish remainders of the repudiated gender. Patients are required to be on hormone therapy for a certain period of time and assume the dressing and role of the desired gender for at least 2 years. This trial period allows time for the patient to reassess his or her decision for the sex change, while the physicians will have ample time to gauge the suitability of the patient for the surgical change. Hormone therapy also leads to the development of somatic sex characteristics of the desired gender both before and after gonadectomy, and ensures their maintenance.

There are rarely any studies that systematically evaluate the efficacy of hormone therapy in achieving the desired effects, as well as the side-effects, associated with therapy. In a recent report various forms and doses of hormone therapy used in the treatment of non-castrate transsexuals were compared (Meyer et al, 1981). They found that ethinyl oestradiol (EE) is more effective in suppressing gonadotrophin and testosterone but equally as effective in inducing breast growth as conjugated oestradiol. Since 100 μg of EE was found to be as effective as 500 μg, they advocate that the lower dose be used. Our experience with hormone therapy for male transsexuals has shown similar conclusions.

It is important to bear in mind that most male transsexuals have a misguided concept of hormone therapy. They erroneously and persistently believe that the higher the oestrogen dose, the more feminine they will become. In their desperate drive towards attainment of femininity they often resort to self-prescription. Many patients have already experienced several years of hormone therapy before they register at a gender identity clinic. It is not uncommon to come across patients taking 500 μg of EE plus 5 mg of a progestin, supplemented with weekly oestrogen injection (depot preparation). It is worth noting that chronic oestrogen treatment is held responsible for several cancer deaths of male transsexuals (Symmers, 1968) and a case of pulmonary embolism (Lehrman, 1976). Pulmonary embolism is a risk of any major surgery, but those patients who have been on oestrogens are more likely to suffer from it (Lehrman, 1976; Felstein, 1983). For this reason the hormone treatment is usually stopped at least 1 month preoperatively and not resumed postoperatively for another month in our centre.

In the management of more than 200 male transsexuals over the past few years we had encountered several side-effects which may be attributed to the hormone therapy used by patients. Several cases of hyperprolactinaemia (>4000 mIU/l), pill-induced jaundice and diabetes, oedema and pigmentation (usually on the face) were noted. A more general but often overlooked side-effect is malaise, and it is more evident in patients on higher doses. The prevention of these side-effects varies from the reduction of the doses to changing the type of hormone preparations, or to stopping the therapy altogether.

To help reduce the risks associated with higher doses, our efforts have been directed towards educating transsexuals in the proper use of hormone therapy and recruiting them to participate in our controlled hormone therapy regime. One of the hardest things to do, in this respect, is to get male transsexuals to accept the minimum dose and at the same time to convince them that the efficacy, and their desire for femininity, are not being compromised.

The problem of over-dosing in transsexuals is often compounded by the existence of a black market for these sex steroid hormones. Many general practitioners have unknowingly been the suppliers of such hormones to transsexuals. Since most of the practitioners lack the facilities to meet the need for close monitoring of these patients it would be beneficial that their involvement in the management of transsexual patients be carried out in conjunction with an established gender identity clinic (Imber, 1976).

Hormone therapy for female transsexuals usually is less problematic; this is at least true for us in Singapore. Almost all of the patients participate in the androgen therapy scheme of our clinic. We have found that an intramuscular injection of 100 mg of testosterone cypionate in oil, given once every fortnight, is sufficient to initiate the desired amenorrhoea, hirsutism and beard growth within 1–2 months, and the maintenance of these somatic changes thereafter. Similar regimes were suggested by Meyer and co-workers (1981) except that they proposed the use of 200 mg of testosterone cypionate. Side-effects with this regime of androgen therapy for female transsexuals are few, the most common ones being severe acne, and in very few patients, general body erythema. These are often prevented by reducing the dose.

Total management

It is useful to remember that clinicians and their patients share the same goal—attainment of a sexual identity that no longer interferes with the patient's capacity to live a full and meaningful life (Levine & Shumaker, 1983). To achieve a higher level of success in this aim, it is timely that both patients and their doctors be aware of the need for total management, not merely surgical and hormonal treatments. A team approach to the total management is advocated. As mentioned earlier, many transsexuals also suffer from other psychological disturbances. Apart from endocrinologists, surgeons, and clinical behavioural scientists, psychotherapists are needed to help alleviate patients from stresses other than those of gender dysphoria. Finally, regular counselling should be instituted as part of the programme in the management of transsexualism. Pre-surgery counselling should include topics such as advice on the need to change jobs, and the requirements and possible problems associated with the surgery. Other personal and practical help should include training in personal make-up, dressing, hair-do and speech therapy. All these will give additional support to the patients in adapting to their new role, and hopefully to live a more personally satisfying and socially acceptable life (Campbell, 1983).

REFERENCES

Abraham F 1931 Genitalumwandlung an zwei maenlichen transvestiten. Zeitschrift fur Sexualwissenschaft 18 : 223–226

Ball J R B 1981 Thirty years experience with transsexualism. Australian and New Zealand Journal of Psychiatry 15 : 39–43

Bell A P, Weinberg M S, Hammersmith S K 1981 Sexual preference: its development in men and women. Indiana University Press, Bloomington

Benjamin H 1966 The transsexual phenomenon. Julian Press, New York

Berger J, Green R, Laub D et al 1977 Standards of care: the hormonal and surgical sex reassignment of gender dysphoric persons. University of Texas Medical Branch, Janus Information Centre, Galveston, Texas

Brady J, Brodie H 1978 Controversy in psychiatry. Saunders, Philadelphia

Campbell C 1983 A woman in the making. Nursing Mirror 157: 20–22

Dorner G 1976 Hormones and brain differentiation. Elsevier, Amsterdam

Dorner G 1981 Sex hormones and neurotransmitters as mediators for sexual differentiation of the brain. Endokrinologie 78 : 129–138

Dorner G, Staudt J 1968 Structural changes in the preoptic anterior hypothalamic area of the male rat, following neonatal castration and androgen substitution. Neuroendocrinology 3 : 131–140

Dorner G, Staudt J 1969 Structural changes in the hypothalamic ventromedial nucleus of the male rat, following neonatal castration and androgen treatment. Neuroendocrinology 4 : 278–281

Dorner G, Staudt J 1972 Vergleichende morphologische Untersuchungen der Hypothalamusdifferenzierung bei Ratte und Mensch. Endokrinologie 59 : 152–155

Dorner G, Rohde W, Stahl F, Krell L, Masins W-G 1975 A neuroendocrine predisposition for homosexuality in men. Archives of Sexual Behavior 4(1) : 1–8

Edgerton Jr M T, Langman M W, Schmidt J S, Sheppe Jr W 1982 Psychological considerations of gender reassignment surgery. Clinics in Plastic Surgery 9(3) : 355–366

Ehrhardt A A 1979 Psychosexual adjustment in adolescence in patients with congenital abnormalities of their own sex organs. In: Vallet H L, Porter I H (eds) Genetic mechanisms of sexual development (Birth Defects Institute Symposia). Academic Press, New York, pp 473–484

Ehrhardt A A, Meyer-Bahlburg H F L 1979 Psychosexual development: an examination of the role of prenatal hormones. In: Poter B, Whelan J (eds) Ciba Foundation Symposium on sex, hormone, and behaviour. Excerpta Medica, Amsterdam, vol. 62, pp 41–57

Eicher W, Spoljar M, Cleve H, Murken J-D, Richter K, Stangel-Rutkowski S 1979 H-Y antigen in transsexuality. Lancet ii: 1137–1138

Eicher W, Spoljar M, Cleve H, Murken J-D, Eiermann W, Richter K, Stangel-Rutkowski S 1981 H-Y antigen in transsexuality. Manuscript for presentation at the Annual Meeting of the International Academy of Sex Research, Haifa, Israel, 17–20 June

Fallowell F, Ashley A 1982 April Ashley's odyssey. Jonathan Cape, London

Felstein I 1983 Clinical comment. In: Campbell C (ed) A woman in the making. Nursing Mirror 157(7): 20–22

Forest M G, de Peretti E, Bertrand J 1980 Testicular and adrenal androgens and their binding to plasma proteins in the perinatal period: development patterns of plasma testosterone, 4-androstenedione, dehydroepiandrosterone and its sulfate in premature and small-for-date infants as compared with that of full-term infants. Journal of Steroid Biochemistry 12: 25–36

Friedman R C, Green R, Spitzer R L 1976 Reassignment of homosexuality and transsexualism. Annual Review of Medicine 7: 57–62

Futterweit W 1980 Endocrine management of transsexual. Hormone profiles of serum prolactin, testosterone, and oestradiol. New York State Journal of Medicine 80: 1260–1264

Gajdusek D C 1977 Urgent opportunistic observations: the study of changing, transient and disappearing phenomena of medical interest in disrupted primitive human communities. In Health and disease in tribal society. Ciba Foundation Symposium 49 (new series), pp 69–94. Elsevier, Amsterdam

Gartrell N K, Loriaux D L, Chase T N 1977 Plasma testosterone in homosexual and heterosexual women. American Journal of Psychiatry 134: 1117–1119

Goh H H 1980 The effect of oestradiol and luteinizing hormone releasing hormone on the secretion of gonadotrophins in castrated male transsexuals. Singapore Journal of Obstetrics and Gynaecology 11(2): 17–30

Goh H H, Karim S M M, Ratnam S S 1979 Endocrine profile of 'virgin' male transsexuals. Singapore Journal of Obstetrics and Gynaecology 10(3): 67–71

Goh H H, Karim S M M, Ratnam S S 1981 Recovery of hypophyseal–testicular function from sex steroid treatment and the pituitary response to castration in male transsexuals. Clinical Endocrinology 15: 519–523

Goh H H, Ratnam S S, London D R 1984 The feminization of gonadotrophin response in intact male transsexual. Clinical Endocrinology 20: 591–596

Gorski R A, Gordon J H, Shryne J E, Southam A M 1978 Evidence for a morphological sex difference within the medial preoptic area of the rat brain. Brain Research 148: 333–346

Gorski R A, Harlan R E, Jacobson C D, Shryne J E, Southam A M 1980 Evidence for the existence of a sexually dimorphic nucleus in the preoptic area of the rat. Journal of Comparative Neurology 193: 529–540

Goy R W, McEwen B S 1980 Sexual differentiation of the brain. MIT Press, Cambridge

Green R 1969 Mythological, historical and cross-cultural aspects of transsexualism. In: Green R & Money J (eds) Transsexualism and sex reassignment. The Johns Hopkins Press, Baltimore, pp 13–22

Green R 1974 Adults who want to change sex; adolescents who cross-dressed and children called 'Sissy and Tomboy'. In: Green R (ed) Human sexuality. Williams and Wilkins, Baltimore, pp 83–95

Green R 1976 One-hundred ten feminine and masculine boys: behavioral contrasts and demographic similarities. Archives of Sexual Behavior 5: 425–446

Hamburger C 1953 Desire for change of sex as shown by personal letters from 465 men and women. Acta Endocrinologica (Copenh) 14: 361–375

Hoenig J, Kenna J C 1974 Prevalence of transsexualism in England and Wales. British Journal of Psychiatry 124: 181–190

Hore B D, Phil M, Nicolle F V, Chir B, Calnan J S 1973 Male transsexualism: two cases in a single family. Archives of Sexual Behavior 2: 317–321

Hunt D D, Hampson J L 1980 Follow-up of 17 biologic male transsexuals after sex-reassignment surgery. American Journal of Psychiatry 137: 432–438

Imber H 1976 The management of transsexualism. Medical Journal of Australia 2: 676–678

Imperato-McGinley J, Peterson R E, Gautier T, Sturla E 1979 Androgens and the evolution of male-gender identity among male pseudohermaphrodites with 5a-reductase deficiency. New England Journal of Medicine 300: 1233–1237

Jorgenson C 1967 A personal autobiography. Paul E Ericson, New York

Karsch F J, Ierschke D J, Knobil E 1973 Sexual differentiation of pituitary function: apparent difference between primates and rodents. Science 179: 484–486

Kolata G B 1979 Sex hormones and brain development. Science, 205: 985–987

Laub D R, Fisk N 1974 A rehabilitation program for gender dysphoria syndrome by surgical sex change. Plastic Reconstruction Surgery 53: 388–403

Lehrman K L 1976 Pulmonary embolism in a transsexual man taking diethylstilbestrol. Journal of American Medical Association 235: 532–533

Levine S B, Shumaker R 1983 Increasing Ruth: toward understanding sex reassignment. Archives of Sexual Behavior 12: 247–261

Lothstein L 1980 The postsurgical transsexual: empirical and theoretical considerations. Archives of Sexual Behavior 9: 547–564

Lothstein L M 1982 Sex reassignment surgery: historical, bioethical, and theoretical issues. American Journal of Psychiatry 139(4): 417–425

MacCulloch M J, Waddington J L 1981 Neuroendocrine mechanisms and the aetiology of male and female homosexuality. British Journal of Psychiatry 139: 341–345

MacLusky N J, Naftolin F 1981 Sexual differentiation of the central nervous system. Science 211: 1294–1303

McConaghy N 1982 Current status of behavior therapy in homosexuality. Proceedings of the Fifth World Congress of Sexology. Jerusalem, Israel, 21–26 June

McEwen B S 1981 Neural gonadal steroid actions. Science 211: 1303–1311

Meyer W J III, Finkelstein J W, Stuart C A, Webb A, Smith E R, Payer A F, Walker P A 1981 Physical and hormonal evaluation of transsexual patients during hormone therapy. Archives of Sexual Behavior 10: 347–356

Meyer J, Reter C 1979 Sex reassignment: follow-up. Archives of General Psychiatry 36: 1010–1015

Meyer-Bahlburg H F L 1980 Hormones and homosexuality. In: Advances in psychoneuroendocrinology. The Psychiatric Clinics of North America 3(2): 349–364. Saunders, Philadelphia

Meyer-Bahlburg H F L 1982 Hormones and psychosexual differentiation: implications for the management of intersexuality, homosexuality and transsexuality. Clinics in Endocrinology and Metabolism, 11(3): 681–701

Money J 1977 Determinants of human gender identity/role. In: Money J, Musaph H (eds) Handbook of sexology. Elsevier, Amsterdam, pp 57–79

Money J, Ehrhardt A A 1972 Man, woman, boy and girl: the differentiation and dimorphism of gender identity from conception to maturity. Johns Hopkins University Press, Baltimore

Money J, Primrose C 1968 Sexual dimorphism with psychology of male transsexuals. Journal of Nervous and Mental Diseases 147: 472–485

Money J, Hampson J G, Hampson J L 1955 An examination of some basic sexual concepts: the evidence of human hermaphroditism. Bulletin of the Johns Hopkins Hospital 97: 301–319

Money J, Hampson J G, Hampson J L 1956 Sexual incongruities and psychopathology: the evidence of human hermaphroditism. Bulletin of the Johns Hopkins Hospital 98: 43–57

Newman L E 1970 Transsexualism in adolescence: problems in evaluation and treatment. Archives of General Psychiatry 23: 112–121

Newman L E, Stoller R J 1974 Nontranssexual men who seek sex reassignment. American Journal of Psychiatry 131: 437–441

Opitz J M, Simpson J L, Sario G E, Summitt R L, New M, German J 1971 Pseudovaginal perineoscrotal hypospadia. Clinical Genetics 3: 1–26

Pauly I B 1968 The current status of change of sex operation. Journal of Nervous and Mental Diseases 147: 460–471

Raisman G, Field P M 1973 Sexual dimorphism in the neurophil of the preoptic area of the rat and its dependence on neonatal androgen. Brain Research 54: 1–29

Randell J B 1969 Preoperative and postoperative status of male and female transsexuals. In: Green R, Money J (eds) Transsexualism and sex reassignment surgery. Johns Hopkins University Press, Baltimore

Rekers G A, Crandall B F, Rosen A C, Bentler P M 1979 Genetic and physical studies of male children with psychological gender disturbances. Psychological Medicine 9: 373–375

Rollin H R 1982 Transsexualism observed. British Medical Journal 285: 461

Ross M W, Walinder J, Lundstrom B, Thuwe I 1981 Cross-cultural approaches to transsexualism: a comparison between Sweden and Australia. Acta Psychiatrica Scandinavica 63: 75–82

Rubin R T, Reinisch J M, Haskett R F 1981 Postnatal gonadal steroid effects on human behavior. Science 211: 1318–1324

Saenger P, Goldman A S, Levine L S, Korth-Schutz S, Muecke E C, Katsumata M, Doberne Y, New M I 1978 Prepubertal diagnosis of steriod 5a-reductase deficiency. Journal of Clinical Endocrinology and Metabolism 46: 627–634

Seyler L E, Canalis E, Spare S, Reichlin S 1978 Abnormal gonadotropin secretory responses to LRH in transsexual women after diethylstibestrol priming. Journal of Clinical Endocrinology and Metabolism 47: 176–183

Short R 1979 Discussion of Dorner's paper on hormones and sexual differentiation of the brain. In: Ciba Foundation Symposium on Sex, Hormone, and Behaviour. Excerpta Medica, Amsterdam, vol. 62, pp 81–112

Spoljar M, Eicher W, Eiermann W, Cleve H 1981 H-Y antigen expression in different tissues from transsexuals. Human Genetics 57: 52–57

Staudt J, Dorner G 1976 Structural changes in the medial and central amyldala of the male rat, following neonatal castration and androgen treatment. Endokrinologie 67: 296–300

Stoller K J, Baker J H 1973 Two male transsexuals in one family. Archives of Sexual Behavior 2: 323–328

Sturup G K 1976 Male transsexuals: a long-term follow-up after sex reassignment operations. Acta Psychiatrica Scandinavica 53: 51–63

Symmers W C 1968 Carcinoma of breast in transsexual individuals after surgical and hormonal interference with the primary and secondary sex characteristics. British Medical Journal ii: 83–85

Tsoi W F, Kok L P, Long F Y 1977 Male transsexualism in Singapore: a description of 56 cases. British Journal of Psychiatry 131: 405–409

Volkin V 1979 Transsexualism: as examined from the viewpoint of internalized object relations. In: Karasu T B, Socarides C (eds) On sexuality: psychoanalytic observations. International University Press, New York

Walinder J 1967 Transsexualism: a study of forty-three cases. Scandinavian University Books, Copenhagen, Denmark

Walinder J 1968 Transsexualism: definition, prevalence and sex distribution. Acta Psychiatrica Scandinavica Supplement 203: 255–257

Walinder J 1971 Incidence and sex ratio of transsexualism in Sweden. British Journal of Psychiatry 119: 195–196

Walsh P C, Madden J D, Harrod M J, Goldstein J L, MacDonald P C, Wilson J D 1974 Familial incomplete male pseudohermaphroditism, Type 2. Decreased dihydrotestosterone formation in pseudovaginal perineoscrotal hypospadia. New England Journal of Medicine 291: 944–949

Wilson G D, Fulford K W M 1977 Sexual behavior; personality and hormonal characteristics of heterosexual, homosexual and bisexual men. In: Cook M, Wilson G (eds) Love and attraction. Pergamon Press, Oxford, pp 387–394

Premalignant lesions of the lower genital tract

CERVICAL INTRA-EPITHELIAL NEOPLASIA

The incidence of cervical intra-epithelial neoplasia (CIN) has more than doubled over the past decade in England and Wales (Draper & Cook, 1983) and is becoming more common in younger women (Wolfendale et al, 1983; Roberts, 1982). It is believed that if CIN can be detected and treated, this will significantly reduce the mortality rate from cervical cancer. This concept is supported by results from cytology screening programmes in Canada (Walton, 1976), the United States (Cramer, 1974), Finland (Hakama, 1985), Iceland (Johannesson et al, 1978), Scotland (Macgregor & Teper, 1978), and England and Wales (Parkin et al, 1985). All of these studies have shown significant reductions in the incidence of cervical cancer in screened populations.

The CIN classification is gradually replacing the World Health Organisation classification (1975); CIN I, II and III corresponding to mild, moderate and severe dysplasia/carcinoma in situ respectively.

The association of human papillomavirus and cervical neoplasia

It is now accepted that sexual transmission is a factor in the aetiology of cervical neoplasia (Rotkin, 1973; Kessler, 1974) and many epidemiological studies point to the involvement of an infectious agent.

Herpes simplex virus (HSV) was the first virus to be extensively investigated as a possible aetiological agent in cervical carcinogenesis. The ability of partially inactivated HSV to transform rodent cells has been demonstrated (Duff & Rapp, 1973). Seroepidemiological studies have shown an association between HSV and cervical cancer (Rawls et al, 1968). HSV-specific structural and non-structural antigens have been identified in premalignant and malignant tissues (Aurelian et al, 1981). McDougall et al (1980) have demonstrated HSV-specific RNA in cervical cancer biopsies. Some investigators have found varying amounts of HSV-specific DNA in cervical cancer tissue (Frenkel et al, 1972) although others have failed to find any. This has led to the 'hit-and-run' theory, which suggests that HSV may act as an initiator of the transformation process, the continuation of which is not dependent on further replication of the viral genome.

In 1976 Zur Hausen suggested that human papillomavirus (HPV) warranted investigation as a possible agent in the aetiology of genital neoplasia, as it belongs to a well-characterised group of oncogenic DNA viruses. Papillomaviruses are the aetiological agents of papillomas or benign warts; malignant transformation of papillomavirus-induced lesions has been documented in animals (Kreider, 1980) and in man (Jablonska et al, 1972). Since the cytological and colposcopic appearances of cervical HPV infection were documented (Meisels & Fortin, 1976; Meisels et al, 1977) cytological and histological evidence of cervical HPV infection is being reported with increasing frequency, although this in part may reflect an increased awareness of the condition.

Forty-one distinct genotypes of HPV have now been identified; types 6, 10, 11, 16 and 18 appear to be associated with genital tract neoplasia.

HPV type 6 (Gissmann & Zur Hausen, 1980) and HPV type 11 (Gissmann et al, 1983) have been isolated from genital warts. McCance et al (1983) demonstrated the presence of HPV DNA type 6 in 60 per cent of 22 biopsies of CIN. Zur Hausen (1985) reports the presence of HPV 6 and HPV 11 in 40 per cent of biopsies of CIN, the majority of which were graded as CIN I/II and contained koilocytotic cells, 20 per cent of CIN lesions contained HPV 16 or 18, most of these lesions were graded as CIN II/III and failed to reveal evidence of a high degree of koilocytosis. HPV 16 (Durst et al, 1983) and HPV 18 (Boshart et al, 1984) have been isolated from cervical cancer tissue, but the majority of these biopsies are negative when tested for DNA of type 6 and 11.

Zur Hausen suggests that the available data point to the existence of two risk groups of genital papillomavirus infectin; HPV type 6, 10 and 11 representing a low-risk group, HPV types 16 and 18 representing a high-risk group although recent data reported by McCance et al (1985) do not fully support this hypothesis: they detected HPV 16 DNA in 50 per cent of CIN I, 70 per cent of CIN 3 and 90 per cent of invasive cervical cancers.

While this evidence of association does not prove causation, and although Koch's postulates cannot be completely satisfied, there is nevertheless a great deal of circumstantial evidence incriminating HPV in genital tract carcinogenesis.

Malignant potential of CIN

The treatment of all women with proven CIN is now established practice, based on the premise that a significant number of cases will ultimately progress to invasive cancer if left untreated. Reporting on a series of 948 women with untreated CIN III, McIndoe et al (1984) concluded that women with cytological evidence of continuing neoplasia after initial diagnosis of carcinoma in situ of the cervix had an 18 per cent chance of developing invasive cancer of the cervix or vaginal vault at 10 years, and a 36 per cent chance at 20 years.

While there is little doubt that the more severe forms of CIN have significant malignant potential, the treatment of lesser grades of CIN, particularly in association with HPV infection, is controversial. The RCOG Study Group (Jordan et al, 1982) recommended that CIN should be regarded as a continuum, CIN I being taken as seriously as CIN III, and advised that all grades of CIN should be treated even in the presence of HPV infection.

There appears to be a significant spontaneous regression of disease in patients with histological evidence of HPV infection. We have documented the spontaneous regression of cytological and colposcopic evidence of histologically proven cervical HPV infection without associated CIN in 58 per cent of 45 patients after a median follow-up of 28 months; four patients developed CIN (Woodman et al, 1985a).

Singer et al (1984) believe that these types of lesions should be destroyed because of the increased risk of developing CIN and invasive cancer. The lesions are easily treated with local destructive methods and the psychological trauma caused to such women by regular cytological review far outweighs the inconvenience of immediate treatment.

Cone biopsy

Cone biopsy of the cervic is mandatory for the evaluation of cytological abnormality and treatment of CIN when:

1. colposcopic examination is not available;
2. the whole of the transformation zone cannot be visualised colposcopically;
3. colposcopic, histological or cytological examination suggests the presence of an invasive lesion;
4. cytological examination suggests the presence of a glandular endocervical lesion.

Complications

The main complications are haemorrhage, cervical stenosis, increased pregnancy loss and incomplete excision of the lesion.

1. Haemorrhage. Reported incidences of postoperative haemorrhage vary between 4 and 21 per cent (Rubio et al, 1975; Jones & Buller, 1980; Larsson et al, 1983). Attempts to quantify the extent of haemorrhage are notoriously unreliable; thus complication rates might be more appropriately discussed in relation to the frequency with which further haemostatic intervention is required.

Luesley et al (1985a) found that 101 of 788 patients who had a cone biopsy performed had a postoperative haemorrhage; 46 occurred within 24 hours of surgery, 55 between 24 hours and 12 days postoperatively. Further intervention in the form of hysterectomy, packing or resuturing was required in 75 patients. The incidence of primary and secondary haemorrhage is related to both the base width (Claman & Lee, 1974), and the length of the cone (Luesley et al, 1985a).

2. *Cervical stenosis.* There is no standard definition of postoperative cervical stenosis. Reported incidences vary between 3 and 31 per cent (Byrne, 1966; Hollyhock & Chanen, 1972; Larsson, 1983). A recent study performed in our unit has shown that, in 788 women who had a cone biopsy performed, the incidence of cervical stenosis was related to the length of the cone; if the cone was 25 mm or less in length the stenosis rate was 12·8 per cent, while the stenosis rate was 24·2 per cent when the cone length was greater than 25 mm (Luesley et al, 1985a). Cervical stenosis can be symptomatic or asymptomatic. Symptoms include dysmenorrhoea, irregular bleeding, and rarely amenorrhoea with an associated haematometra if the stenosis is complete. The presence of cervical stenosis after cone biopsy, even if symptomless, may frustrate adequate colposcopic and cytological examination and postpone the detection of residual or recurrent disease.

A number of claims have been made as to the influence of a variety of suture techniques on the incidence of postoperative complications. There is a dearth of prospective studies evaluating haemostatic sutures. However, when comparing two methods of suturing—one of which inverted the cone bed, the other leaving it open—Luesley et al (1985b) found no difference in the stenosis rate but the frequency of visibility of the squamocolumnar junction was higher using the latter technique.

Laser vaporisation has been successfully used to excise the stenotic segment and thus relieve post-cone cervical stenosis (Luesley et al, 1985c). We await with interest the outcome of a study comparing this technique with more traditional dilatation of the cervix.

3. *Pregnancy complications.* The effect of cone biopsy on subsequent fertility and pregnancy is uncertain. Weber & Obel (1979) were unable to find any effect on subsequent pregnancies, but others have found an increased incidence of preterm delivery and second-trimester abortion (Larsson et al, 1982; Moinian & Andersch, 1982). If stenosis impedes cervical dilatation in labour incision of the cervix or Caesarean section may be necessary.

4. *Incomplete excision.* Incomplete excision of the lesion can occur at the proximal and/or distal end of the cone. Reported rates of incomplete excision are variable; Larsson (1981) found an incomplete excision rate of 5·5 per cent in a series of 1013 patients, while McIndoe et al (1984) reported an incomplete excision rate of 32 per cent in 667 patients. The management of patients with an incompletely excised lesion following cone biopsy is controversial. Histological examination of hysterectomy specimens often fails to detect residual disease; it is possible that the healing process may in some way destroy the remaining neoplastic cells. McIndoe et al (1984) showed that the risk of invasive carcinoma after incomplete excision is

related to the presence of cytological abnormality following treatment. The results of this study suggest that a persistent cytological abnormality after cone biopsy is a good indicator of residual disease; such patients require further treatment.

Microcolpohysteroscopy

The complications following cone biopsy are related to the length of the cone excised. Therefore every effort must be made to remove only as much cervical tissue as is necessary to completely excise the lesion. The Hamou microcolpohysteroscope may be useful in this respect. The instrument can be used as a conventional panoramic hysteroscope with CO_2 as the distending medium. Alternatively it can be used as a contact hysteroscope in combination with tissue-staining techniques in the endocervix. When used as a contact hysteroscope in the endocervical canal before cone biopsy it can accurately locate the squamocolumnar junction (Soutter et al, 1984; Nava et al, 1985). Whether using this finding to tailor the length of the cone biopsy will affect complication rates and rates of incomplete excision has yet to be evaluated.

Laser excision cone biopsy

The carbon dioxide laser is now being used to excise cone biopsies as an alternative to cold knife surgery. Preliminary reports are encouraging, and suggest that the complication rates may be reduced (Dorsey & Diggs, 1979; Wright et al, 1984; Baggish, 1985). We are currently evaluating this technique.

Glandular atypia

Cytologists are increasingly recognising glandular abnormalities on cervical smears. The natural history and topography of these lesions is not yet fully established; therefore optimal management is uncertain. A cone biopsy removing most of the endocervical canal is usually advocated. This may well be overtreatment or undertreatment depending on the site and severity of the lesion. Contact hysteroscopy in the endocervical canal may in the future prove helpful. It must be stressed that cytological suspicion of a glandular lesion is an absolute contraindication to local destructive therapy (Woodman et al, 1985c).

Local destructive therapy

Local destructive therapy is an alternative to surgical excision for the treatment of CIN. The rationale for local destructive therapy is based on our understanding of the cervical transformation zone and its role in the development of cervical neoplasia. Cervical squamous neoplasia develops only within the limits of the transformation zone when immature metaplastic epithelium is exposed to oncogenic stimuli. If the whole of the transformation zone can be seen and destroyed to an adequate depth, CIN should be successfully eradicated. Four types of local destructive therapy are available:

1. Cold coagulation

The misleading term 'cold coagulation' was coined by Semm, the inventor of the instrument, in 1966. The instrument consists of a small portable apparatus which gives a range of temperatures between 50 and 120°C. The heat is conveyed to the tissues via a Teflon-coated thermosound. The whole of the transformation zone is destroyed by overlapping applications of the thermosound for 20 seconds at 100°C per area. A depth of destruction of 3–4 mm is achieved (Duncan, 1983). The treatment is carried out as an outpatient procedure, usually without anaesthesia, although a paracervical block may be used. In many patients no discomfort is felt, but some complain of crampy lower abdominal pain during the procedure; this resolves almost as soon as the thermosound is removed. In a series of 1005 patients with CIN of all grades, a single treatment was effective in restoring cervical cytology to normal in 96·6 per cent of cases after 6 months follow-up, and 93·7 per cent after 7 years (Duncan, 1985).

2. Electrodiathermy

Although electrodiathermy has the disadvantage of requiring general anaesthesia it is an effective method of treating CIN, and in contrast to other forms of local destructive therapy it requires no specialised or expensive equipment as the apparatus is available in most operating theatres. The whole of the transformation zone and adjacent columnar epithelium is destroyed to a depth of 1–1·5 cm using needle-and-ball electrodes (Chanen, 1982).

The results of electrodiathermy are comparable to those achieved with other forms of local destructive therapy—cure rates ranging from 88 to 98 per cent have been reported (Woodman et al, 1985b; Chanen & Rome, 1983).

3. Cryocautery

Cryocautery can be performed as an outpatient procedure, requires no anaesthesia and has few complications.

Earlier reports on the use of cryocautery employed a continuous freeze technique (Townsend, 1979). A more recent innovation employs the use of a 3-minute freeze, 3-minute thaw, 3-minute freeze technique (DiSaia &

Creasman, 1984). When the probe is removed any area not adequately frozen should be retreated again immediately; an overlapping technique may be required for larger lesions. Tissue destruction to a depth of 3–4 mm is usually achieved.

Cure rates after cryotherapy vary considerably, ranging from 27 to 96 per cent in one review (Charles & Savage, 1980). In a prospective randomised trial comparing cryocautery with laser vaporisation in the treatment of CIN, Townsend & Richart (1983) found no significant difference in the failure rates for cryocautery (7 per cent) and laser therapy (11 per cent). A randomised study comparing single- and double-freeze techniques was reported by Schantz & Thormann (1984), who found a statistically significant better cure rate in those patients treated with a double-freeze technique.

Some reservation has been expressed about the adequacy of this form of local destructive therapy because of the limited depth of destruction, and also because of the inability of the operator to assess the achieved depth of destruction.

4. The carbon dioxide laser

The laser generates a parallel, coherent, synchronous beam of light energy which can be focused to vaporise tissue accurately under colposcopic control with minimal thermal damage to the surrounding tissue. The majority of women can be treated as outpatients without anaesthesia, although a paracervical block may be used. Healing is rapid with minimal fibrosis.

Because laser treatment is a relatively recent innovation in the management of CIN there are no reports on long-term follow-up, although early results from the major centres are encouraging. In a series of 423 patients treated with the carbon dioxide laser, 32 of whom required a second treatment, Evans & Monaghan (1983) reported a 96 per cent success rate. Jordan et al (1985) reported that 95 per cent of 711 women with CIN treated by laser vaporisation remained colposcopically and cytologically free of disease after a median follow-up of 20 months. In this series a single laser vaporisation to a depth of 5–9 mm eradicated the lesion in 90 per cent of patients. About half of those with residual disease were successfully treated by a further laser vaporisation, giving an overall cure rate of 95 per cent.

The depth of tissue destruction is important. Early results of treatment of CIN with the laser were poor because tissue was vaporised to an inadequate depth. Anderson & Hartley (1980), measuring the depth of crypt involvement with CIN, reported that destruction to a depth of 3·80 mm would eradicate disease in 99·7 per cent of cases. It is now generally accepted by those using laser therapy that a depth of destruction of between 5 and 8 mm is required (Baggish, 1980; Burke, 1982; Evans & Monaghan, 1983; Jordan et al, 1985).

Local destructive therapy failures

Success rates of approximately 95 per cent can be achieved in the treatment of CIN using laser vaporisation, cryocautery, electrodiathermy, and cold coagulation. However, cases of invasive carcinoma have been described following all of these treatment modalities. In a collaborative study Townsend et al (1981) reported 24 cases of invasive cancer in patients who were treated with either cryocautery, electrodiathermy or laser vaporisation. Sevin et al (1979) reported eight cases of invasive cervical carcinoma following cryocautery. There have been four cases of invasive squamous carcinoma in patients treated with the CO_2 laser at the Women's Hospital, Birmingham. More worrying, however, is the occurrence of cervical adenocarcinoma following local destructive therapy. Two such cases have been reported by Woodman et al (1985c). Regardless of the type of treatment used, invasive carcinoma will develop in a few patients; Coppleson (1981) has reported the occurrence of invasive disease after both conisation and hysterectomy. Nevertheless these cases of invasive disease following local destructive therapy serve as a reminder that careful patient selection is required before local destructive therapy is used; many of the reported cases of invasive disease following local destructive therapy probably reflect operator error rather than failure of a correctly applied technique.

In 1981 the RCOG Study Group proposed a list of criteria which should be strictly adhered to before a patient has local destructive therapy:

1. The patient is seen and assessed by an expert colposcopist.
2. The colposcopist is able to see the entire lesion, i.e. can see the squamocolumnar junction.
3. Invasive carcinoma has been excluded by colposcopically directed biopsy or biopsies.
4. The destructive therapy is carried out by the colposcopist.
5. There is adequate cytology and/or colposcopic follow-up.

To this list of criteria should be added a sixth: there should be no suspicion of an endocervical glandular abnormality, reported by either the cytologist or pathologist.

VAGINAL INTRA-EPITHELIAL NEOPLASIA

While vaginal intra-epithelial neoplasia (VAIN) may be found in association with cervical and vulval neoplasia or as a primary lesion it is most frequently discovered after hysterectomy for CIN.

Incidence

The recurrence rate after hysterectomy for CIN has been reported to be between 0·7 and 8 per cent.

Table 20.1   Outcome of 7722 cases of CIN treated by hysterectomy

Reference	No. of cases	VAIN	Invasive cancer	Recurrence rate (%)
Fennell, 1956	71	2	1	4·2
Mussey et al, 1960	670	3	2	0·8
Parker et al, 1960	267	1	2	0·8
Carter et al, 1961	275	0	2	0·7
Gusberg & Marshall, 1962	310	3	3	1·9
Funnell & Merrill, 1963	74	4	2	8·0
McIndoe & Green 1969	175	4	0	2·3
Boyes et al, 1970	2849	20	3	0·8
Creasman & Rutledge, 1972	608	27	7	5·6
Brudenell et al, 1973	352	4	2	1·7
Lee & Symonds, 1976	1290	3	0	0·2
Kolstad & Klemm, 1976	233	3	5	3·4
Burghardt & Holzer, 1980	418	13	3	3·8
Woodman, 1986	123	6	0	4·9
Total	7722	93 (1·2%)	32 (0·41%)	

Table 20.1 summarises the outcome in 7722 cases of CIN treated by hysterectomy as reported by 14 authors. There were 93 (1.2 per cent) cases of VAIN and 32 (0·41 per cent) of invasive cancer.

Aetiology

VAIN is thought to occur after hysterectomy for CIN because an atypical transformation zone extending onto the vagina has been incompletely excised. Three observations support this concept:

1. Colposcopic examination has demonstrated an atypical transformation zone extending onto the vagina.
2. Histological examination has shown the cervical lesion to extend to the line of resection in patients who subsequently develop VAIN.
3. Colposcopic examination demonstrates the vast majority of these lesions to involve the vaginal angles or vault suture line.

However not all cases of VAIN after hysterectomy can be explained by inadequate excision of a cervical lesion. Multifocal neoplasia of the genital tract is well described and these cases may only be discovered when cytological examination shows abnormality to persist after hysterectomy.

Factors relating to the development of VAIN

1. Length of follow-up

The incidence of VAIN after hysterectomy for CIN would appear to reflect the duration of follow-up. Boyes et al (1970) reported the recurrence rate to be 1·9 per cent after 5 years, 8·2 per cent after 10 years and 13 per cent in those who had been followed for longer than 15 years.

2. Route of hysterectomy

Unfortunately only a few authors report whether the uterus was removed by the abdominal or vaginal route. Burghardt & Holzer (1980), Creasman & Rutledge (1972) and Parker et al (1960) have found the incidence of vault recurrences to be lower if the uterus was removed vaginally. However, paucity of numbers, possibe differences in case selection and lack of information relating to the depth of vaginal cuff removed may confound the significance of this observation.

3. Presence or absence of a vaginal cuff

Burghardt (1980) reported a vault recurrence in 7 of 177 patients treated by hysterectomy alone, but in 0 of 60 where a vaginal cuff had also been removed.

4. Depth of vaginal cuff

It might therefore be expected that the incidence of VAIN would vary inversely with the amount of vaginal epithelium removed at hysterectomy. However, Creasman & Rutledge (1972) could demonstrate no relationship between the size of the cuff removed and the recurrence rate. This lack of difference might be explained if the vaginal extension of the transformation zone were to consistently extend beyond the maximum depth of cuff removed (3 cm) in this study.

5. Extent of cervical lesion

We have examined the outcome of 123 patients with CIN treated by hysterectomy.

Histological examination of the hysterectomy specimen showed the cervical lesion to extend to the line of resection in five cases; three of these were found to have VAIN less than 1 year after hysterectomy. Examination was frustrated by extensive epithelial stripping in nine cases; two were subsequently found to have VAIN. In 109 cases histological examination has shown the line of resection to be free of disease; two were subsequently found to have VAIN, 4 and 11 years after hysterectomy (Table 20.2).

Thus VAIN was significantly more likely to occur if histological examination had shown the cervical lesion to extend to the line of resection ($p < 0.001$; Chi-square test).

Diagnosis

VAIN is suspected if cytological examination shows abnormality to persist after hysterectomy. The patient should be referred for colposcopic

Table 20.2 Outcome in 123 cases of CIN treated by hysterectomy (Woodman et al, 1985)

	No. of cases	No. developing VAIN
Line of resection free	109	2
Line of resection indeterminable	9	2
Line of resection involved	5	3
Total	123	7

assessment, which should be performed under general anaesthesia. This facilitates the manipulation which is often necessary to adequately expose the epithelium 'pocketed' in the vaginal angles and provides the opportunity to perform a wide excision biopsy where possible.

Treatment

A variety of treatment modalities have been used in this condition.

5-Fluorouracil

Woodruff et al (1975) and Daly & Ellis (1980) have reported this antimitotic agent to cause regression of the lesion in some patients, but these had been followed for only a short time after treatment.

Carbon dioxide laser

Considerable success has been claimed for the CO_2 laser and the combined results of four series (Stafl et al, 1977; Capen et al, 1982; Townsend et al, 1982; Petrilli et al, 1980) suggest it had been successful in 60 of 67 patients treated. However, this claim was based on limited follow-up; only seven patients were followed for more than 12 months.

The Birmingham Group have used the CO_2 laser to treat 14 patients with VAIN after hysterectomy; six remain free of disease after a median follow-up of 30 months; six required other forms of treatment to eradicate VAIN, and two were subsequently found to have invasive carcinoma (Woodman et al, 1984).

We believe the disappointing results obtained following local destructive treatment to be attributable to atypical epithelium being inaccessible as a result of sequestration above the vault suture line, or hidden in the angles of the vaginal vault. This would appear to be an inevitable sequel to the usual method of closing the vaginal vault, which results in a variable amount of vaginal epithelium being retained above the suture line (Fig. 20.1).

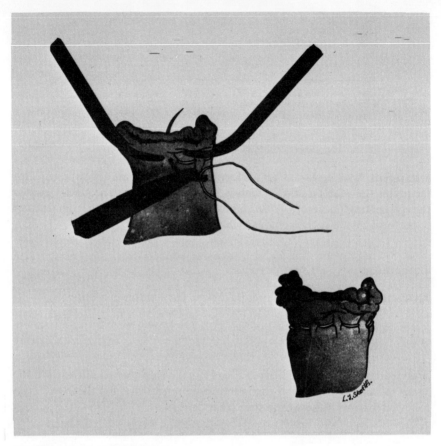

Fig. 20.1   Closure of vaginal vault

Surgical excision, partial or total vaginectomy

We have not evaluated these procedures, but have found the considerable morbidity associated with their occasional use to make them an unattractive first line of treatment.

Vault radiotherapy

The usefulness of vault radiotherapy in the treatment of these lesions is currently being evaluated in our unit. Following radiotherapy the patient is encouraged to use vaginal dilators. Preliminary results are encouraging and suggest that sexual function is not seriously impaired, and that adequate cytological and colposcopic assessment of the vault epithelium remains possible.

Recommendations

1. Preoperative colposcopic assessment of the vaginal epithelium should be performed in all patients undergoing hysterectomy for CIN. Only in this way can the size of vaginal cuff requiring excision be determined.
2. Careful inspection of the entire vaginal epithelium and vulva is necessary to identify those patients with multifocal intra-epithelial neoplasia.
3. Histological examination of the extent of the cervical lesion in the hysterectomy specimen will identify those patients who are at greatest risk of developing VAIN.
4. VAIN may occasionally occur *de novo* when the cervical lesion has been completely excised. The genital epithelium of these patients may have an increased susceptibility to squamous intra-epithelial neoplasia; therefore all women undergoing hysterectomy for CIN should have lifelong cytological review.
5. Local destructive therapy is contraindicated when VAIN follows incomplete excision of a cervical lesion. Its use in the treatment of VAIN occurring *de novo* after hysterectomy, while conceptually attractive, remains to be evaluated.

VULVAL INTRA-EPITHELIAL NEOPLASIA

Classification

Three grades of vulval intra-epithelial neoplasia (VIN) are recognised; VIN I is equivalent to mild atypia/dysplasia which is limited to the lower third of the epithelium; VIN II represents moderate atypia/dysplasia with extension of the abnormal cells into the middle third of the epithelium; VIN III is diagnosed when there is extension of abnormal cells into the outer third of the epithelium, this includes both severe atypia/dysplasia and carcinoma in situ.

The International Society for the Study of Vulvar Disease recommended that Bowen's disease, erythroplasia of Queyrat and carcinoma simplex should be classified as a single category of carcinoma in situ (Friedrich, 1976) as there was no difference in the biological behaviour of the three conditions and their treatment and progress were considered to be the same. While Paget's disease and melanoma in situ now fall within the most recent VIN classification (Kneale, 1984) they are grouped separately from the squamous type of VIN.

Although definitions of VIN have been standardised, different varieties of VIN III are recognised. Buckley et al (1984) describes two distinct patterns of VIN III; the basaloid type in which atypical cells of basal or parabasal type extend into the upper layers of the epidermis, and the Bowenoid type in which the key features are premature cellular maturation with variable retention of stratification and pleomorphism.

Incidence

VIN is uncommon; the Third National Cancer Survey in the United States estimated the incidence rate for VIN III was 0·53 per 100 000 white women, based on a sample of 157 reported cases (Hensen & Tarone, 1977). The most common presenting symptom is pruritus, reported in up to 73 per cent of cases (Iversen et al, 1981). It is interesting to note that in one series 48 per cent of patients were asymptomatic (Freidrich et al, 1980), the disease being detected during gynaecological examination in women with other complaints. This figure, however, reflects a specialised interest in the condition; all patients examined by these authors have a detailed vulval assessment. The disease is reported more frequently, especially in younger women, with between 38 and 58 per cent of cases being diagnosed in women under 40 (Buscema et al, 1980; Townsend et al, 1982b; Caglar et al, 1982; Bernstein et al, 1983).

Clinical features

VIN lesions may be white, grey, pink, dull red or brown. The lesion is invariably papular with a roughened surface, although this may be appreciated only with the aid of low-power magnification. The lesions are commonly pigmented and often parakeratotic (i.e. retention of nuclear chromatin in the usually acellular layer of the epithelium). Although the identification of parakeratotic epithelium by toluidine blue dye staining has been described (Collins et al, 1966), further critical evaluation of this technique is required. VIN lesions may be unifocal or multifocal; Townsend et al (1982b) reported that 65 per cent of lesions in a series of 33 were multifocal. A careful gynaecological assessment of the whole of the lower genital tract is essential in women who present with VIN, as there is a significant association with neoplasia of the cervix and vagina (Caglar et al, 1982; Townsend et al, 1982; Bernstein et al, 1983).

VIN has many features of an infectious disease. Woodruff et al (1973) suggested that the majority of lesions in younger women represented proliferative responses to an infectious agent, particularly HPV. There appears to be an association between vulval warts and neoplasia; Daling et al (1984), reporting on a group of women with in situ and invasive vulval lesions, found that 16·6 per cent had a history of vulval warts, while none of the patients with non-squamous vulval neoplasia had a similar history.

Diagnosis

The role of exfoliative cytology in the diagnosis of VIN is limited. Although cell samples from the vulva may predict the presence of VIN and invasive carcinoma, cytological evaluation of the degree of abnormality in cases of VIN is unreliable. This is due to the prevention of exfoliation of cells by the surface layer of hyperkeratosis, and due to difficulty in interpretation if an inflammatory process is present. A better yield of cells may be obtained if a double-scrape technique is used, the first scrape removing the hyperkeratotic layer of cells, the second sampling the underlying and possibly dysplastic cells. Nevertheless, exfoliative cytology contributes little to the diagnosis and treatment of the condition.

When compared to its use in the diagnosis of CIN, colposcopy is of limited value in the diagnosis of VIN. The epithelium of the labia majora is thick and cornified, thus rendering the underlying terminal vasculature invisible. Application of normal saline or oil may improve visualisation of the vascular pattern. The vascular pattern may also be obscured as many lesions are covered by dry hyperkeratotic epithelium and some are inflamed due to scratching, although lesions which are situated in the moist medial aspect of the labia minora often reveal patterns of mosaic, punctation and atypical vessels (Kolstad & Stafl, 1977). These lesions may become white after application of acetic acid.

Treatment

Although spontaneous regression of the disease has been reported (Friedrich et al, 1980) there are no methods which can predict those lesions most likely to regress. Therefore it is generally, although not universally, accepted that all patients with a histological diagnosis of VIN should be treated. Over the past 20 years the management of the condition has become less radical. Various approaches have been reported; vulvectomy (Parry-Jones, 1976); 'skinning vulvectomy' (Rutledge & Sinclair, 1968); wide local excision (Forney et al, 1977); topical 5-fluorouracil (Carson et al, 1976); di-nitno chlorobenzene (DNCB) (Weintraub and Lagasse 1973), cryosurgery (Forney et al, 1977) and carbon dioxide laser vaporisation (Baggish & Dorsey, 1981). The trend towards less radical management is partly due to the realisation that there is a very small, although uncertain, risk of progression to invasive cancer, and partly because the disease is occurring in younger women who wish to avoid mutilating surgery and thus preserve sexual function.

Carbon dioxide laser vaporisation is a relatively new treatment for VIN, first reported simultaneously by Baggish & Dorsey (1981) and Valentine (1981). Under colposcopic control the neoplastic tissue can be located accurately and vaporised, preserving as much normal tissue as possible. Reid (1985) advises that those using the carbon dioxide laser for the ablation of large areas of vulval epithelium must learn to recognise four surgical planes by the characteristic appearance of the tissue vaporised at each level. Tissue is destroyed to the third plane, which consists of the upper reticular dermis. The third surgical plane is the deepest level from which optimal healing will occur; vaporisation to the fourth plane causes a third-degree burn which results in delayed healing and the formation of scar tissue due to full-thickness epithelial destruction. Smaller lesions can be treated on an outpatient basis using local anaesthesia, but larger areas require general anaesthesia. The main disadvantage of laser therapy is postoperative pain, although this can be limited by the use of a suprapubic catheter for 2 weeks, which prevents urinary soiling of the operation site. This form of treatment is suitable for the majority of patients with VIN provided invasive disease has been excluded by prior biopsy. Success rates of 91–94 per cent have been reported following a single treatment (Baggish & Dorsey, 1981; Townsend et al, 1982b), but long-term follow-up studies are required in order to determine the recurrence rate.

REFERENCES

Anderson M C, Hartley R B 1980 Cervical crypt involvement by intraepithelial neoplasia. British Journal of Obstetrics and Gynaecology 55: 546–550

Aurelian L, Manak M M, MacKinlay M, Smith C C, Klacsmann K T, Gupta P K 1981 The Herpes virus hypothesis—are Koch's postulates satisfied? Gynecological Oncology 12: 56–87

Baggish M S 1980 High power density carbon dioxide laser therapy for early cervical neoplasia. American Journal of Obstetrics and Gynecology 136: 117–125

Baggish M S 1985 Carbon dioxide laser for combination excisional-vaporisation conization. American Journal of Obstetrics and Gynecology 151: 23–27

Baggish M S, Dorsey J H 1981 Carbon dioxide laser treatment of vulvar carcinoma in situ. Obstetrics and Gynecology 57: 371–375

Bernstein S G, Kovacs B R, Townsend D E, Morrow P 1983 Vulvar carcinoma in situ. Obstetrics and Gynecology 61: 304–307

Boshart M, Gissmann L, Ikenberg H, Kleinheinz A, Scheurlen W, zur Hausen H 1984 A new type of papillomavirus DNA, it's presence in genital cancer biopsies and in cell lines derived from cervical cancer. EMBO Journal 3: 1151–1157

Boyes D A, Worth D A, Fidler H K 1970 The results of treatment of 4389 cases of pre-clinical cervical squamous carcinoma. Journal of Obstetrics and Gynaecology of the British Commonwealth 77: 769–780

Brudenell M, Cox B S, Taylor L N 1973 The management of dysplasia, carcinoma in situ and microinvasive carcinoma of the cervix. Journal of Obstetrics and Gynaecology of the British Commonwealth 80: 673

Buckley C H, Butler E B, Fox H 1984 Vulvar intraepithelial neoplasia and microinvasive carcinoma of the vulva. Journal of Clinical Pathology 37: 1201–1211

Burghardt E, Holzer E 1980 Treatment of carcinoma in situ: evaluation of 1609 cases. Obstetrics and Gynecology 55: 539–545

Burke L 1982 The use of the carbon dioxide laser in the treatment of CIN. American Journal of Obstetrics and Gynecology 144: 337–340

Buscema J, Woodruff J D, Parmley T H, Genadry R 1980 Carcinoma in situ of the vulva. Obstetrics and Gynecology 55: 225–230

Byrne G D 1966 Cone biopsy: a survey of 100 cases. Australian and New Zealand Journal of Obstetrics and Gynaecology 6: 266–268

Caglar H, Tamer S, Hreshchyshyn M M 1982 Vulvar intraepithelial neoplasia. Obstetrics and Gynecology 60: 346–349

Capen C V, Masterson J, Magrina Javier F, Calkins J W 1982 Laser therapy of vaginal intraepithelial neoplasia. American Journal of Obstetrics and Gynecology 142: 973–976

Carson T E, Hoskins W J, Wurzel J F 1976 Topical 5-fluorouracil in the treatment of carcinoma in situ of the vulva. Obstetrics and Gynecology 47: 59s–62s

Carter E R, Salvaggio A T, Karkowski T I 1961 Squamous cell carcinoma of the vagina following vaginal hysterectomy for intrapithelial carcinoma of the cervix. American Journal of Obstetrics and Gynecology 82: 401

Chanen R 1982 Radical electrocoagulation diathermy. In : Coppleson M (ed) Gynecologic oncology. Churchill Livingstone, Edinburgh, pp 82–85

Chanen W, Rome R M 1983 Electrocoagulation diathermy for cervical dysplasia and carcinoma in situ : a 15 year experience. Obstetrics and Gynecology 61 : 673–679

Charles E H, Savage E W 1980 Cryosurgical treatment of cervical intraepithelial neoplasia. Obstetrical and Gynecological Survey 35 : 539–541

Claman A D, Lee N 1974 Factors that relate to complications of cone biopsy. American Journal of Obstetrics and Gynecology 120 : 124–128

Collins C G, Hansen L H, Theriot E 1966 A clinical stain for use in selecting biopsy sites in patients with vulvar disease. Obstetrics and Gynecology 28 : 158–163

Coppleson M (ed) 1981 Cervical intraepithelial neoplasia : clinical features and management. In Gynecologic oncology—fundamental principles and clinical practice. Churchill Livingstone, Edinburgh, vol 1, pp 408–433

Cramer D W 1974 The role of cervical cytology in the declining morbidity and mortality of cervical cancer. Cancer 34 : 2018–2027

Creasman W T, Rutledge F 1972 Carcinoma in situ of the cervix : an analysis of 861 patients. Obstetrics and Gynecology 39 : 373–380

Daling J R, Chu J, Weiss N S, Emel L, Tamini H K 1984 The association of condylomata acuminata and squamous carcinoma of the vulva. British Journal of Cancer 50 : 533–535

Daly J, Ellis G F 1980 Treatment of vaginal dysplasia and carcinoma in situ with topical 5-fluorouracil. Obstetrics and Gynecology 55 : 530–532

DiSaia P J, Creasman W T (eds) 1984 Clinical gynecological oncology. C V Mosby, St Louis, pp 22–25

Dorsey J M, Diggs E S 1979 Microsurgical conization of the cervix by carbon dioxide laser. Obstetrics and Gynecology 54 : 565–570

Draper G J, Cook G A 1983 Changing patterns of cervical cancer. British Medical Journal 287 : 510–512

Duff R, Rapp F 1973 Oncogenic transformation of hamster embryo cells after exposure to inactivated herpes simplex virus type 1. Journal of Virology 12 : 209–217

Duncan I D 1983 The Semm cold coagulator in the management of cervical intraepithelial neoplasia. Clinical Obstetrics and Gynecology 26 : 996–1006

Duncan I 1985 Destruction of cervical intraepithelial neoplasia at 100°C with the Semm 'cold coagulator'. Proceedings from the Eleventh World Congress in Obstetrics and Gynecology. Springer-Verlag, Berlin

Durst M, Gissmann L, Ikenberg H, Zur Hausen H 1983 A new type of papillomavirus DNA from a cervical carcinoma and it's prevalence in genital cancer biopsies from different geographical areas. Proceedings of the National Academy of Science of the USA 80 : 3812–3815

Evans A S, Monaghan J M 1983 The treatment of cervical intraepithelial neoplasia using the carbon dioxide laser. British Journal of Obstetrics and Gynaecology 90 : 553–556

Fennell R H 1956 Carcinoma in situ of the uterine cervix. Cancer 9 : 374–384

Forney J P, Morrow C P, Townsend D E, DiSaia P J 1977 Management of carcinoma in situ of the vulva. American Journal of Obstetrics and Gynecology 127 : 801–806

Franklin E W, Rutledge F D 1972 Epidemiology of epidermoid carcinoma of the vulva. Obstetrics and Gynecology 39 : 165–172

Frenkel N, Roizman B, Cassai E, Nahmias A 1972 A DNA fragment of Herpes simplex2 and its transcription in cervical cancer tissues. Proceedings of the National Academy of Science of the USA 69 : 3784–3789

Friedrich E G 1976 International Society for the Study of Vulvar Disease. Report of the Committee on Terminology. Obstetrics and Gynecology 47 : 122–124

Friedrich E G, Wilkinson E J, Yao S F 1980 Carcinoma in situ of the vulva : a continuing challenge. American Journal of Obstetrics and Gynecology 136 : 830–843

Funnell J D, Merrill J A 1963 Recurrence after treatment of carcinoma in situ of the cervix. Surgery in Gynecology and Obstetrics 117 : 15–19

Gissmann L, zur Hausen H 1980 Partial characterisation of viral DNA from human genital warts (Condylomata acuminata). International Journal of Cancer 25 : 605–609

Gissmann L, Wolnick L, Ikenberg H et al 1983 Human papillomavirus type 6 and 11 DNA sequences in genital and laryngeal papillomas and in some cervical cancers. Proceedings of the National Academy of Science (USA) 80 : 560–563

Gusberg S B, Marshall D 1962 Intraepithelial carcinoma of the cervix: A clinical reappraisal. Obstetrics and Gynecology 19: 713

Hakama M 1985 Effects of population screening for carcinoma of the uterine cervix in Finland. Maturitas 7: 3–10

Hensen D, Tarone R 1977 An epidemiological study of cancer of the cervix, vagina and vulva based on the Third National Cancer Survey in the United States. American Journal of Obstetrics and Gynecology 129: 525–532

Hollyhock V E, Chanen W 1972 Colposcopy in patient selection for cone biopsy. American Journal of Obstetrics and Gynecology 40: 23–27

Iversen T, Abeler V, Kolstad P 1981 Squamous cell carcinoma in situ of the vulva: a clinical and histopathological study. Gynecologic Oncology 11: 224–229

Jablonska S, Dabrowski J, Jakubowitz K 1972 Epidermodysplasia verruciformis as a model in studies on the role of papovaviruses in oncogenesis. Cancer Research 32: 583–589

Johannesson G, Geirsson G, Day N 1978 The effects of mass screening in Iceland, 1965–1974, on the incidence of mortality of cervical cancer. International Journal of Cancer 21: 418–425

Jones H W, Buller R E 1980 The treatment of cervical intraepithelial neoplasia by cone biopsy. American Journal of Obstetrics and Gynecology 137: 882–887

Jordan J A, Sharp F, Singer A (eds) 1982 In: Preclinical neoplasia of the cervix. Proceedings of the Ninth Study Group of the Royal College of Obstetricians and Gynaecologists. RCOG, London, p 185

Jordan J A, Woodman C B J, Mylotte M J et al 1985 The treatment of cervical intraepithelial neoplasia by laser vaporisation. British Journal of Obstetrics and Gynaecology 92: 394–398

Kessler I I 1974 Perspectives on the epidemiology of cervical cancer with special reference to the Herpesvirus hypothesis. Cancer Research 34: 1091–1110

Kneale B L 1984 Microinvasive cancer of the vulva; report of the ISSVD Task Force. Journal of Reproductive Medicine 29: 454–456

Kolstad P, Klemm V 1976 Long term follow-up of 1121 cases of carcinoma in situ. Obstetrics and Gynecology 48: 125–129

Kolstad P, Stafl A 1977 Atlas of colposcopy, 2nd edn. University Park Press, Baltimore, p 228

Kreider J W 1980 Neoplastic progression of the Shope rabbit papilloma. Cold Springs Harbor Conference, Cold Springs Harbor, New York, pp 283–300

Larsson G 1981 Conization for cervical dysplasia and carcinoma in situ: long term follow-up of 1013 women. Annales Chirurgiae et Gynaecologiae (Helsinki) 70: 79–85

Larsson G 1983 Conization for preinvasive and early invasive carcinoma of the uterine cervix. Acta Obstetrica Gynecologica Scandinavica 114: 19s–21s

Larsson G, Grundsell H, Gullberg B, Svennerud S 1982 Outcome of pregnancy after conization. Acta Obstetrica Gynecologica Scandinavica 61: 461–466

Larsson G, Gullberg B, Grundsell H 1983 A comparison of complications of laser and cold knife conization. Obstetrics and Gynecology 62: 213–217

Lee R A, Symmonds R E 1976 Recurrent carcinoma in situ of the vagina in patients previously treated for in situ carcinoma of the cervix. Obstetrics and Gynecology 48: 61–64

Luesley D M, McCrum A, Terry P B et al 1985a Complications of cone biopsy related to the dimensions of the cone and the influence of prior colposcopic assessment. British Journal of Obstetrics and Gynaecology 92: 158–164

Luesley D M, Williams D R, Woodman C B J, Gee H, Chan K K 1985b The influence of suture technique on the outcome of cone biopsy. Obstetrics and Gynecology (In press)

Luesley D M, Williams D R, Gee H, Chan K K, Jordan J A 1985c The management of post cone cervical stenosis by laser vapourisation. Journal of Obstetrics and Gynaecology (In press)

Macgregor J E, Teper S 1978 Mortality from carcinoma of the cervix uteri in Britain. Lancet ii: 774–776

McCance D J, Walker P G, Dyson J L, Coleman D V, Singer A 1983 Presence of Human Papillomavirus DNA in cervical intraepithelial neoplasia. British Medical Journal 287: 784–788

McCance D J, Campion M J, Clarkson P K, Chesters P M, Jenkins D, Singer A 1985 Prevalence of HPV type 16 DNA sequences in cervical intraepithelial neoplasia and carcinoma of the cervix. British Journal of Obstetrics and Gynaecology 92: 1101–1105

McDougall J K, Galloway D A, Fenoglio C M 1980 Cervical carcinoma: detection of herpes simplex virus RNA in cells undergoing neoplastic change. International Journal of Cancer 25: 1–8

McIndoe W A, Green G H 1969 Vaginal carcinoma in situ following hysterectomy. Acta Cytologica 13: 158–162

McIndoe W A, McLean M R, Jones R W, Mullins P R 1984 The invasive potential of carcinoma of the cervix. Obstetrics and Gynecology 64: 451–458

Meisels A, Fortin R 1976 Condylomatous lesions of the cervix and vagina. I. Cytologic patterns. Acta Cytologica 20: 505–509

Meisels A, Fortin R, Roy M 1977 Condylomatous lesions of the cervix: II. Cytologic, colposcopic and histopathologic study. Acta Cytologica 21: 379–390

Moinian M, Andersch B 1982 Does cervic conisation increase the risk of subsequent pregnancies? Acta Obstetrica et Gynecologica Scandinavica 61: 101–103

Mussey E, Soule E H 1959 Carcinoma in situ of the cervix: A clinical review of 842 cases. American Journal of Obstetrics and Gynecology 77: 957–972

Nava G, Jordan J A, Chan K K, Wade-Evans T 1985 Microcolopohysteroscopy and cone biopsy of the cervix in the management of cervical intraepithelial neoplasia. Archives of Gynaecology 237: 40s

Parker R T, Cuylor W K, Kaufman L A et al (1960) Intraepithelial (stage 0) cancer of the cervix (485 patients). American Journal of Obstetrics and Gynecology 80: 693–710

Parkin D M, Nguyen-Dinh X, Day N E 1985 The impact of screening on the incidence of cervical cancer in England and Wales. British Journal of Obstetrics and Gynaecology 92: 150–157

Parry-Jones E 1976 The management of pre-malignant and malignant conditions of the vulva. Clinics in Obstetrics and Gynecology 3: 217–227

Petrilli E S, Townsend D E, Morrow C P, Nakao C Y 1980 Vaginal intraepithelial neoplasia. Biologic aspects and treatment with 5-fluorouracil and the carbon dioxide laser. American Journal of Obstetrics and Gynecology 138: 321–328

Rawls W E, Tompkins W A F, Figueroa M E, Melnick J L 1968 Herpes simplex virus type 2: association with carcinoma of the cervix. Science 161: 1255–1256

Reid R 1985 Superficial laser vulvectomy. III. A new surgical technique for appendage-conserving ablation of refractory condylomas and vulvar intraepithelial neoplasia. American Journal of Obstetrics and Gynecology 152: 504–509

Richart R M, Townsend D E, Crisp W 1980 An analysis of 'long term' follow-up results in patients with cervical intraepithelial neoplasia treated by cryotherapy. American Journal of Obstetrics and Gynecology 137: 823–826

Roberts A 1982 Cervical cytology in England and Wales 1965–80. Health Trends 14: 41–44

Rotkin I D 1973 A comparison review of the key epidemiologic studies in cervical cancer related to current searches for transmissible agents. Cancer Research 33: 1353–1367

Rubio C A, Thomassen P, Koch Y 1975 The influence of the size of cone specimens on post-operative haemorrhage. American Journal of Obstetrics and Gynecology 122: 939–944

Rutledge F, Sinclair M 1968 Treatment of intraepithelial cancer of the vulva by skin excision and graft. American Journal of Obstetrics and Gynecology 102: 806–818

Schantz A, Thormann L 1984 Cryosurgery for dysplasia of the uterine cervix: a randomised study of the single and double freeze techniques. Acta Obstetrica Gynecologica Scandinavica 63: 417–420

Semm K 1966 New approaches for the 'cold coagulation' of benign cervical lesions. American Journal of Obstetrics and Gynecology 95: 963–966

Sevin B, Ford J H, Girtanner R D et al 1979 Invasive cancer of the cervix after cryosurgery. Obstetrics and Gynecology 53: 456–471

Singer A, Walker P G McCance D 1984 Genital wart virus infection: a nuisance or potentially lethal? British Medical Journal 288: 735–737

Soutter W P, Fenton D W, Gudgeon P, Sharp F 1984 Quantitative microcolopohysteroscopic assessment of the extent of the endocervical involvement by cervical intraepithelial neoplasia. British Journal of Obstetrics and Gynaecology 91: 712–715

Stafl A, Wilkinson E J, Mattingly R J 1977 Laser treatment of cervical and vaginal neoplasia. American Journal of Obstetrics and Gynecology 128: 128–136

Townsend D E 1979 Cryosurgery for cervical intraepithelial neoplasia. Obstetrical and Gynecological Survey 34: 838–840

Townsend D E, Richart R M 1983 Cryotherapy and carbon dioxide laser management of cervical intraepithelial neoplasia: a controlled comparison. Obstetrics and Gynecology 61: 75–78

Townsend D E, Richart R M, Marks E, Nielsen J 1981 Invasive cancer following outpatient evaluation and therapy for cervical disease. Obstetrics and Gynecology 57: 145–149

Townsend D E, Levine R U, Crum C P, Richart R M 1982a Treatment of vaginal carcinoma in situ with the carbon dioxide laser. American Journal of Obstetrics and Gynecology 143: 565–568

Townsend D E, Levine R U, Richart R H, Crum C P, Petrilli E S 1982b Management of vulvar intraepithelial neoplasia by carbon dioxide laser. Obstetrics and Gynecology 60: 49–52

Valentine B H 1981 Outpatient laser therapy for vulval intraepithelial neoplasia: a case report. Journal of Obstetrics and Gynaecology 1: 260–262

Walton R J 1976 Canadian Task Force Report 1976, Cervical cancer screening programs. Canadian Medical Association Journal 114: 1003–1033

Weber T, Obel E B 1979 Pregnancy complications following conization of the uterine cervix (II). Acta Obstetrica et Gynecologica Scandinavica 58: 348–351

Weintraub I, Lagasse L D 1973 Reversibility of vulvar atypia by DNCB-induced delayed hypersensitivity. Obstetrics and Gynecology 41: 195–199

Wolfendale M R, King S, Usherwood M M 1983 Abnormal cervical smears: are we in for an epidemic? British Medical Journal 87: 526–528

World Health Organisation 1975 International histological classification of tumours 13. (Poulson H E, Taylor C W in collaboration with Sobin L H and other pathologists from nine countries). WHO, Geneva

Woodman C B J, Jordan J A, Wade-Evans T 1984 The management of vaginal intraepithelial neoplasia after hysterectomy. British Journal of Obstetrics and Gynaecology 91: 707–711

Woodman C B J, Byrne P, Fung S Y, Wade-Evans T, Jordan J A 1985a Human papillomavirus infection of the uterine cervix—a self limiting disease? Colposcopy and Gynecologic Laser Surgery 2: 9–13

Woodman C B J, Jordan J A, Mylotte M J, Gustafeson R, Wade-Evans T 1985b The management of cervical intraepithelial neoplasia by coagulation electrodiathermy. British Journal of Obstetrics and Gynaecology 92: 751–755

Woodman C B J, Williams D, Waddell C, Wade-Evans T 1985c Adenocarcinoma following laser vaporisation of squamous intraepithelial neoplasia. Obstetrics and Gynecology (In press)

Woodruff J D, Julian C, Paray T, Mermut S, Katayama P 1973 The contemporary challenge of carcinoma in situ of the vulva. American Journal of Obstetrics and Gynecology 115: 677–686

Woodruff J D, Parmley T H, Julian C G 1975 Topical 5-fluorouracil in the treatment of vaginal carcinoma in situ. Gynecologic Oncology 3: 124–132

Wright V C, Davies E, Riopelle M A 1984 Laser cylindrical excision to replace conization. American Journal of Obstetrics and Gynecology 150: 704–709

zur Hausen H 1985 Genital Papillomavirus Infections. In: Rigby P W J, Wilkie N M (eds) Viruses and cancer, Thirty-Seventh Symposium of the Society for General Microbiology. Cambridge University Press, Cambridge

Staging in gynaecological cancer

A discussion of tumours of any part of the body including the female pelvis without reference to staging would be akin to catching an aeroplane at Heathrow without reference to a flight timetable—an uncomfortable experience with an uncertain ending. A thorough understanding of the principles and rules involved in the classification and staging of gynaecological tumours is essential for anyone involved in the treatment of patients with genital cancer. It facilitates the planning of treatment, gives some idea of the likely result of such treatment and permits the exchange of information between individuals and centres similarly involved both nationally and internationally. To this end, the rules for the classification and staging of malignant tumours of the female pelvis adopted by the International Federation of Gynaecology and Obstetrics (FIGO) are generally accepted all over the world. These originated in the late 1920s when the Cancer Commission of the League of Nations initiated the work which led to an international classification. FIGO has a standing Cancer Committee which deals with all questions concerning classification, stage grouping and reporting of treatment results in gynaecological cancer, and these are published in the *Annual Report on the Results of Treatment in Gynaecological Cancer*. The latest eight reports have appeared at 3-yearly intervals in connection with FIGO World Congresses, the nineteenth and latest Report having been issued in 1985.

In 1954 the Research Commission of the International Union Against Cancer (UICC) set up a special committee on clinical stage classification and applied statistics to pursue studies in this field and to extend the general technique of classification to cancer at all sites. This committee has promoted the TNM classification of malignant tumours, but there has been close collaboration with the Cancer Committee of FIGO. Readers requiring details of this classification as it applies to the uterus, ovary and vagina are referred to the UICC's handbook. In gynaecological oncology the TNM system has been most widely adopted in carcinoma of the vulva and will be described in this chapter under that heading.

GENERAL GUIDELINES

The classification and staging of carcinoma of the uterus, vagina, vulva and urethra should be based on careful clinical examination and should be performed under anaesthesia by an experienced examiner. Ovarian cancer differs from the others in that surgical exploration is permitted but the staging must be decided before definitive treatment is carried out. The clinical stage must under no circumstances be changed on the basis of subsequent findings. When it is doubtful to which stage a particular case should be allotted, a case must be referred to an earlier stage. If this were not the case, an institution could improve its results, for example, for any stage II carcinoma by calling all its stage I cases stage II.

Difficulties may be encountered in determining the primary site; for instance if a clear decision cannot be made when cancer involves both the corpus and the cervix uteri, then an adenocarcinoma should be allotted to carcinoma of the corpus and an epidermoid carcinoma to carcinoma of the cervix. It is similarly accepted that when an apparent vaginal carcinoma has extended to the portio and reached the area of the external os, it should be allotted to carcinoma of the cervix. Classification of a tumour as carcinoma of the urethra is restricted to either those tumours limited to the urethra or to those in which it is evident that the primary site of growth is in the urethra. More commonly, the urethra is secondarily involved in carcinomas of the vulva.

CARCINOMA OF THE CERVIX

The clinical staging of carcinoma of the cervix should be based on examinations which can be carried out in any hospital. It is generally accepted that these include palpation, inspection, colposcopy, endocervical curettage, cystoscopy, proctoscopy, intravenous urography and X-ray examination of the lungs and skeleton. A conisation or amputation of the cervix should also be regarded as a clinical examination.

Definitions of the clinical stages in carcinoma of the cervix uteri

Pre-invasive carcinoma

Stage 0   Carcinoma in situ, intraepithelial carcinoma
Cases of Stage 0 should not be included in any therapeutic statistics for invasive carcinoma.

Invasive carcinoma

Stage I   Carcinoma strictly confined to the cervix (extension to corpus
                should be disregarded).
Stage Ia   Microinvasive carcinoma (early stromal invasion).

Stage Ib   All other cases of stage I. Occult cancer should be marked 'occ'.

Stage II   The carcinoma extends beyond the cervix, but has not extended on to the pelvic wall. The carcinoma involves the vagina, but not the lower third.

Stage IIa   No obvious parametrial involvement.

Stage IIb   Obvious parametrial involvement.

Stage III   The carcinoma has extended on to the pelvic wall. On rectal examination there is no cancer-free space between the tumour and the pelvic wall. The tumour involves the lower third of the vagina. All cases with a hydronephrosis or non-functioning kidney should be included, unless they are known to be due to other cause.

Stage IIIa   No extension on to the pelvic wall, but involvement of the lower third of the vagina.

Stage IIIb   Extension on to the pelvic wall and/or hydronephrosis or non-functioning kidney.

Stage IV   The carcinoma has extended beyond the true pelvis or has clinically involved the mucosa of the bladder or rectum.

Stage IVa   Spread of the growth to adjacent organs.

Stage IVb   Spread to distant organs.

Extension to the corpus should be disregarded in the clinical staging of carcinoma of the cervix although involvement of the cervix by a carcinoma of the corpus alters the stage of that tumour (see below). When a cervical carcinoma is fixed to the pelvic wall by a short, indurated, but smooth parametrium the case should be allotted to stage IIb since it is impossible at clinical examination to distinguish between truly cancerous and inflammatory change in such cases. A case should only be allocated to stage III if the parametrium is nodular out on the pelvic wall or the growth itself extends out on the pelvic wall. When intravenous pyelography reveals a non-functioning kidney due to stenosis of the ureter by cancer, then the case should be allotted to stage III even if according to the other findings it would seem to be only stage I or stage II. Bullous oedema *per se* does not permit a case to be allotted to stage IV and the finding of malignant cells in washings from the urinary bladder warrants bladder biopsy.

    Readers should be aware that controversy exists with regard to microinvasive carcinoma of the cervix. According to FIGO, stage Ia (microinvasive carcinoma) represents those cases of epithelial abnormalities in which histological evidence of early stromal invasion is unambiguous, the diagnosis being based on microscopic examination of tissue removed by biopsy, conisation, amputation of the cervix or hysterectomy. Occult cancer is described as a histologically invasive cancer which cannot be diagnosed by routine clinical examination and is more than early stromal invasion. As a rule, it is diagnosed on cone biopsy, the amputated cervix or the removed uterus. Such cases are described as Ib occult. The above definition begs the question 'how early is "early" invasion?'. In an attempt to shed some light on this, the following working definition was arrived at by a Committee of the Ninth Royal College of Obstetricians and Gynaecologists Study Group in London in 1981. This working definition has been accepted in principle by the Cancer Committee of FIGO at the XIth World Congress in Berlin in September 1985.

> Microinvasive carcinoma: this is a histological diagnosis which should be made on a large biopsy which removes the whole lesion, preferably a cone biopsy. Two groups should be recognized:
>
> 1. Early stromal invasion in which invasive buds are present, either in continuity with an in situ lesion or apparently separated cells not more than 1 mm from the nearest surface or crypt basement membrane.
> 2. Measurable lesions should be measured in two dimensions; the depth should be measured from the base of the epithelium from which it develops and should not exceed 5 mm and the largest diameter should not exceed 10 mm on the section that shows the greatest extent. When reporting Stage Ia lesions, the chosen depth and diameter for including the cases in the statistics should be given. Furthermore, the percentage of confluent lesions and of cases with involvement of endothelial lined spaces should also be stated.

CARCINOMA OF THE CORPUS

The following examination methods are permitted for clinical staging of carcinoma of the corpus: palpation, inspection, fractional curettage, cystoscopy, proctoscopy and X-ray examination of the lungs and skeleton.

Definitions of the clinical stages in carcinoma of the corpus uteri

Stage 0   Atypical endometrial hyperplasia (carcinoma in situ). Histological findings suspicious of malignancy.
Cases of stage 0 should not be included in any therapeutic statistics

Stage I   The carcinoma is confined to the corpus.
Stage Ia   The length of the uterine cavity is 8 cm or less.
Stage Ib   The length of the uterine cavity is more than 8 cm.

Stage II   The carcinoma has involved the corpus and the cervix, but has not extended outside the uterus.

Stage III   The carcinoma has extended outside the uterus, but not outside the true pelvis.

Stage IV   The carcinoma has extended outside the true pelvis or has obviously involved the mucosa of the bladder or rectum.
Stage IVa   Spread of the growth to adjacent organs as urinary bladder, rectum, sigmoid or small bowel.

Stage IVb Spread to distant organs.

Cases of carcinoma of the corpus should be grouped with regard to the degree of differentiation of the adenocarcinoma as follows:

G1 highly differentiated adenomatous carcinoma;

G2 moderately differentiated adenomatous carcinoma with partly solid areas;

G3 predominantly solid or entirely undifferentiated carcinoma;

GX grade not assessed.

The extension of the carcinoma to the endocervix is confirmed by fractionated curettage. Scraping of the cervix should be the first step of the curettage and the specimens from the cervix should be examined separately. Occasionally it may be difficult to decide whether the endocervix is involved by the cancer or not. In such cases the simultaneous presence of normal cervical glands and cancer in the same fragment of tissue will give the final diagnosis.

The presence of metastases in the vagina or in the ovary is sufficient evidence as such to allot a case to stage III.

CARCINOMA OF THE VAGINA

The rules for staging are similar to those for carcinoma of the cervix.

Definitions of the clinical stages in carcinoma of the vagina

Pre-invasive carcinoma

Stage 0 Carcinoma in situ, intra-epithelial carcinoma.

Invasive carcinoma

Stage I The carcinoma is limited to the vaginal wall.

Stage II The carcinoma has involved the subvaginal tissue, but has not extended on to the pelvic wall.

Stage III The carcinoma has extended on to the pelvic wall.

Stage IV The carcinoma has extended beyond the true pelvis or has involved the mucosa of the bladder or rectum.

Stage IVa Spread of the growth to adjacent organs.

Stage IVb Spread to distant organs.

CARCINOMA OF THE OVARY

The term 'ovarian carcinoma' encompasses more than one tumour. Therapeutic statistics of ovarian cancer are of limited value, therefore, if attention is not paid to the histological type of the growth. Cases should be classified as carcinoma of the ovary only when the primary growth is a malignant epithelial tumour. It should be noted that cases of germ cell tumours, hormone-producing neoplasms and metastatic carcinomas should be excluded from therapeutic statistics on ovarian epithelial tumours. The widely accepted FIGO histological classification of the common primary epithelial ovarian tumours is as follows:

1. *Serous cystomas*
   (a) serous benign cystadenomas;
   (b) serous cystadenomas with proliferating activity of the epithelial cells and nuclear abnormalities, but with no infiltrative destructive growth (borderline cases; low potential malignancy);
   (c) serous cystadenocarcinomas.
2. *Mucinous cystomas*
   (a) mucinous benign cystadenomas;
   (b) mucinous cystadenomas with proliferating activity of the epithelial cells and nuclear abnormalities, but with no infiltrative destructive growth (borderline cases; low potential malignancy);
   (c) mucinous cystadenocarcinomas.
3. *Endometrioid tumours* (similar to adenocarcinoma in the endometrium)
   (a) endometrioid benign cysts;
   (b) endometrioid tumours with proliferating activity of the epithelial cells and nuclear abnormalities, but with no infiltrative destructive growth (borderline cases; low potential malignancy);
   (c) endometrioid adenocarcinomas.
4. *Clear cell tumours* (mesonephroid tumours)
   (a) benign mesonephroid tumours;
   (b) mesonephroid tumours with proliferating activity of the epithelial cells and nuclear abnormalities, but with no infiltrative destructive growth (borderline cases; low potential malignancy);
   (c) mesonephroid cystadenocarcinomas.
5. *Undifferentiated carcinoma*
   A malignant tumour of epithelial structure that is too poorly differentiated to be placed in any of the groups 1–4 or 6.
6. *Mixed epithelial tumours*
   Tumours composed of a mixture of two or more of the malignant groups 1c, 2c, 3c or 4c described above, and where none of them is predominant. Thus a case should be listed as 'mixed epithelial tumour' only if it is not possible to decide which is the predominant structure. The pathologist should always try to find out which is the leading structure and classify the case according to that element.
7. *No histology or unclassifiable*
   Cases where explorative surgery has shown that obvious ovarian epithelial malignant tumour is present, but where no biopsy has been taken, or where the specimen is unclassifiable because of, for instance, necrosis.

In some cases of anaplastic inoperable widespread malignant tumour it may be difficult for the gynaecologist to decide the origin of the growth. Such cases should not be included in therapeutic statistics on carcinoma of the ovary. They should be classified as carcinoma abdominis.

Stage-grouping for primary carcinoma of the ovary

This is based on findings at clinical examintaion and/or surgical examination. The histology is to be considered in the staging, as is cytology as far as effusions are concerned. It is desirable that a biopsy be taken from suspicious areas outside of the pelvis.

Stage I	Growth limited to the ovaries
Stage Ia	Growth limited to one ovary; no ascites:

(i) no tumour on the external surface; capsules intact;
(ii) tumour present on the external surface and/or capsule ruptured.

Stage Ib   Growth limited to both ovaries; no ascites:
    (i) no tumour on the external surface; capsules intact;
    (ii) tumour present on the external surface and/or capsule(s) ruptured.
Stage Ic   Tumour either stage Ia or stage Ib, but with obvious ascites* present or positive peritoneal washings.

Stage II   Growth involving one or both ovaries with pelvic extension.
Stage IIa   Extension and/or metastases to the uterus and/or tubes.
Stage IIb   Extension to other pelvic tissues.
Stage IIc   Tumour either stage IIa or stage IIb, but with obvious ascites* present or positive peritoneal washings.

Stage III   Growth involving one or both ovaries with intraperitoneal metastases outside the pelvis and/or positive retroperitoneal nodes. Tumour limited to the true pelvis with histologically proven malignant extension to small bowel or omentum.

Stage IV   Growth involving one or both ovaries with distant metastases.

If pleural effusion is present there must be positive cytology to allot a case to stage IV. When parenchymal liver involvement is present then the case should be allotted to stage IV.
A sub-division of stage III and also minor modifications of stages I and II have recently been agreed by the Cancer Committee of FIGO and will appear in a future FIGO publication.

---

*Ascites is peritoneal effusion which in the opinion of the surgeon is pathological and/or clearly exceeds normal amounts

CARCINOMA OF THE VULVA

The rules for staging are similar to those for carcinoma of the cervix.

TNM classification of the vulva

T—Primary tumour

Tis Pre-invasive carcinoma (carcinoma in situ).
T1   Tumour confined to the vulva—2 cm or less in larger diameter.
T2   Tumour confined to the vulva—more than 2 cm in diameter.
T3   Tumour of any size with adjacent spread to the urethra and/or vagina and/or perineum and/or to the anus.
T4   Tumour of any size infiltrating the bladder mucosa and/or the rectal mucosa, including the upper part of the urethral mucosa and/or fixed to the bone.

N—Regional lymph nodes

N0   No nodes palpable
N1   Nodes palpable in either groin, not enlarged, mobile (not clinically suspicious of neoplasm)
N2   Nodes palpable in either one or both groins, enlarged, firm and mobile (clinically suspicious of neoplasm)
N3   Fixed or ulcerated nodes

M—Distant metastases

M0   No clinical metastases.
M1a Palpable deep pelvic lymph nodes.
M1b Other distant metastases.

Definitions of the clinical stages in carcinoma of the vulva (FIGO)

Stage 0   Carcinoma in situ, intraepithelial carcinoma.

Stage I
T1 N0 M0 Tumour confined to the vulva—2 cm or less in the larger
T1 N1 M0 diameter. Nodes are not palpable, or are palpable in either groin, not enlarged, mobile (not clinically suspicious of neoplasm).

Stage II
T2 N0 M0 Tumour confined to the vulva—more than 2 cm in diameter.
T2 N1 M0 Nodes are not palpable, or are palpable in either groin, not enlarged, mobile (not clinically suspicious of neoplasm).

Stage III

T3 N0 M0   Tumour of any size with:
T3 N1 M0   (1) adjacent spread to the lower urethra and/or the vagina,
T3 N2 M0   and/or the perineum, and/or the anus, and/or
T1 N2 M0   (2) nodes palpable in either one or both groins, enlarged, firm
T2 N2 M0   and mobile, not fixed (but clinically suspicious of neo-
               plasm).

Stage IV

T4 N0 M0   Tumour of any size
T4 N1 M0   (1) infiltrating the bladder mucosa and/or the upper part of
T4 N2 M0   the urethral mucosa and/or the rectal mucosa, and/or
All condi- (2) fixed to the bone or other distant metastases fixed or
tions con-   ulcerated nodes in either one or both groins.
taining
N3 or M1a
or M1b

Normally, the clinical presentation will allow the diagnosis of carcinoma of the cervix, corpus, vagina or vulva to be made with reasonable certainty. Thus, clinical staging under anaesthesia can normally be carried out by an experienced examiner with a sound knowledge of the staging sub-groups. This is not always the case with ovarian cancer, which typically presents once the disease has become advanced and with symptomatology less readily recognisable as due to a gynaecological problem. The individual performing the diagnostic laparotomy, although a skilled surgeon, may not be a gynaecologist and may be unfamiliar with the sub-stages of ovarian cancer. Checklists, such as that shown in Figure 21.1, available in the operating theatre help to improve the accuracy of recording of the extent of disease while illustrations such as Figure 21.2 are an adjunct to narrative description.

Clinical staging, as described above, permits broad comparisons between groups of patients and between one institution and another, but it cannot always be used as a prescription for treatment in the individual case. It is evident that despite a similar stage and a similar treatment, a dissimilar outcome may result. It is incumbent upon the doctor to strive to improve the efficacy of treatment while minimising the risk of complications or side-effects. While the clinical stage once made cannot be changed, refinements in diagnostic techniques may improve the outlook and shed more light on the biological behaviour of the gynaecological cancer.

A concentration of surgical expertise and case material has permitted recent reports on surgical staging of carcinoma of the cervix (Averette & Jobson, 1981; Berman et al, 1984), cancer of the corpus (Chen & Lee, 1983; Boronow et al, 1984), cancer of the vulva (Monaghan & Hammond, 1984; Boyce et al, 1985). These workers, in company with others, have demonstrated the superior accuracy of surgical staging over clinical staging. Thus, sub-groups of individuals may be recognised for whom departures

Ward   Hospital
Consultant

Surname   D.O.B.
First name   Unit no.

Date:

1. Ascites   YES/NO
                    Amount   ....
                    Cytology ....

2. Peritoneal Washings   YES/NO
   N.B. Should always be taken for
   cytology when ascites is absent

3. Macroscopic Ovarian Tumour   LEFT/RIGHT/BILATERAL

4. Extracapsular Tumour   YES/NO

5. Capsule Ruptured   YES/NO

6. Tumour involving Fallopian Tube   LEFT/RIGHT/BOTH/NEITHER

7. Tumour on Uterus   YES/NO

8. Tumour on Visceral Peritoneum   YES/NO

9. Extra Genital Pelvic Tumour   BLADDER/BOWEL/PELVIC SIDE WALL
   Details

10. Other Intraperitoneal Tumour Detail   YES/NO
    Details

11. Omental Tumour   YES/NO

12. Diaphragmatic Tumour   RIGHT/LEFT/BOTH

13. Liver Tumour   YES/NO

14. Para-aortic Lymph Nodes   ENLARGED/NOT ENLARGED
                               BIOPSY/NO BIOPSY

15. Pelvic Lymph Nodes   ENLARGED/NOT ENLARGED
                               BIOPSY/NO BIOPSY

16. Operative Procedure
    Summarise   ⟨o⟩   Pre-op

17. Residual Disease
    Summarise   Sites & Volume   ⟨o⟩   Post-op
                     Nil < 2 cm > 2 cm
                     (Largest deposits)

Fig. 21.1 Ovarian cancer staging sheet—operative findings.

from the routine therapy may result in increased survival. Not all patients are fit to undergo surgical staging, and not all gynaecologists have the expertise for the demanding surgery. Looking to the future, it is to be hoped that such studies can draw important correlations with other diagnostic procedures.

Lymphography has been available for many years and may be useful in the individual patient. The detection rate is low in early-stage disease. The

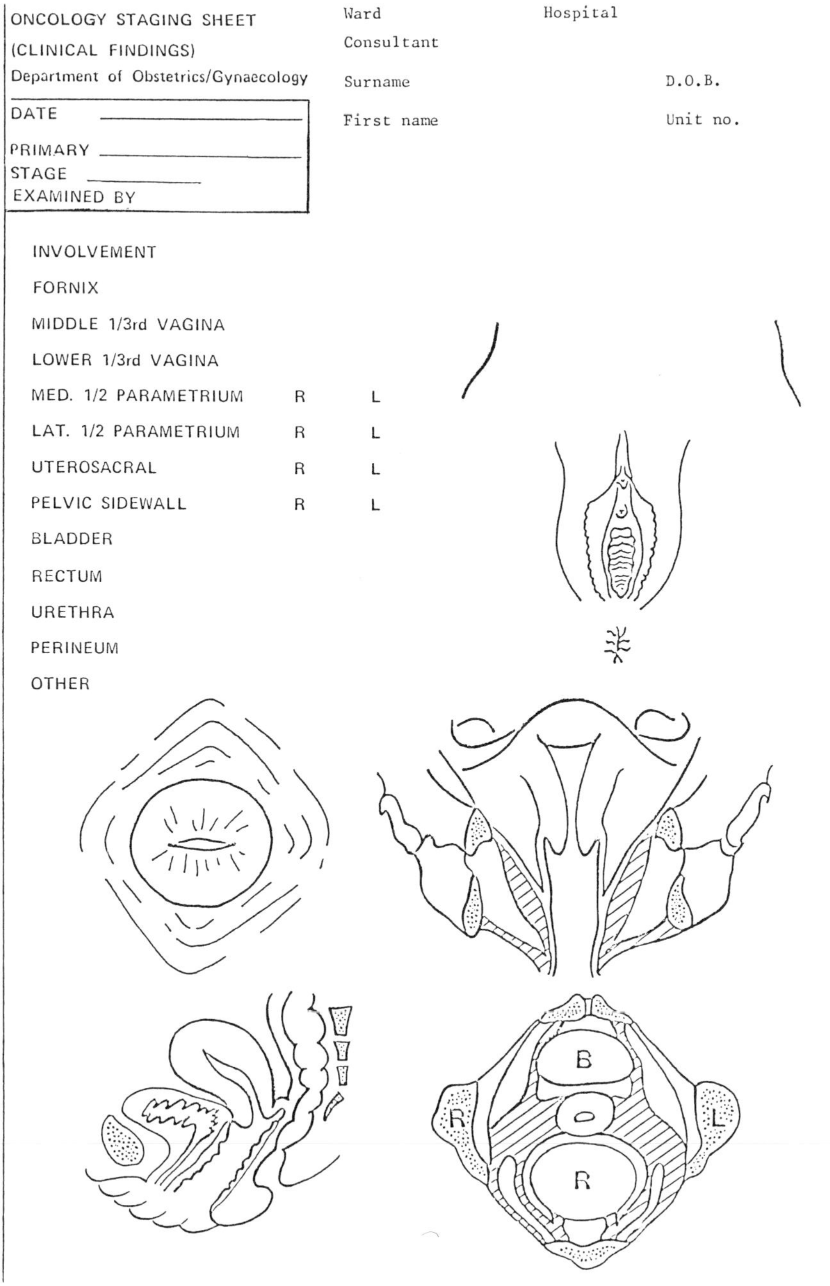

ONCOLOGY STAGING SHEET

(CLINICAL FINDINGS)

Department of Obstetrics/Gynaecology

DATE _____

PRIMARY _____
STAGE _____
EXAMINED BY

Ward   Hospital

Consultant

Surname   D.O.B.

First name   Unit no.

INVOLVEMENT

FORNIX

MIDDLE 1/3rd VAGINA

LOWER 1/3rd VAGINA

MED. 1/2 PARAMETRIUM   R   L

LAT. 1/2 PARAMETRIUM   R   L

UTEROSACRAL   R   L

PELVIC SIDEWALL   R   L

BLADDER

RECTUM

URETHRA

PERINEUM

OTHER

Fig. 21.2   Oncology staging sheet—clinical findings.

technique suffers from the disadvantages of being invasive and having low but recognised complication rates. In addition, interpretation of the findings is difficult with both false positive and false negative results occurring. Despite the duration of its availability, lymphography has not received general acceptance. The newer non-invasive techniques of computerised tomography and nuclear magnetic resonance are becoming available in some centres. Evaluations of the usefulness of these extremely expensive facilities are beginning to appear in the literature (Johnson et al, 1984; Kerr-Wilson et al, 1984; Kormano & Gronroos, 1984; van Engelshoven et al, 1984). Results so far would suggest that the value of such procedures is limited, but improvements in the technology and interpretation may give better results, for instance when accompanied by fine-needle aspiration (Bandy et al, 1985; Fortier et al, 1985). Tumour markers may be of use in two ways. Circulating blood levels of substances such as CA 125, CA 19-9, and carcinoembryonic antigen may be of prognostic significance while the labelling of monoclonal antibodies directed against tumour cells allows radioimmunoscintography which may also provide important information in the determination of tumour status, localisation, extent and spread (Pateisky et al, 1984). Ultrasound is widely available and may be used in the initial characterisation of ovarian tumours and in the follow-up of patients with known residual disease after surgery.

In addition to clinical staging it is apparent that a battery of techniques can be brought to bear on the problem of accurate initial assessment of the patient with malignant disease. Close co-operation between scientists, physicians, surgeons, radiologists and pathologists should improve her prognosis.

REFERENCES

Annual report on the results of treatment in gynecological cancer, vol 19. International Federation of Gynecology and Obstetrics, 1985

Averette H E, Jobson V W 1981 Surgical staging—new approaches. In: Coppleson M (ed) Gynaecologic oncology: fundamental principles and clinical practice. Churchill Livingstone, Edinburgh, ch 20, p 265

Bandy L C, Clarke-Pearson D L, Silverman P M, Creasman W T 1985 Computed tomography in evaluation of extra-pelvic lymphadenopathy in carcinoma of the cervix. Obstetrics and Gynecology 65(1): 73–76

Berman M L, Keys H, Creasman W T 1984 Survival and patterns of recurrence in cervical cancer: metastatic to peri-aortic lymph nodes (a gynecologic oncology study). Gynecologic Oncology 19(1): 8–16

Boronow R C, Morrow C P, Creasman W T 1984 Surgical staging in endometrial cancer: clinical pathologic findings of a prospective study. Obstetrics and Gynecology 63(6): 825–832

Boyce J, Freuchter R G, Kasambilides E 1985 Prognostic factors in carcinoma of the vulva. Gynecologic Oncology 20(3): 364–377

Chen S S, Lee L 1983 Retroperitoneal lymph node metastases in stage I carcinoma of the endometrium: correlation with risk factors. Gynecologic Oncology 16(3): 319–325

Fortier K J, Clarke-Pearson D L, Creasman W T, Johnston W W 1985 Fine needle aspiration in gynecology : evaluation of extra-pelvic lesions in patients with gynecologic malignancy. Obstetrics and Gynecology 65(1) : 67–72

Harmer M M (ed) 1978 TNM classification of malignant tumours, 3rd edn. International Union Against Cancer, Geneva

Johnson I R, Symonds E M, Worthington B S 1984 Imaging ovarian tumours by nuclear magnetic resonance. British Journal of Obstetrics and Gynaecology 91(3) : 260–264

Kerr-Wilson R H J, Shingleton H M, Orr J W Jr., Hatch K D 1984 The use of ultrasound and computed tomography scanning in the management of gynecologic cancer patients. Gynecologic Oncology 18(1) : 54–61

Kormano M, Gronroos M 1984 Computer-tomographic evaluation of gynecologic tumors. Acta Obstetrica et Gynecologica Scandinavica 63(6) : 509–516

Monaghan J M, Hammond I G 1984 Pelvic node dissection in the treatment of vulval carcinoma : is it necessary ? British Journal of Obstetrics and Gynaecology 91(3) : 270–274

Pateisky N, Philipp K, Burchell J, Skodler W 1984 Visualization of malignant tumours in the abdomen using radio-labelled monoclonal antibodies. Geburtshilfe und Frauenheilkunde 44(10) : 623–626

Pre-clinical neoplasia of the cervix. Proceedings of the Ninth Study Group of the Royal College of Obstetricians and Gynaecologists, 1981 (ed. Jordan J A, Sharp F, Singer A).

Van Engelshoven J M A, Versteege C W M, Ruys J H J 1984 Computed tomography in staging untreated patients with cervical cancer. Gynecologic and Obstetric Investigations 18(6) : 289–295

Improving the prognosis in ovarian cancer

Discussion of ovarian cancer usually commences with a catalogue of the horrors of the disease. Unfortunately there is a wealth of evidence with which to paint such a bleak picture.

Two particularly depressing characteristics of ovarian cancer are worthy of special emphasis. First it is a disease which presents late, with approximately 75 per cent of cases having stage III or stage IV disease at the initial laparotomy (Table 22.1). Secondly, the success of treatment of disseminated disease has been extremely poor; 5-year survival of about 10 per cent amongst patients with disease outside the pelvis at presentation (Table 22.1). This combination of late presentation and poor response to treatment accounts for the fact that, although less common than endometrial cancer and cancer of the cervix, ovarian cancer causes more deaths than both combined, and has a diagnosis to death ratio of 1·6 : 1 (American Cancer Society, 1982).

Table 22.1　Five-year survival rates by stage at presentation for epithelial ovarian cancer (modified from Kottmeier, 1982)

Stage	Percentage incidence (no. of patients)	5-year survival (%)
Ia	17·9　(940)	69·7
Ib	4·3　(227)	63·9
Ic	3·0　(157)	50·3
Total stage I	25·2　(1324)	67·1
IIa	4·8　(251)	51·8
IIb+c	12·8　(672)	42·4
III	39·5　(2074)	13·3
IV	17·7　(993)	4·1
Total stages III and IV	57·2　(3067)	10·4
Total all stages	100·0　(5254)	30·6

Although this appalling background cannot be disputed there are now grounds for some optimism that the pattern of the disease can be changed and survival figures improved. During the past decade the combined efforts of a variety of disciplines have greatly increased our understanding of ovarian cancer. A great deal of information has become available concerning the epidemiology and accurate staging of ovarian malignancy. Progress has been made towards defining and improving management for different stages of the disease. Enormous efforts aimed at producing a technique for early diagnosis are beginning to yield useful results.

It would be naive to suggest that a revolution in the pattern of ovarian cancer is about to occur, but there is a basis for believing that some improvement in ovarian cancer statistics is possible now through consistent application of available information. In all too many cases of ovarian cancer women suffer unnecessarily because established knowledge has not been transformed into established practice. Opportunity for improvement exists in several areas:

1. Earlier diagnosis: greater awareness of the women at risk, prompt investigation of suspicious symptoms, and further development of screening techniques.
2. Prevention: prophylactic oophorectomy at surgery for benign disease and in women with a strong family history of ovarian cancer.
3. Improved use of existing therapeutic techniques: accurate staging, maximum surgical effort, and optimal adjuvant therapy.
4. Further development of experimental therapies.

This chapter will discuss these areas with an emphasis on epithelial ovarian cancer.

TOWARDS EARLY DIAGNOSIS

Identifying the woman at risk

Although the aetiology of epithelial cancer of the ovary remains obscure modern epidemiological studies have identified risk factors and associations which describe the most susceptible groups of the population.

Some of these factors are either too vague or too difficult to identify to be useful in clinical practice. For example studies have shown an increased occurrence of subclinical mumps and lower persistent mumps antibody titres, among ovarian cancer patients (Mencer et al, 1979) and a 3·9-fold increase in risk of developing ovarian cancer in women who contracted rubella between ages 12 and 18, compared to controls infected before age 12 (McGowan et al, 1979). Other associations are easily identifiable and clinically more valuable.

Ovarian cancer is a disease of western industrialised nations, but even in these countries the incidence was low until this century (Woodruff, 1979). Epithelial ovarian cancer is now 3 to 5 times more common in industrialised populations than in developing countries (Waterhouse et al, 1976) although to some extent this reflects differences in registration and reporting. Age-adjusted incidence rates range from 14·9 per 100 000 in Sweden to intermediate levels in the USA and UK, and a rate of just 2·8 per 100 000 in some areas of Japan (Fig. 22.1). That country of residence is of greater importance than race is shown by studies of rates among immigrants from developing countries to industrialised areas (Dunn, 1975; Muir & Mectoux, 1978). However Japanese, Chinese, Hispanic and black women in the United States do have incidence rates to a variable degree lower than those of white women (Weiss & Peterson, 1978) and one case study found Jewish women to be at increased risk (Hildreth et al, 1981). (These findings may be a reflection of family size.) The women at greatest risk are white and north European.

Age is an important criterion of risk assessment for all histological types

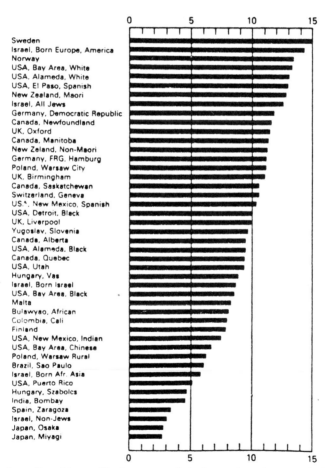

Fig. 22.1   Age-adjusted (to world reference population) annual ovarian cancer incidence rates per 100 000 women reported to selected international cancer registries. (From Green et al, 1984)

Table 22.2 Ovarian carcinoma: age distribution
by decade of life (from Morrow, 1981)

Age group (years)	Total cases	Percentage of total
0–9	9	0·2
10–19	35	0·9
20–29	161	4·1
30–39	439	11·3
40–49	1064	27·3
50–59	1187	30·5
60–69	729	18·7
70–79	235	6·0
80+	32	0·8

of ovarian cancer. Epithelial ovarian cancer is most frequent in peri- and postmenopausal women with a median age in the sixth decade (Table 22.2). The age-specific incidence of ovarian cancer is low until the fifth decade but gradually increases, to peak in the eighth decade.

Considerable weight of evidence suggests that events of reproductive life are key factors in development of ovarian cancer (Table 22.3). Case–control studies consistently reveal that women with ovarian cancer are less likely to have been pregnant than are matched controls. The same studies also suggest that if they have been pregnant they are less likely to have had an early age of first pregnancy and are less likely to have had multiple pregnancies than matched controls. Most reports demonstrate that oral contraceptive use confers a significant decrease in the risk of developing ovarian cancer in later life; the degree of protection is proportional to duration of use and persists long after contraceptive use ceases.

Table 22.3 Summary of case control studies of ovarian cancer: relative risk of reproductive and endocrine factors in ovarian cancer versus controls (modified from Green et al, 1984)

Reference	Pregnancy (ever)	Total pregnancies			Age first pregnancy		OCC use (ever)
		0	1–2	3 or more	<25 years	>25 years	
Joly et al, 1978		1·0	0·83	0·42			
Annegers et al, 1979	0·54						0·5
Casagrande et al, 1979, 1983		1·0	0·75	0·59		N.S.	N.S.
Risch et al, 1983; Weiss et al, 1981		1·0	0·97	0·76			0·68
Cramer et al, 1982a							0·38
Rosenberg et al, 1982	0·7					N.S.	0·6
Hildreth et al, 1981	0·47	1·0	0·62	0·37	0·46	0·85	0·5
Franceschi et al, 1982; La Vecchia et al, 1983	0·66	1·0	0·85	0·48	0·43	0·90	0·7
Newhouse et al, 1977	0·41						0·3
McGowan et al, 1979	0·45	1·0	0·52	0·41	0·44	0·92	N.S.
Dicker et al, 1983	0·41	1·0	0·49	0·35			0·6

Such data are consistent with the 'incessant ovulation' hypothesis first proposed by Fathalla (1972) and expanded by Casagrande et al (1979) and Henderson et al (1982). They suggested that the trauma of ovulation may be responsible for neoplastic change, and developed the concept of 'ovulatory age' (time from menarche to cessation of ovulation minus time of anovulation due to pregnancy, lactation, oral contraceptive use, etc.) as an index of ovarian cancer risk. This model has been criticised on the grounds that relating risk of ovarian cancer to simple duration of ovulatory activity is inconsistent with the fact that age at first birth is more strongly associated with the risk of ovarian cancer than actual number of births.

There are many case reports of familial aggregation of ovarian cancer. These associations are supported by several case–control studies (Casagrande et al, 1979; McGowan et al, 1979; Hildreth et al, 1981). Hildreth et al (1981) reported an 18-fold increased risk among women who had a mother or sister with epithelial ovarian cancer. A cancer family syndrome in which ovarian cancer is associated with colon, endometrial, breast and other adenocarcinomas has been described (Lynch & Lynch, 1979; Lynch et al, 1981). These same malignancies also occur significantly more often as double primaries in the same women. Women with an initial primary malignancy of the breast, endometrium or colon have a two to four times greater risk of developing a subsequent ovarian cancer than women of comparable age and race who have not had these malignancies (Table 22.4).

An aetiological role for talc in ovarian cancer has been postulated, based on its similarity with peritoneal mesotheliomas and the fact that consumer talc is known to be contaminated with asbestos (Rohl et al, 1976), which is a cause of peritoneal mesotheliomas. Talc particles have been observed in both normal and neoplastic ovarian tissue (Henderson et al, 1979). A cohort

Table 22.4 Studies linking ovarian cancer with carcinoma of the breast, endometrium and colon (modified from Green et al, 1984)

Reference	First cancer	Second cancer	Relative risk	
Schoenberg et al, 1969	Ovary	Colon	2·4	
	Breast	Ovary	1·9	
Schottenfeld et al, 1969	Ovary	Colon	3·3	
	Colon	'Female genitals'	2·1	
Schottenfeld and Berg, 1971	Ovary	Breast	4·4	
	Breast	Ovary	2·1	
Newell et al, 1974	Breast	Ovary (whites	2·2	
	Breast	Ovary (blacks)	1·1	
Reimer et al, 1978	Ovary	Endometrium	3·7*	5·9†
	Ovary	Breast	1·1*	2·2†
	Ovary	Colon	1·6*	2·8†
Annegers and Malkasian, 1981	Endometrium	Ovary	1·4‡	
Prior and Waterhouse, 1981	Ovary	Breast	1·5	
	Breast	Ovary	1·2	

*Data from NCI end-results programme.
†Data from Reimer survey.
‡Relative risk underestimated: many women had oophorectomy when treated for their endometrial cancer.

study of women occupationally exposed to talc did not show an increased ovarian cancer rate (Newhouse, 1979) but a case–control study controlled for age, parity and menopausal status showed a relative risk of 1·9 among women regularly using talc on sanitary pads or the perineum and a large risk of 3·4 associated with both of these practices (Cramer et al, 1982b).

Studies have failed to confirm a significant association between ovarian cancer and socioeconomic status, obesity, thyroid disease, smoking and alcohol. An increased risk of endometrioid ovarian cancer in women taking non-contraceptive oestrogens has been reported in two studies (Weiss et al, 1982; Trichapoulos et al, 1981). There have been two reports of increased risk of ovarian cancer among coffee-drinkers (Trichapoulos et al, 1981; Hartge et al, 1982).

In summary the woman most likely to develop ovarian cancer is white, of north European origin and in her 40s or older. She is nulliparous or of low parity with a late age of first pregnancy, and has not used oral contraceptives. Her family history or past medical history is more likely to include a previous breast, colon or endometrial cancer than a control group of women (Table 22.5).

Table 22.5   Risk factors for epithelial ovarian cancer

1. Age	> 45 years
2. Race	Caucasian, Jewish
3. Geography	North European, urban areas
4. Reproductive history	Low parity, late age first pregnancy
5. Past medical history	Breast, endometrial, colon cancer
6. Family history	Ovarian, endometrial cancer
7. Cosmetic talc	Regular use on sanitary pad, perineum

Possible risk factors   Coffee drinking, adolescent rubella infection, subclinical premenarchal mumps infection, non-contraceptive oestrogens

Symptomatology

Not surprisingly there are few studies of symptoms in patients with localised ovarian cancer. The majority of patients complain of abdominal pain or swelling at presentation (Table 22.6), and this is a reflection of their advanced-stage disease.

A striking feature of many women presenting with advanced ovarian malignancy is their delay in seeking help despite the gross nature of their symptoms and signs. There is evidence of a relationship between duration of symptoms and prognosis (Holme, 1963; Kent & Mackay, 1960), which suggests that improved public education to seek prompt medical advice may make a significant contribution to improving ovarian cancer statistics.

It is often claimed that non-specific symptoms such as bloating, dyspepsia, nausea, intermittent mild abdominal discomfort and slight loss of appetite are present several months before diagnosis in early disease. However it is

Table 22.6 Ovarian carcinoma: symptoms at the time of diagnosis based on 2099 patients from several series (from Morrow, 1981)

Symptom	Percentage of total	Symptom	Percentage of total
Abdominal pain	50·8	Urinary	16·4
Abdominal swelling	49·5	Pelvic pressure	5·0
Gastrointestinal	21·6	Backache	4·9
Weight loss	17·5	Mass felt by patient	2·8
Abnormal bleeding	17·1	None	0·4

unclear whether they are more common in women with early ovarian cancer than healthy women, or women with other medical conditions, and it is also unclear at which stage of the disease they occur. Nevertheless a higher index of suspicion when such symptoms are present is warranted, particularly in women thought to be at risk on epidemiological grounds.

This non-specific symptomatology accounts for the fact that 50 per cent of women with ovarian cancer present to the wrong doctor, being investigated by general surgeons for abdominal pain or general physicians for ascites. Delay in appropriate treatment is inevitable.

Screening tests

Tumours that most readily lend themselves to screening techniques are those which are a significant cause of morbidity and mortality, and in which the natural history of the disease is well understood and has revealed a high prevalence of preclinical disease in the population. Ovarian cancer cannot at present be said to fall within this category: although certainly a cause of significant mortality it does not fulfil the latter criterion. In contrast to cancers of the cervix, vulva, vagina and endometrium almost nothing is known about precancerous conditions of the ovary (Scully, 1981). The incidence of cervical cancer has never been exceptionally high, but it is suitable for screening because it has a long natural history resulting in a relatively high prevalence of detectable premalignant disease in the population. There is little evidence of a similar natural history in ovarian cancer. If the preclinical phase in ovarian cancer is short the screening interval required in individual women may be so demanding that a screening test, even if available and effective, is impracticable (Fig. 22.2).

The screening test itself must be comfortable and convenient for the patient, economical, easy to perform and have a low incidence of side-effects. Test performance must combine high specificity, to avoid needless diagnostic work-up in healthy individuals (with resultant morbidity and cost), with high sensitivity to prevent failure of detection of preclinical disease.

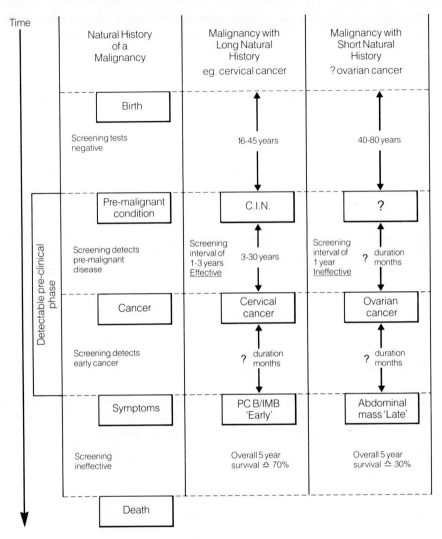

Fig. 22.2   Natural history of ovarian malignancy

Tumour markers

Tumour markers may be detected biochemically as proteins, hormones or enzymes, or immunologically as antigens. There are currently four main categories of potential tumour marker for ovarian cancer:

1. oncodevelopmental markers,
2. carcinoplacental markers,
3. metabolic markers,
4. tumour-specific or tumour-associated antigens.

None of the potential markers investigated in relation to ovarian cancer appears to have a sufficiently high specificity to be useful as a screening test. Figure 22.3 summarises the information available on the sensitivity of a number of marker substances, but should be interpreted with caution. Many of the potential markers are at an early stage of evaluation; often studies suggesting encouraging sensitivity and specificity have involved small

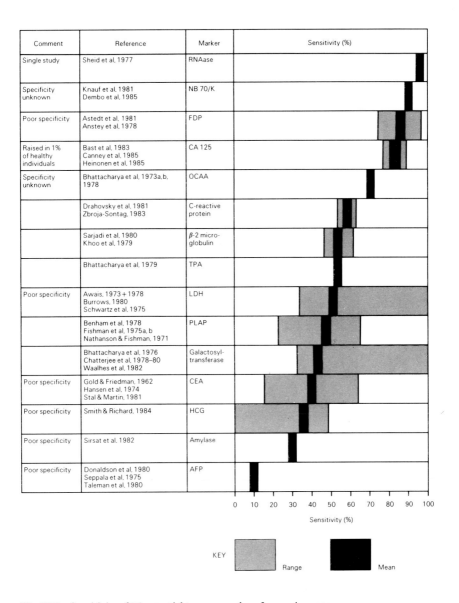

Fig. 22.3   Sensitivity of 15 potential tumour markers for ovarian cancer

numbers of patients and have not been followed up, so that their clinical value remains obscure. In addition, because of the difficulty of demonstrating the sensitivity of screening tests estimates have been based on their application to symptomatic patients. It is important to note that such estimates may not apply to an asymptomatic population with preclinical disease. There have been few prospective studies among groups of asymptomatic women.

A number of the tests may be useful in monitoring response to treatment and recurrence of disease in known ovarian cancer patients. However a correlation between the marker and tumour bulk is not necessarily an indication of its value; it may provide no more information than clinical examination or other easily available tests.

Recent advances in immunological techniques have raised hopes that an ovarian cancer-specific antigen may be identified. The lack of antibody specificity inherent in polyclonal antibodies restricts their use as diagnostic reagents. Antibody specificity can be achieved by production of monoclonal antibodies reacting with a single epitope on surface membrane tumour-associated antigens. However most of the tumour-associated antigens which have been described are present on other tumour cells and some normal cells, and represent tumour-associated differentiation antigens.

One of the most encouraging tumour-associated antigens investigated in relation to ovarian cancer is CA 125. CA 125 is a high molecular weight glycoprotein expressed in coelomic epithelium during embryonic development and defined by murine monoclonal antibody raised against a serous ovarian cancer cell line OVCA 433. A radioimmunoassay to detect CA 125 has been developed by Bast et al (1983a) and is now available commercially.

Bast et al. found serum levels of CA 125 > 35 U/ml in 82 per cent of 101 patients with surgically demonstrated ovarian cancer and correlation with disease course in 93 per cent of 45 patients. One per cent of healthy individuals and 6 per cent with non-malignant disease had elevated levels. Other investigators have found similar results (Table 22.7).

The sensitivity of CA 125 is good, and seems to include all histological types of ovarian epithelial neoplasm except mucinous tumours. Unfortunately the specificity with respect to other epithelial neoplasms is poor, and limits its use in diagnosis. The studies have shown significant correlation between CA 125 and the regression, stability or progression of epithelial ovarian carcinoma and a progressive increase in serum levels prior to clinically evident relapse has been shown for patients who have completed therapy.

CA 125 therefore has potential value for monitoring disease. Its poor specificity precludes its use as a screening method in asymptomatic patients but the diagnostic and prognostic significance of raised levels preoperatively have not yet been determined.

NB/70K is a glycoprotein described by Knauf & Urbach (1981). Preliminary data showed measurable levels in 89 per cent of 127 patients

Table 22.7 Frequency of elevation serum CA 125 level (> 35 U/ml) in several groups of individuals and correlation with disease course

Reference	Post-operative ovarian cancer patients	Non-ovarian cancer patients	Benign diseases	Healthy individuals	Correlation with disease course
Bast et al, 1983	82·0% (101)	28·5% (200)	6·3% (143)	1·0 (888)	93·0% (45)
Canney et al, 1984	83·0% (58)	41·0% (27)	—	—	91·0% (23)
Heinonen et al, 1985	75·0% (12)	—	10·0% (10)	—	—
Crombach et al, 1985	78·0% (95)	—	17·0% (41)	—	90·0% (30)
Total	80·4%	29·9%	8·7%	1·0%	91·8%

Number of patients in parentheses

with epithelial cancer, 60 per cent having levels > 11 kU/ml compared with 5 per cent of 181 gynaecologic controls and none of 55 healthy normal volunteer adults (Dembo et al, 1985). Only 12 patients with ovarian cancer had preoperative levels assayed but all had higher levels than any postoperative group studied. A third of patients with other malignancies, and patients with hepatic and renal failure, also had elevated levels. There was no apparent dependence on histologic type or tumour differentiation. Plasma levels appeared to correlate well with tumour burden.

Bhattacharya & Barlow (1973a,b, 1978) described ovarian cancer-associated antigens (OCAA and OCCAA-1) purified from polyclonal antisera. In tissue extracts OCAA appeared to be significantly selective for ovarian cancer and a radioimmunoassay was developed. Serum elevations were found in two of four patients with early stage, and 67 per cent of 56 patients with late-stage, epithelial cancer. However, up to 30 per cent of patients with other malignancies also had increased serum levels.

Carcinoembryonic antigen (CEA) is a glycoprotein first detected by Gold and Friedman in carcinoma of the colon (Gold & Friedman, 1962). Since then high levels have been found in a variety of malignancies including ovarian cancer and in a non-malignant conditions. Levels of 2·5–5 ng/ml were found in 10·2 per cent of individuals in a study of 10 000 patients (Hansen et al, 1974). A review of the literature has shown levels > 5 ng/ml in 39·5 per cent of 400 ovarian cancer patients of all stages and histology (Stall & Martin, 1981). Although a serum level of CEA > 5 ng/ml suggests the presence of malignant disease, CEA levels in early ovarian cancer are less than this in the majority of cases, and it is unlikely to be useful in early detection of the disease. Serum alpha-fetoprotein (AFP) and human chorionic gonadotrophin (hCG) are reliable markers for germ cell cancers containing endodermal sinus or trophoblastic elements respectively. However although both have been detected in the sera of patients with epithelial ovarian cancer the levels are low and they are not effective markers in these patients. Four studies have found a raised placental alkaline phosphatase (Regan isoenzyme) in an average of 47 per cent of patients with ovarian carcinoma (Benham et al, 1978; Fishman et al, 1975a,b; Nathanson & Fishman, 1971). However the enzyme is also elevated in other malignant disease, a variety of inflammatory conditions, and smokers, and its specificity is unsatisfactory for early detection.

Serum ribonuclease levels were significantly raised in 21 of 22 ovarian cancer patients studied by Sheid et al (1977), including four of five with stage I disease, but not in any with benign ovarian disease. There was a good correlation with tumour bulk.

Galactosyltransferase serum levels were initially reported as significantly raised in all of 30 ovarian cancer patients by Chatterjee et al (1978, 1979) and levels correlated well with clinical course and tumour burden (Chatterjee et al, 1980). Raised levels have since been found in 64 per cent of 25 postoperative patients with other malignant disease. The specificity of galactosyltransferase for a subset of malignancies appears to be relatively good.

Hyperamylassaemia occurs in a wide variety of cancers and non-malignant conditions including about one-third of ovarian cancer patients. An isoenzyme with a different amino acid composition and substrate specificity from pancreatic and salivary isoenzymes has been described in association with ovarian malignancy, and may be useful in diagnosis (Takeuchi et al, 1981).

Multiparametric testing has been assessed in several studies but sacrifices the already limited specificity of individual markers to obtain greater sensitivity and does not appear to be useful in screening asymptomatic women for ovarian cancer.

Imaging

Ultrasound has been used to monitor the response of tumours to chemotherapy, to identify malignant features in an ovarian mass and to delineate changes in tumour size. However the use of real-time ultrasonography as a screening procedure has not yet been fully evaluated. Preliminary data from a study at King's College Hospital are interesting (Campbell et al, 1982). In a series of 42 patients the measurement of ovarian volume by ultrasound was compared with measurements at subsequent laparotomy and a correlation coefficient of 0·97 was obtained. Further, an increase in ovarian volume to twice that of the mean volume was more than two standard deviations above the mean, and an ovary which was twice the volume of its fellow was also more than two standard deviations above the percentage mean difference. Volume increases of this magnitude should therefore be regarded with suspicion.

The technique also demonstrated the presence of cystic ovaries which were not evident on clinical examination. This finding may well be of early diagnostic importance, as although the initial morphological changes during the early development of ovarian cancer are poorly documented, it is known that 94 per cent of all ovarian cancers have cystic spaces, and that most epithelial tumours, which account for 85 per cent of all malignant ovarian neoplasms, are cystic.

The King's group have yet to report the results of their long-term study but this information is awaited with considerable interest. It is feared, however, that these data will not help to resolve the problem of frequency of examination in a disease that does not readily lend itself to screening.

Successful radionucleide imaging requires an antibody of suitable class, affinity and specificity, an accessible antigenic site, a radioactive label with safe half-life and emission energy, a labelling method not causing loss of antigenic activity, and a reliable method of subtracting blood pool activity. Nevertheless successful imaging of ovarian tumours has been achieved with antibodies to CEA (Goldenberg et al, 1978; Van Nagell et al, 1980), AFP (Kim et al, 1980), HCG (Goldenberg et al, 1980) and human milk fat globulin-2 (HMFG-2) (Epenetos et al, 1982). The ovaries are situated away from the central blood pool, making images easier to interpret. In the case of HMFG-2 the antibody has good affinity and there are a large number of antigenic sites on tumour cells which are only exposed to the bloodstream in malignant change, when normal architecture is disrupted. Although HMFG-2 is tumour-associated rather than tumour-specific, and probably of limited use in diagnosis of ovarian cancer, with improvements in antibody specificity and technique this approach may be extremely valuable.

Cytology

The routine Papanicalou smear is abnormal in only 10–30 per cent of advanced ovarian cancers (Shapiro & Nunez, 1983) and is therefore unsuitable as a screening test for this disease.

Peritoneal cytology does not appear to be sufficiently specific or sensitive, and is too time-consuming and painful a procedure to be useful in screening for ovarian cancer in the general population. Keetel reviewed 3014 cases in six studies of cul-de-sac lavage; 35 per cent of the specimens were insufficient and only 1·2 per cent (37) were positive. He concluded that cul-de-sac lavage was of questionable value in early detection of ovarian cancer (Keetel et al, 1974).

Pelvic examination

At present radioimmune scanning remains largely experimental, ultrasound and peritoneal cytology are not of proven value, and no tumour marker possesses sufficient specificity to be useful in screening asymptomatic women. As a consequence it is sadly true that the identification of a pelvic mass on vaginal examination may be the most sensitive means currently available for the detection of early ovarian cancer. Unfortunately a tumour volume of 1 cm³, which is about the smallest clinically detectable, contains about a billion cancer cells and may already be associated with widespread intra-abdominal seeding (Barber, 1979). MacFarlane, Sturgis and Fetterman discovered only six ovarian cancers during 18 753 routine pelvic examinations performed on 1319 women aged 30–80 years from 1938 to 1952 (MacFarlane et al, 1955). Despite these limitations it is important to recognise that palpable ovaries in the postmenopausal women are abnormal and require prompt investigation.

Prevention: the case for prophylactic oophorectomy

Until the promise of early detection of ovarian cancer is realised, or prognosis for established disease is greatly improved, the question of whether or not to remove apparently normal ovaries during the course of laparotomy will remain both relevant and controversial.

Table 22.8 shows that of 4051 women with ovarian cancer reported in the literature, 7·0 per cent (284) had undergone previous laparotomy. Of 30 555 patients with retained ovary/ovaries after operations for benign gynaecological disorders and followed up (for 5–40 years), 0·2 per cent (68) developed an ovarian carcinoma (Table 22.9). Thus although about 500 prophylactic oophorectomies are needed to save one woman from ovarian cancer, if this were to be performed routinely up to 7·0 per cent of cases of ovarian cancer (and the deaths of approximately 300 women a year in England and Wales), could be prevented. A review of 407 patients treated for ovarian cancer at the London Hospital between 1961 and 1985 has revealed that 14·7 per cent had a history of a previous laparotomy at which oophorectomy could have been performed (Jacobs & Oram, 1986, unpublished data). To this benefit of prophylactic oophorectomy must be added removal of risk of re-operation for benign ovarian disease, pain or

Table 22.8 Elimination of risk of ovarian cancer

Reference	No. of patients with ovarian cancer	Percentage with previous pelvic surgery
Speert, 1949	260	9·6
Golub, 1953	211	7·6
Counsellor et al, 1955	1500	4·5
Fagan et al, 1956	172	4·7
Bloom, 1962	141	9·9
Terz et al, 1967	264	8·0
Gibbs, 1971	236	16·0
Kofler, 1972	556	8·1
Grundsell et al, 1981	352	6·0
Total, 1949–81	4051	7·0

Table 22.9   Incidence of ovarian cancer in retained ovaries

Reference	No. of patients with con-served ovaries	Percentage developing ovarian cancer (no. of patients)
Reycraft, 1955	4500	0·2% (9)
Grogan & Duncan, 1956	391	0·0% (0)
Funck-Bretano, 1958	580	0·2% (1)
Whitelaw, 1959	1215	0·0% (0)
Schaburt, 1960	169	0·0% (0)
Randal et al, 1963	915	0·2% (2)
De Neef & Hollenbeck, 1966	207	0·0% (0)
Mackenzie, 1968	252	0·0% (0)
Palovcek, 1969	4981	0·5% (18)
Gibbs, 1971	8398	0·3% (28)
Christ & Loetze, 1975	6188	0·1% (6)
Ranney & Abou-Ghazalem, 1977	2132	0·2% (4)
Total, 1955–77	30 555	0·2% (68)

suspicion of malignancy (reported variously as between 0·3 and 8·9 per cent), and the ill-defined but nevertheless real incidence of morbidity associated with abnormal cyclical function of retained ovaries. There is also evidence of impaired ovarian function after hysterectomy, possibly due to compromised blood flow (Siddle, 1986, unpublished data).

In spite of these data, no consistent clinical practice has emerged. Presumably this is due to an inherent reluctance to remove healthy gonadal tissue in premenopausal women, doubts about the efficacy and practicality of long-term hormone replacement therapy, and concern about psychological sequelae.

The presentation of patients with advanced ovarian cancer who have experienced previous pelvic surgery at which time prophylactic oophorectomy was not even considered is both frustrating and lamentable. The following approach is suggested:

1. Prophylactic oophorectomy should always be performed at the time of pelvic surgery (by gynaecologists and general surgeons) in postmenopausal women.
2. In the premenopausal woman who has completed her family the pros and cons of oophorectomy should be discussed, and a decision made before surgery, taking into account any risk factors present in the woman concerned. The age of the patient is irrelevant if she has completed her family and has no contraindications to long-term hormone replacement therapy.
3. Grossly abnormal ovaries should be removed in all women irrespective of menopausal status or age.
4. In women with a strong family history of ovarian cancer prophylactic oophorectomy as a primary surgical procedure should be considered after completion of childbearing.

IMPROVING THE USE OF EXISTING TREATMENTS

Overall 5-year survival rates in ovarian cancer are of the order of 30 per cent and have been virtually unchanged for the past 30 years (Tobias & Griffiths, 1976; Smith & Day, 1979). Nevertheless, present-day techniques can, if appropriately applied, achieve a prolongation of disease-free and progression-free intervals. In addition there is potential for improving the prognosis of some groups of patients by stricter adherence to principles of management which have been defined during the past decade.

Surgery

Surgery remains the cornerstone of treatment of established disease, and successful primary laparotomy represents the woman's best chance of a cure. It is depressing therefore to note that approximately 50 per cent of patients with ovarian cancer present to the wrong doctor, and 25 per cent are initially treated by specialists other than gynaecologists (Wijnen & Rosensheim, 1980). Further, among gynaecologists the least experienced surgeon frequently has first opportunity of surgical resection. In a retrospective study of 100 consecutive patients undergoing surgery for ovarian cancer Piver et al. (1976) reported that only 17 per cent had an adequate incision allowing for accurate staging and establishment of a primary site. Nine per cent of operative notes had no description of specific pelvic structures and 29 per cent had no description of the abdominal viscera. The liver was not described in 59 per cent, the stomach in 76 per cent, the pancreas in 76 per cent, the colon in 76 per cent, the diaphragm in 84 per cent and the aortic nodes in 92 per cent.

Inadequate surgical exploration sadly remains commonplace. Understaging is the consequence, leading inevitably to undertreatment and the familiar poor attendant prognosis. This practice must surely stop. Principles concerning the process of staging and the mode and sites of spread of the disease have been defined in recent years, and it is essential that surgeons are aware of and adhere strictly to these principles.

Staging

Accurate staging allows appropriate choice of adjuvant therapy and improved assessment of prognosis. Inadequate exploration has often made it necessary to perform repeat operations with 20–30 per cent of patients being assigned to a higher stage as a result (Piver et al, 1976; Young et al, 1983). A consensus has emerged concerning adequate exploration for ovarian cancer (Young et al, 1983; Schwartz, 1981; Wharton & Herson, 1981; Castaldo et al, 1981; Averette & Sevin, 1982; Piver, 1983).

1. Surgery should start with a vertical abdominal incision.

2. Immediately after the peritoneal cavity is opened a specimen for cytology should be obtained either by aspiration of free fluid or by saline washing. Positive peritoneal cytology is found in approximately 30 per cent of patients with disease apparently localised to the ovaries (Piver et al, 1978; Keetel et al, 1974). The finding of positive peritoneal washings indicates a significantly worsened prognosis and is an indication for adjunctive therapy in early-stage lesions (Tobias & Griffiths, 1976; Creasman & Rutledge, 1971).

3. Careful examination of all serosal surfaces and parietal and visceral peritoneum should be carried out. This part of the examination is commonly inadequate. The surface of the liver and right hemidiaphragm are important areas to examine as lymphatics from the peritoneal cavity drain to the inferior surface of the diaphragm before entering mediastinal nodes and the right thoracic trunk (Feldman & Knapp, 1974). The incidence of diaphragmatic metastases in apparent stage I and apparent stage II ovarian cancer has been reported as 11·4 and 23 per cent respectively (Piver et al, 1978).

The paracolic gutters, stomach, small and large bowels, the mesentery and omentum and all other abdominal organs must be examined. The omentum has been shown to be involved in a small but significant percentage of apparent stage I patients on microscopic examination (Piver et al, 1978; Young et al, 1979).

4. The frequency of para-aortic lymph node involvement in apparent stage I ovarian cancer has been reported at between 7 and 25 per cent (Piver et al, 1978; Knapp & Freidman, 1974; Delgado et al, 1978; Knipscheer, 1982; Chen & Lee, 1983). It is therefore clear that women with stage I or II ovarian cancer should have para-aortic lymph node sampling performed.

Surgical procedure

Once accurate staging has been performed, maximum surgical effort is required to achieve total tumour clearance with no residual disease or, failing this, cytoreductive surgery in order to reduce residual disease to a minimum. This often requires persistent, time-consuming and aggressive surgery by an experienced surgeon. Many authors have emphasised the importance of not giving up too readily in the face of what initially appears to be unresectable disease.

As a general rule a total abdominal hysterectomy, bilateral salpingo-oophorectomy, omentectomy and apendicectomy should be performed.

The principle of cytoreductive surgery is well recognised and widely accepted. Griffiths et al (1979) have demonstrated that survival times, disease-free and progression-free intervals are all improved if residual disease is less than 1·6 cm diameter following bulk resection.

Greco et al (1981) found that patients with tumour <3 cm responded better to chemotherapy than patients with residual tumours >3 cm at largest diameter; they reported complete clinical response rates of 100 and 53 per cent respectively and no evidence of residual disease at second-look laparotomy in 11 and 86 per cent respectively. Table 22.10 summarises some of the studies which have used pathological restaging to assess response. In all there is a higher complete response rate in patients starting chemotherapy with minimal residual disease.

Whether primary surgery should include bowel resection and resection of the lower urinary tract is controversial. Castaldo et al (1981) performed intestinal resections to debulk residual disease to masses less than 2 cm in 12 of 419 patients treated for ovarian carcinoma. Colostomy was necessary in seven of these patients and their mean survival was 16 months (range 2–55 months). Berek et al (1983) reported resections of the lower urinary tract including partial cystectomies and partial ureteral resection with restoration of continuity in most cases. Only patients with optimal resection (less than 2 cm tumour) had improved survival. Significant complications occurred in 25 per cent of patients. Limited resection of lower urinary tract and bowel may therefore be appropriate if performed as part of a procedure which can achieve optimal surgical reduction or total disease clearance.

Such radical surgery is usually only justifiable in stage III disease. The frequency with which total tumour clearance or optimal cytoreduction can be achieved in stage III disease has been examined by Delgado et al (1984). In a study of 75 patients with stage III ovarian cancer they found that in spite of an aggressive surgical approach optimum results were obtained in only 28 per cent of cases. This figure is lower than reported in other studies. The discrepancy may be due to the wide variation in disease spread within FIGO stage 3. It has been suggested that tumours that lend themselves to surgical clearance are inherently less virulent. Nevertheless survival in the group of patients who have optimum surgical resection is invariably improved.

Table 22.10 Effect of residual disease on response to chemotherapy (from Ozols & Young, 1984)

Chemotherapy regime	References	Percentage of pathologically complete remissions (no. patients)	
		Non-bulky	Bulky
Hexa-CAF	Young et al, 1978	100 (8/8)	16 (5/32)
CHex-UP	Young et al, 1981	36 (5/14)	14 (5/37)
H-CAP	Greco et al, 1981	86 (18/21)	11 (3/29)
A-C	Parker et al, 1983	92 (11/12)	4 (1/24)
PAC	Ehrlich et al, 1979	30 (5/17)	13 (5/39)
Mean (range)		69 (30–100)	11 (4–16)

Postoperative treatment

Prognostic indicators

A significant advance in a rational approach to postoperative treatment of ovarian cancer has been the establishment of prognostic factors which help to define the probability of successful therapy. This knowledge has been gained from studies using careful surgical staging followed by chemotherapy or radiotherapy.

The evidence suggests that extent of residual disease and tumour grade are the most predictive variables for survival, followed by stage, age and histological type.

The extent of residual tumour and stage are independent prognostic indicators and the former may be the better predictor of therapeutic outcome.

Histological grade is particularly important in early-stage disease (Decker et al, 1972; Day et al, 1975) and more significant in patients with serous tumours than in those with endometrioid or clear-cell tumours (Dembo & Bush, 1982).

Adjuvant therapy options

One of the few favourable statements that can be made about ovarian cancer is that it is relatively chemosensitive. Chemotherapeutic regimens vary between the use of single-agent alkylating agents and combinations of newer and more potent drugs. The most widely used preparation is cisplatinum or its less toxic analogues, either singly or in combination.

There is some evidence that combination chemotherapy regimens are superior to single-agent therapy in terms of overall tumour response rates, but this must be set in the context of the increased morbidity associated with such potent preparations. The literature on this subject is abundant and confusing, and has to be read with great care as different authors quote different response rates for different regimes. Notwithstanding this, pathologically documented complete remission rates for most combination regimes are similar (Ozols & Young, 1984).

It is essential therefore that the choice of chemotherapy for an individual patient is made with great thought, taking into account the characteristics of the tumour as outlined above and not least the nature and wishes of the patient herself.

Although chemotherapy is not the ultimate solution to the problem of this disease, in order to achieve a progressive improvement in prognosis it is essential that the quest for new more potent drugs with low toxicity should continue until such time as an effective screening test is identified.

Radiotherapy as an adjuvant therapy in ovarian cancer has not met with widespread popularity in this country. Part of the reason for this is the frequently disseminated nature of the disease process and the recognition, therefore, that to be effective the treatment field should include the whole of the abdomen and pelvis. The effectiveness of radiotherapy is dependent upon the fact that the tumoricidal dose is less than the toxic dosage to neighbouring normal tissues, and dosage restrictions necessitated by the liver and kidneys have led to disagreement amongst radiotherapists as to the best method of delivery and the extent of adequate therapy.

It is clear now, however, from the work of Bush and Dembo in Toronto, that there is no place in any stage of this disease for pelvic radiation alone. Their study of stage I, II and asymptomatic stage III patients (Dembo et al, 1979) suggests that whole abdominal irradiation may have a role as adjuvant therapy. Whether it is a better option than chemotherapy is doubtful, although no data currently exist directly comparing these modalities.

Intraperitoneal radiocolloid therapy is, in theory, a method of applying high doses of radiation to tumour and omental surfaces with low dose to liver and kidneys, and should therefore be well suited to treating a disease which commonly involves the peritoneal surfaces of the entire abdominal cavity. A review of the literature (Rosenshein, 1983) showed that although no prospective, randomised, well-controlled study has demonstrated the effectiveness of radiocolloids, the available evidence suggests that the role of ^{32}P in early-stage disease is worthy of further investigation. ^{196}Au has largely been discarded due to problems of intraperitoneal adhesions and the main problem that has to be overcome with any intraperitoneal technique is distribution throughout the whole peritoneal cavity.

As the isotopes have a limited penetration, probably no more than 5 mm, they are of no value in the treatment of bulk disease. However it is reasonable to think that they would have a place in the management of stage Ic disease and cases of cyst rupture or capsule perforation. The isotope is picked up by macrophages within the peritoneal cavity and transported via the thoracic duct to the retroperitoneal nodes where microscopic disease might also be ablated. A study to evaluate the effectiveness of these theories is currently being performed by the GOG, and its results are awaited with interest.

It is clear that improving the prognosis for established disease will depend on accurate surgical staging, maximal surgical effort and individualisation of adjuvant therapy according to the prognostic indicators.

Monitoring the course of disease

A clinical diagnosis of complete response is not an accurate predictor of disease status. The number of patients in which this impression is confirmed histologically has varied in different studies (72 per cent Stuart et al, 1982; 63 per cent Curry et al, 1981; 60·2 per cent Smirz et al, 1985; 57 per cent Podratz et al, 1985 and Roberts et al, 1982; 46 per cent Webb et al, 1983), but the false negative rate is rarely less than 25 per cent.

An accurate indicator of disease status in patients who are undergoing or have completed a course of treatment is desirable for several reasons:

1. to confirm a complete response and allow prompt cessation of therapy, thereby limiting short- and long-term toxicity;
2. to avoid premature discontinuation of therapy when residual disease, though not clinically apparent, is present;
3. to confirm the presence of residual tumour requiring resection or the modification of treatment regimens;
4. as a research procedure to assess the efficacy of different treatment modalities.

The most commonly used method of assessment is surgery but less invasive techniques would be preferable if equally reliable.

CT scanning

CT scanning has been evaluated (Stern et al, 1981; Brenner et al, 1983) but the studies show a high level of false negative scans, making it an unreliable method for determining disease status.

Laparoscopy

Laparoscopy also has a high false negative rate varying from 20 to 77 per cent (Smith et al, 1977; Mangiani et al, 1979; Piver et al, 1980; Quinn et al, 1980; Ozols et al, 1981). In addition it is technically unsatisfactory in some patients, has a significant complication rate, and is unsuitable for the assessment of retroperitoneal structures. A positive finding at laparoscopy may spare the patient a laparotomy but a negative finding is not reliable enough to do so.

Tumour markers

A biochemical or immunological marker is more likely to be useful in monitoring disease than in diagnosis, as the need for absolute specificity is less, provided the marker is sufficiently sensitive and provides a clinically useful lead time.

Two recent studies suggest that serum CA 125 levels are a good reflection of bulk of disease and disease course is epithelial ovarian cancer. In the study by Canney et al (1984) 20 patients were assessed for response to chemotherapy and correlation of CA 125 with clinical response. CA 125 levels in patients with a good response to chemotherapy fell exponentially to a plateau within the normal range. Three patients in whom disease progressed following an initial transient response to chemotherapy showed a rising antigen level several weeks before clinical evidence of progression. No patients responding to chemotherapy showed such increases. A falling level of antigen indicated either a response to treatment or disease stabilisation, and these two groups could be distinguished by the half-life of the antigen which was much shorter (9·2 days v. 22·6 days) in the former. A response to chemotherapy was associated with an acute rise in serum CA 125 before falling probably due to tumour lysis.

Dodd et al. (1985) made a longitudinal assessment of 25 women with ovarian cancer. In nine of the patients who died of the disease serum levels of CA 125 were low after initial surgical debulking for a variable period, but in every case death was preceded by a consistent increase in detectable levels. Patients responding to treatment and remaining in remission (13) showed a dramatic decrease in CA 125 post-operatively, which usually remained low during follow-up. In two other patients who died, both with a history of numerous metastatic deposits not accessible to surgery, CA 125 levels remained elevated for 15 months after tumour debulking.

Second-look laparotomy

Second-look laparotomy was introduced into the management of ovarian cancer in the early 1960s, gained momentum with the advent of effective combination chemotherapy and is now an established part of the treatment regime in the USA. In the UK the procedure is usually reserved for therapeutic trials. As there are no randomised studies available the impact of second-look exploration on the overall survival of patients with ovarian cancer is speculative. However there have been a number of studies from which useful information has emerged concerning the reliability of the procedure and the patients most likely to benefit.

The finding of a negative second-look laparotomy is correlated with original stage of disease, thoroughness of primary tumour reduction and in some studies (Berek et al, 1984) but not all (Smirz et al, 1985; Raju et al, 1982; Cohen et al, 1983), with initial tumour grade. Using these criteria it is possible to define a group of patients with a low incidence of incorrect clinical assessment in which clinical impression of complete response may be adequate and re-exploration unnecessary. A pathologically confirmed negative second-look laparotomy is a good predictor of survival. Recurrence does, however, occur in a significant number of these patients (Table 22.11) and is most commonly associated with advanced stage and large volume of disease at initial operation and the amount of chemotherapy administered

Table 22.11   Recurrent disease after negative second-look laparotomy

Reference	No. of patients	Recurrent disease (%)
Schwartz and Smith, 1980	58	12·1
Phillips et al, 1979	21	4·7
Curry et al, 1981	17	17·6
Roberts et al, 1982	61	9·8
Greco et al, 1981	17	5·8
Podratz et al, 1985	77	15·6
Smirz et al, 1985	30	26·7

prior to second look. These recurrences reflect the limitations of the second-look procedure.

Although therapy is commonly discontinued after a negative second look it is possible that additional treatment such as intraperitoneal chromic phosphorus would reduce recurrence rates.

Prognosis after positive second-look laparotomy is unfavourably influenced by increasing tumour size and increasing histological grade of residual tumour. Schwartz and Smith (1980) advocate volume reduction at second look and report improved survival in these patients. However other studies (Smirz et al, 1985; Podratz et al, 1985) suggest that there is minimal value in further aggressive tumour reduction.

In summary it would appear that there is a group of patients who do not benefit from second-look procedures; those with original early-stage disease completely resected (clinical impression being accurate in most cases), and a group of patients in whom a negative second-look procedure is unreliable; those with original advanced-stage or bulky disease treated with cisplatin (in whom cessation of treatment may be inappropriate). At present there is no satisfactory alternative monitor of disease but serum tumour markers may replace second-look procedures in the near future.

EXPERIMENTAL APPROACHES

New cytotoxic agents

A number of platinum analogues have been developed in attempts to increase efficacy or decrease the toxicity associated with cisplatin. Carboplatin (JM8) has comparable antitumour activity to cisplatin with less ototoxicity and nephrotoxicity and is now in clinical use. Several other drugs which appear to have activity in treatment of ovarian cancer are under evaluation; ifosfamide, prednimustine, galactilol, and mitomycin, but there is no evidence that these agents are more effective than those presently available.

Hormonal therapy

The suggestion that hormonal therapy may have a place in treatment of ovarian cancer was based upon the role of the ovaries as target organs as well as a major source of hormones.

Ten studies involving 176 patients with advanced ovarian cancer have examined the use of progestins (Thigpen et al, 1984). The overall response rate was low, 12 per cent (22 patients).

Few patients with advanced ovarian cancer have been treated with anti-oestrogens. In one series of 13 patients, one had a partial response and four disease stabilisation (Schwartz et al, 1982). A second study described prolonged partial remissions in three women with slowly evolving serous cystadenocarcinomas that had failed previous cytotoxic treatments (Myers et al, 1981). Further investigation is warranted as hormonal therapy has a low incidence of side-effects and is potentially of great value.

Several studies have examined the incidence of oestrogen and progesterone receptors in ovarian cancer: 52 per cent of cases in these series had significant titres of both oestrogen and progesterone receptors and 74 per cent had detectable oestrogen receptors. The presence of receptors correlated with degree of differentiation of the tumour and improved prognosis, but could not be related to response to hormonal therapy on the basis of present data (Thigpen et al, 1984).

Stem cell assay

The development of the human tumour stem cell assay (Hamburger & Salmon, 1977) appeared to provide a method of selecting drugs with specific action in individual patients with the possibility of improving the response rate, decreasing toxicity from ineffective drugs, aiding development of more effective drug combinations and speeding up selection of new drugs for clinical trial. However there have been problems with both the technical and clinical application of the assay. Although ovarian tumours are usually more easily grown in the assay system than other tumours, with greater than 90 per cent colony formation in one study (Welander & Alberts, 1985), there is no evidence to show that the sensitivity data available are of clinical relevance. The assay has a relatively high predictive accuracy for resistance but that for sensitivity is lower (Williams, 1985), with the result that many patients would be denied a potentially active drug if it formed the basis for therapy. At present the assay remains a research tool with possible roles in screening for new drugs and as a biological model for tumours.

Immunotherapy

Immunotherapy is potentially the most specific treatment for cancer. However, as discussed above, although several tumour-associated antigens to ovarian cancer have been identified, a specific antigen remains elusive.

Investigation of the role of immunotherapy in ovarian cancer is proceeding along two avenues. One is based upon the finding that patients with ovarian cancer have impaired immunological status and attempts to stimulate non-specifically cell-mediated immunity with micro-organisms such as BCG and *Corynebacterium parvum.* A randomised controlled trial comparing treatment with cyclophosphamide and adriamycin alone, or with BCG in stage III and IV patients, produced significantly better pathologically proven complete responses in the BCG group (18 v. 3 per cent) and significantly better median survival (22 v. 14 months) (Alberts & Moon, 1980).

Corynebacterium parvum given intravenously with oral melphalan produced better response rates and longer survival than historical controls in previously untreated stage III patients, than did melphalan alone, but the efficacy of *C. parvum* was not confirmed in a randomised controlled trial (Creasman et al, 1979). Intraperitoneal *C. parvum* produced surgically documented regression of tumour in five of 11 patients with poorly differentiated stage III epithelial ovarian cancer persisting as small nodules after chemotherapy with cyclophosphamide, adriamycin and cisplatin. A favourable response to treatment was associated with abdominal pain, fever and chills (Bast et al, 1983b).

Interferon inhibits growth of ovarian carcinoma *in vitro* as well as stimulating antibody-dependent cell-mediated cytotoxicity. Studies in ovarian cancer patients have been disappointing but intraperitoneal therapy has not been investigated.

The second approach is based upon the knowledge that tumour-associated antigens are produced in ovarian cancer, but is limited by the failure as yet to identify a specific antigen. Preliminary reports using heteroantisera from several species have been encouraging.

A combined approach using tumour-directed monoclonal antibodies with active non-specific immunostimulants such as *C. parvum* may prove to be useful.

Biological modifiers

Mullerian inhibiting substance produces regression of the Mullerian duct in male embryos, and has been shown to inhibit the growth of a human ovarian cancer cell line *in vitro* and in nude mice (Donahoe et al, 1981). This is a potentially specific treatment which awaits evaluation in clinical trials.

High-dose chemotherapy

Animal studies suggest that cisplatin nephrotoxicity can be eliminated by administration in hypertonic saline (Lillerst, 1981) allowing high-dose systemic therapy. Preliminary results of a trial using high-dose cisplatin in refractory ovarian cancer patients who had relapsed after previous treatment with standard-dose cisplatin demonstrated a response in 35 per cent of cases (Ozols et al, 1984b).

The theoretical basis to intraperitoneal chemotherapy is that the high intraperitoneal concentrations of therapeutic agents which have been shown to occur for methotrexate, fluorouracil, adriamycin and cisplatin are able to produce a response in cancers resistant to the maximally tolerable systemic dose. The four agents mentioned have been evaluated in phase I–II trials, which show this method to be both safe and practicable, and there have been objective responses to adriamycin and cisplatin. In one study using intraperitoneal cisplatin, 90 mg/m^2 given intraperitoneally produced nephrotoxicity but with an intravenous neutralising agent, sodium thiosulphate, doses as high as 270 mg/m^2 were administered without nephrotoxicity

(Howell et al, 1982). Further studies are currently in progress which hopefully will establish the clinical value of this treatment.

Pharmacological reversal of drug resistance

Many ovarian cancer patients who do not achieve a complete remission with initial chemotherapy are resistant to treatment with a wide spectrum of other drugs. Rogan et al. (1984) noted that adriamycin resistance in ovarian cancer cell lines was reversed following exposure of cells to verapamil. Preliminary results of a clinical trial of verapamil in refractory ovarian cancer patients suggest that sensitisation by verapamil is possible without myelosuppression or gastrointestinal toxicity (Ozols et al, 1984).

SUMMARY

There is no doubt that there have been significant developments in the understanding and management of epithelial ovarian cancer during the past decade. Nevertheless it remains an evil and ominous disease. Progress has occurred over a wide spectrum but at a plodding pace in a disease which awaits a dramatic breakthrough.

There is no foreseeable prospect of a treatment being able to produce long-term remissions or indeed cures in advanced-stage disease. One area of hope for progress is the possibility of early diagnosis. However even the prospects for early detection are uncertain and depend upon the existence of premalignant or early disease of sufficient duration to be detectable by interval screening. If such a stage exists, production of a screening test with sufficient sensitivity and specificity to justify a large-scale prospective study may not be far away.

Until such a breakthrough is made those involved in the management of ovarian cancer have a responsibility to ensure that all available knowledge is utilised. Some degree of improvement in ovarian cancer statistics is possible *now* through consistent application of established principles. General practitioners, as well as specialists, must be aware of risk factors for the disease and suspicious of gastrointestinal symptoms in the high-risk group of women. General surgeons and gynaecologists must be prepared to ensure that thorough staging and optimum surgery is performed, and to request assistance from specialists who are skilled in this field. Adjuvant chemo-therapy and radiotherapy must be performed in specialist centres supported by accurate staging, a clear report of surgical findings, and close collaboration with surgeons and pathologists. Finally, prevention by prophylactic oophorectomy and hormone replacement therapy should be considered and discussed with all women who have completed their family and are undergoing an elective laparotomy.

The ultimate hope must be that developments in the management of ovarian cancer will follow the pattern of progress in cervical malignancy, with introduction of effective screening techniques to clearly identify the women at risk at a premalignant stage and provide the opportunities for preventive measures. For as long as this remains a dream, and opportunities for prevention are confined to women undergoing surgery for benign desease, the clinician must concentrate upon improving the prognosis for established disease by conscientious adherence to recognised principles of management.

REFERENCES

Alberts D S, Moon T E 1980 Randomized trial of chemotherapy versus chemoimmunotherapy for advanced ovarian carcinoma: a preliminary report of a southwest oncology study group. In: National Cancer Institute Second International Conference on Immunotherapy of Cancer: Present status of trials in man. New York, p 13

American Cancer Society 1982 Cancer facts and figures. New York

Annegers J F, Malkasian G D 1981 Patterns of other neoplasia in patients with endometrial carcinoma. Cancer 48: 856–859

Annegers J F, Strom H, Decker D G, Dokerty M B, O'Fallon W M 1979 Ovarian cancer: incidence and case control study. Cancer 43: 723–729

Anstey J T, Blythe J G 1978 Fibrin degradation products and the diagnosis of ovarian carcinoma. Obstetrics and Gynecology 52: 605

Astedt B, Svanberg L, Nilsson I M 1971 Fibrin degradation products and ovarian tumours. British Medical Journal 4: 458

Averette H E, Seven B V 1982 Debulking surgery and second look operation. International Journal of Radiation, Oncology, Biology, Physics 8: 891–892

Awais G M 1973 Serum lactic dehydrogenase levels in the diagnosis and treatment of carcinoma of the ovary. American Journal of Obstetrics and Gynecology 116: 1053

Awais G M 1978 Carcinoma of the ovary and serum lactic acid dehydrogenase levels. Surgery, Gynecology and Obstetrics 146: 893

Barber H R K 1979 Ovarian Cancer, Part 1. Ca—A Cancer Journal for Clinicians 29: 341

Bast R C, Klug T L, St John E, Jenison E, Niloff J M, Lazarus H et al 1983a A radioimmunoassay using a monoclonal antibody to monitor the course of epithelial ovarian cancer. New England Journal of Medicine 309: 883–887

Bast R C Jr, Berek J S, Obrist R, Griffiths C T, Berkowitz R S, Hacker R F et al 1983b Intraperitoneal immunotherapy of human ovarian carcinoma with *Corynebacterium parvum*. Cancer Research 43: 1395–1401

Benham F J, Povey M S, Harris H 1978 Placenta-like alkaline phosphatase in malignant and ovarian tumours. Clinica Chimica Acta 86: 201

Berek J S, Hacker N F, Lagasse L D et al 1983 Lower urinary tract resection as part of cytoreduction surgery for ovarian carcinoma. Gynecology and Oncology 13: 87–92

Berek J S, Hacker N F, Lagasse L D, Poth T, Resnick G, Nieberg R K 1984 Second look laparotomy in stage III epithelial ovarian cancer: clinical variables associated with disease status. Obstetrics and Gynecology 64: 207–212

Bhattacharya M, Barlow J J 1973a An immunologic comparison between serous cystadenocarcinoma of the ovary and other human gynecologic tumours. American Journal of Obstetrics and Gynecology 117: 849

Bhattacharya M, Barlow J J 1973b Immunologic studies of human serous cystadenocarcinoma of ovary; demonstration of tumor-associated antigens. Cancer 31: 588

Bhattacharya M, Barlow J J 1978 Ovarian tumour antigens. Cancer 42: 1616

Bhattacharya M, Barlow J J 1979 Tumor markers for ovarian cancer. International Advances in Surgical Oncology 2: 155

Bhattacharya M, Chatterjee S K, Barlow J J 1976 Uridine 5'-diphosphate-galactose: glycoprotein galactosyltransferase activity in the ovarian cancer patient. Cancer Research 36: 2096

Bloom L M 1962 Certain observations based on a study of 141 cases of primary adenocarcinoma of the ovaries (1950–1959). South African Medical Journal 36: 714

Brenner D E, Grosh W W, Jones H W 1983 An evaluation of the accuracy of computed tomography in patients with ovarian carcinoma prior to second look laparotomy. ASCO Proceedings 2: 149

Burrows S 1980 Serum enzymes in the diagnosis of ovarian malignancy. American Journal of Obstetrics and Gynecology 137: 140

Campbell S, Goessens L, Goswamy R, Whitehead M 1982 Real time ultrasonography for determination of ovarian morphology and volume: a possible early screening test for ovarian cancer? Lancet 1: 425

Canney P A, Moore M, Wilkinson P M, James R D 1984 Ovarian cancer antigen CA 125: a prospective clinical assessment of its role as a tumour marker. British Journal of Cancer 50: 765–769

Casagrande J T, Lovie E W, Pike M C, Roy S, Ross R K, Henderson B E 1979 'Incessant ovulation' and ovarian cancer. Lancet 2: 170–173

Casagrande J T, Pike M C, Henderson B E 1983 Oral contraceptives and ovarian cancer (letter). New England Journal of Medicine 308: 843–844

Castaldo T W, Petrilli E S, Ballou S, Lagasse L D 1981 Intestinal operations in patients with an ovarian carcinoma. American Journal of Obstetrics and Gynecology 139: 80–84

Chatterjee S K, Bhattacharya M, Barlow J J 1978 Correlation of UDP-galactose glycoprotein: galactosyltransferase levels in the sera with the clinical status of ovarian cancer patients. Cancer Letters 5: 238

Chatterjee S K, Bhattacharya M, Barlow J J 1979 Glycosyltransferase and glycosidase activities in ovarian cancer patients. Cancer Research 39: 1943

Chatterjee S K, Bhattacharya M, Barlow J J 1980 Determination of serum galactosyltransferase levels in ovarian cancer patients for the evaluation of the effectiveness of therapeutic programs. Cancer Letters 8: 247

Chen S S, Lee L 1983 Incidence of paraaortic and pelvic lymph node metastases in epithelial carcinoma of the ovary. Gynecologic Oncology 16: 95–100

Christ J E, Loetze E C 1975 The residual ovary syndrome. Obstetrics and Gynecology 46: 551

Cohen C J, Goldberg J D, Holland J F, Bruckner H W, Deppe G, Gusberg S B, et al 1983 Improved therapy with cisplatin regimens for patients with ovarian carcinoma (FIGO stages III and IV) as measured by surgical end-staging (second look operation). American Journal of Obstetrics and Gynecology 145: 955

Counsellor V S, Hunt W, Haigue F M 1955 Carcinoma of the ovary following hysterectomy and oophorectomy. American Journal of Obstetrics and Gynaecology 69: 538

Cramer D W, Hutchison G B, Welch W R, Scully R E, Knapp R C 1982a Factors affecting the association of oral contraceptives and ovarian cancer. New England Journal of Medicine 307: 1047–1057

Cramer D W, Welch S R, Scully R E, Wojciechowski C A 1982b Ovarian cancer and talc: a case control study. Cancer 50: 372–376

Creasman W T, Rutledge F 1971 The prognostic value of peritoneal cytology in gynecologic malignant disease. American Journal of Obstetrics and Gynecology 110: 773

Creasman W T, Gall S A, Blessing J A, Schmidt H J, Abu-Ghazaleh S, Whisnant J K et al 1979 Chemoimmunotherapy in the management of primary stage III ovarian cancer: a Gynaecologic Oncology Study Group. Cancer Treatment Reports 63: 319–323

Crombach G, Zippel H H, Wurz H 1985 Experiences with CA 125, a tumour marker for malignant epithelial ovarian tumours. Geburtshilfe Frauenheilkd 45(4): 205–212

Curry S L, Zembo M M, Nahhas W A, Jahshan A E, Whitney C W, Mortel R 1981 Second look laparotomy for ovarian cancer. Gynecologic Oncology 11: 114–118

Day T G, Gallagher H S, Rutledge F 1975 Epithelial carcinoma of the ovary: prognostic importance of histologic grade. National Cancer Institute Monogram 42: 15–18

Decker D G, Musey E, Williams T J 1972 Grading of gynaecologic malignancy: epithelial ovarian cancer. In Proceedings of the 7th National Cancer Congress, J B Lipincott, Philadelphia, pp 232–241

Delgado G, Chun B, Caglar H, Bepko F 1978 Paraaortic lymphadenectomy in gynecologic malignancies confined to the pelvis. Obstetrics and Gynecology 50: 418–423

Delgado G, Oram D H, Petrilli E S 1984 Stage III epithelial ovarian cancer: the role of maximal surgical reduction. Gynecologic Oncology 18: 293–298

Dembo A J, Bush R S 1982 Choice of postoperative therapy based on prognostic factors. International Journal of Radiation, Oncology, Biology, Physics 8: 893–897

Dembo A J, Bush R S, Beale F A, Bean H A, Pringle J F, Sturgeon J F 1979 The Princess

Margaret Hospital study of ovarian cancer: Stage I, II and asymptomatic III presentations. Cancer Treatment Reports 63: 349

Dembo A J, Chang P L, Urbach G I 1985 Clinical correlations of ovarian cancer antigen NB/ 70K: a preliminary report. Obstetrics and Gynecology 65: 710–714

De Neef J C, Hollenbeck C J R 1966 The fact of ovaries preserved at the time of oophorectomy. American Journal of Obstetrics and Gynecology 96: 1088

Dicker R C, Webster L A, Layde P M 1983 Oral contraceptive use and the risk of ovarian cancer. Journal of the American Medical Association 249: 1596–1599

Dodd J, Tyler J P P, Crandon A J, Blumenthal N J, Fay R A, Baird P J et al 1985 The value of the monoclonal antibody (cancer antigen 125) in serial monitoring of ovarian cancer: a comparison with circulating immune complexes. British Journal of Obstetrics and Gynaecology 92: 1054–1060

Donahoe P, Fuller A F, Scully R E, Guy S R, Budzik G P 1981 Mullerian inhibiting substance inhibits growth of a human ovarian cancer in nude mice. Annals of Surgery 194: 477–480

Donaldson E S, van Nagell J R, Pursell S, Gay E C, Meeker W R, Kashmiri R et al 1980 Multiple biochemical markers in patients with gynecologic malignancies. Cancer 45: 948

Drahovsky D, Duzendorfer U, Ziegenhagen G, Drahovsky M, Kellen J A 1981 Reevaluation of C-reactive protein in cancer sera by radioimmunoassay and radial immunodiffusion. Oncology (Basel) 38: 286

Dunn J E 1975 Cancer epidemiology in populations of the United States—with emphasis on Hawaii and California and Japan. Cancer Research 35: 3240

Ehrlich C E, Einhorn L, Williams S D, Morgan J 1979 Chemotherapy for stage III–IV epithelial ovarian cancer with cisplatin, adriamycin and cyclophosphamide: a preliminary report. Cancer Treatment Reports 63: 281–288

Epenetos A A, Britton K E, Mather S, Shepherd J, Granowska M, Taylor-Papadimitriou J 1982 Targeting of iodine-123-labelled tumour-associated monoclonal antibodies to ovarian, breast and gastrointestinal tumours. Lancet 2: 999–1005

Fagan E G, Allan E D, Klahans A M 1956 Ovarian neoplasm and repeat pelvic surgery. Obstetrics and Gynecology 7: 418

Fathalla M F 1972 Factors in causation and incidence of ovarian cancer. Obstetrics, Gynecology and Surgery 27: 757–768

Feldman G B, Knapp R C 1974 Lymphatic drainage of the peritoneal cavity and its significance in ovarian cancer. American Journal of Obstetrics and Gynecology 119: 991

Fishman W H, Inglis N R, Vaitukaitis J 1975a Regan isoenzyme and human chorionic gonadotrophin in ovarian cancer. National Cancer Institute Monograph 42: 63

Fishman W H, Raam S, Stolbach L L 1975b Markers for ovarian cancer: Regan isoenzyme and other glycoproteins. Seminars in Oncology 2: 211

Franceschi S, La Vecchia C, Helmrich S P, Mangioni C, Tognoni G 1982 Risk factors for epithelial ovarian cancer in Italy. American Journal of Epidemiology 115: 714–719

Funck-Bretano P 1958 L'ovaire restant apres hysterectomie. Revue Francaise de Gynecologie et d'Obstetrique 53: 217

Gibbs E K 1971 Suggested prophylaxis for ovarian cancer. American Journal of Obstetrics and Gynecology 11: 756

Gold P, Friedman S O 1962 Demonstration of tumour specific antigens in human colonic carcinoma by immunological tolerance and absorption techniques. Journal of Experimental Medicine 121: 439–462

Goldenberg D M, DeLand F, Kim E, Bennett S, Primus F J, van Nagell J R 1978 Use of radiolabelled antibodies to carcinoembryonic antigen for the detection and localisation of diverse cancers by external photo scanning. New England Journal of Medicine 298: 1384

Goldenberg D M, Kim E, Deland F H, van Nagell J R, Javadpour N 1980 Clinical radioimmunodetection of cancer with radioactive antibodies to human chorionic gonadotrophin. Science 208: 1284

Golub L J 1953 The diagnosis of ovarian cancer. American Journal of Obstetrics and Gynecology 66: 169

Greco F A, Julian C G, Richardson R L, Burnett L, Hande K R, Oldham R K 1981 Advanced ovarian cancer: brief intensive combination chemotherapy and second look operation. Obstetrics and Gynecology 58: 199–205

Green M H, Clark J W, Blayney D W 1984 The epidemiology of ovarian cancer. Seminars in Oncology 11: 209–226

Griffiths C T, Parker L M, Fuller A F Jr 1979 Role of cytoreductive surgical treatment in the management of advanced ovarian cancer. Cancer Treatment Reports 62: 235–240

Grogan R H 1967 Reappraisal of residual ovaries. American Journal of Obstetrics and Gynecology 97: 124

Grogan R H, Duncan C J 1966 Ovarian salvage in routine abdominal hysterectomy. American Journal of Obstetrics and Gynecology 70: 1277

Grundsell H, Ekman G, Gullberg B, Johnsson J E, Larsson G, Lundahl B et al 1981 Some aspects of prophylactic oophorectomy and ovarian carcinoma. Annales Chirurgie et Gynaecologiae 70: 36–42

Hamburger A, Salmon S 1977 Primary bioassay of human tumour stem cells. Science 197: 461–463

Hansen H J, Snyder J J, Miller E 1974 Carcinoembryonic antigen (CEA) assay: a laboratory adjunct in the diagnosis and management of cancer. Human Pathology 3: 139

Hartge P, Lesher L P, McGowan L, Hoover R 1982 Coffee and ovarian cancer (letter). International Journal of Cancer 30: 531

Heinonen P K, Tontti K, Koivula T, Pystynen P 1985 Tumour associated antigen CA 125 in patients with ovarian cancer. British Journal of Obstetrics and Gynaecology 92: 528–531

Henderson B E, Ross R K, Pike M C, Casagrande J T 1982 Endogenous hormones as a major factor in human cancer. Cancer Research 42: 3232–3239

Henderson W J, Hamilton T C, Griffiths K 1979 Talc in normal and malignant ovarian tissue. Lancet 1: 499

Hildreth N G, Kelsey J L, LiVolsi V A, Fischer D B, Holford T R, Mostow E D et al 1981 An epidemiologic study of epithelial carcinoma of the ovary. American Journal of Epidemiology 114: 398–405

Holme G M 1963 Prognostic factors in malignant ovarian disease. Aeta Unio Internat Contra Cancrum 19: 113S

Howell S B, Pfeifle C L, Wung W E, Olshen R A, Lucas W E, Yon J L 1982 Intraperitoneal cisplatin with systemic thiosulfate protection. Annals of Internal Medicine 97: 845–951

Joly D J, Lilienfeld A M, Diamond E L 1978 An epidemiologic study of the relationship of reproductive experience to cancer of the ovary. American Journal of Epidemiology 98: 190–209

Keetel W C, Pixley E E, Buchsbaum H J 1974 Experience with peritoneal cytology in the management of gynecologic malignancies. American Journal of Obstetrics and Gynecology 120: 174–182

Kent S W, Mackay D G 1960 Primary cancer of the ovary: an analysis of 349 cases. American Journal of Obstetrics and Gynecology 94: 766

Khoo S K, Daunter B, Mackay E 1979 Carcinoembryonic antigen and beta-2-microglobulin as serum tumour markers in women with genital cancer. International Journal of Gynaecology and Obstetrics 16: 388

Kim E E, Deland F H, Nelson M O, Bennett S, Simmons G, Alpert E et al 1980 Radioimmunodetection of cancer with radiolabelled antibodies to alpha fetoprotein. Cancer Research 40: 308

Knapp R C, Friedman E A 1974 Aortic lymph node metastases in early ovarian cancer. American Journal of Obstetrics and Gynecology 119: 1013–1017

Knauf S, Urbach G I 1981 Identification, purification and radioimmunoassay of NB/70K, a human ovarian tumour associated antigen. Cancer Research 41: 1351

Knipscheer R J L 1982 Para-aortal lymph node dissection in 20 cases of primary epithelial ovary carcinoma stage I (FIGO). Influence on staging. European Journal of Obstetrics, Gynecology and Reproductive Biology 13: 303–307

Kofler E 1972 The incidence of previous hysterectomies and/or unilateral oophorectomies in women with malignant ovarian tumours. Gubertshilfe frauenheit 32: 873

Kottmeier H (ed) 1982 Annual report on the results of treatment in gynaecological cancer, vol 18. FIGO, Stockholm

La Vecchia C, Liberati A, Franceschi S 1982 Noncontraceptive estrogen use and the occurrence of ovarian cancer (letter). Journal of the National Cancer Institute 69: 1207

La Vecchia C, Franceschi S, Gallus G, Decarli A, Liberati A, Tognoni G 1983 Incessant ovulation and ovarian cancer: a critical approach. International Journal of Epidemiology 12: 161–164

Lillerst C L 1981 Alterations in the toxicity of cis-dichlorodiamine platinum II and in tissue localisation of platinum as a function of NaCl concentration in the vehicle of administration. Toxicology and Applied Pharmacology 61 : 99–108

Lynch H T, Lynch P M 1979 Tumour variation in the cancer family syndrome. American Journal of Surgery 138 : 439

Lynch H T, Albano W, Black L, Lynch J F, Recabaren J, Pierseon R 1981 Familial excess of cancer of the ovary and other anatomic sites. Journal of the American Medical Association 245 : 261

MacFarlane C, Sturgis M C, Fetterman F C 1955 Results of an experiment in the control of cancer of the female pelvic organs and report of a 15 year research. American Journal of Obstetrics and Gynecology 69 : 294

Mackenzie L L 1968 On discussion of the frequency of oophorectomy at the time of hysterectomy. American Journal of Obstetrics and Gynecology 100 : 724

Mangiani C Bolis G, Motteni P 1979 Indications, advantages and limits of laparoscopy in ovarian cancer. Gynecologic Oncology 7 : 47–55

McGowan L, Parent L, Lednar W, Norris H J 1979 The woman at risk for developing ovarian cancer. Gynecologic Oncology 7 : 325–344

Mencer J, Modan M, Ronon L 1979 Possible role of mumps virus in the etiology of ovarian cancer. Cancer 43 : 1375

Morrow C P 1981 Malignant and borderline tumours of the ovary : clinical features and management. In : Coppleson M (ed) Gynecologic oncology, vol. 2. Churchill Livingstone, Edinburgh

Muir C S, Mectoux J 1978 Ovarian cancer : some epidemiological features. World Health Statistics W.31 : 51

Myers M, Moore G E, Major F J 1981 Advanced ovarian carcinoma : response to anti-estrogen therapy. Cancer 48 : 2368–2370

Nathanson L, Fishman W H 1971 New observations on the Regan isoenzyme of alkaline phosphatase in cancer patients. Cancer 27 : 1388

Newell G R, Rawlings W, Krementz E T 1974 Multiple primary neoplasms in blacks compared in whites. III. Initial cancers of the female breast and uterus. Journal of the National Cancer Institute 53 : 369–373

Newhouse M L 1979 Cosmetic talc and ovarian cancer. Lancet 1 : 528

Newhouse M L, Pearson R M, Fullerton J M, Boesen E A, Shannon H S 1977 A case control study of carcinoma of the ovary. British Journal of Preventive and Social Medicine 31 : 148–153

Ozols R F, Fisher R I, Anderson T, Makuch R, Young R C 1981 Peritoneoscopy in the management of ovarian cancer. American Journal of Obstetrics and Gynecology 140 : 611–619

Ozols R F, Young R C 1984 Chemotherapy of ovarian cancer. Seminars in Oncology 11 : 251–263

Ozols R F, Corder B J, Jacob J, Wesley M N, Ostchega Y, Young R C 1984a High dose cisplatin in hypertonic saline. Annals of Internal Medicine 100 : 19–24

Ozols R F, Rogan A M, Hamilton T C 1984b Verapamil plus adriamycin in refractory ovarian cancer : design of a clinical trial on basis of reversal of adriamycin resistance in human ovarian cancer cell lines. Proceedings of the American Association of Cancer Research 28 : 300

Palovcek F P 1969 Cited in : Randall C L (ed) 1970 Background of statistical data on ovarian cancer. Gynaecological oncology. Excerpta Medical Foundation, p 211

Parker L M, Griffiths C T, Yankee R A 1983 Combination chemotherapy with adriamycin-cyclophosphamide for advanced ovarian carcinoma. Cancer 46 : 669–674

Philips B P, Buchsbaum H J, Lifshitz S 1979 Re-exploration after treatment for ovarian carcinoma. Gynecological Oncology 8 : 339

Piver M S 1983 Importance of proper staging in ovarian carcinoma. Clinics in Obstetrics and Gynaecology 10(2) : 223–234

Piver M S, Lele S B, Barlow J J 1976 Preoperative and intraoperative evaluation in ovarian malignancy. Obstetrics and Gynecology 48 : 312–315

Piver M S, Barlow J J, Lele S B 1978 Incidence of subclinical metastasis in stage I and II ovarian carcinoma. Obstetrics and Gynecology 52 : 100–104

Piver M S, Lele S B, Barlow J J, Gamarra M 1980 Second look laparoscopy prior to proposed second look laparotomy. Obstetrics and Gynecology 55 : 571–573

Podratz, K C, Malkasian G D, Hilton J F, Harris E A, Gaffey T A 1985 Second loop laparotomy in ovarian cancer: evaluation of pathologic variables. American Journal of Obstetrics and Gynecology 152: 230–235

Prior P, Waterhouse J A H 1981 Multiple primary cancers of the breast and ovary. British Journal of Cancer 44: 628–636

Quinn M A, Bishop G H, Campbell J J, Rogerson J, Pepperell R J 1980 Laparoscopic follow-up of patients with ovarian carcinoma. British Journal of Obstetrics and Gynaecology 87: 1132–1139

Raju K S, McKina J A, Barker G H, Wiltshaw E, Jones J M 1982 Second look operations in the planned management of advanced ovarian carcinoma. American Journal of Obstetrics and Gynecology 144: 650

Randal C L 1963 Ovarian conservation. In: Meigs, Sturgis (eds) Progress in gynecology, vol. 4: Grune & Stratton, New York, p 457

Ranney B, Abou-Ghazalem S 1977 The future function and fortune of ovarian tissue which is retained in vivo during hysterectomy. American Journal of Obstetrics and Gynecology 128: 626

Reimer R R, Hoover R, Fraumeni J F Jr, Young R C 1978 Second primary neoplasms following ovarian cancer. Journal of the National Cancer Institute 61: 1195–1197

Reycraft J L 1955 Discussion of Counsellor. American Journal of Obstetrics and Gynecology 69: 543

Risch H A, Weiss N S, Lyon J L 1983 Events of reproductive life and the incidence of epithelial ovarian cancer. American Journal of Epidemiology 111: 128–139

Roberts W S, Hodel K, Rich W M, De Saia P J 1982 Second look laparotomy in the management of gynecologic malignancy. Gynecologic Oncology 13: 345–355

Rogan A M, Hamilton T C, Young R C, Klecker R W Jr, Ozols R F 1984 Reversal of adriamycin resistance by verapamil in human ovarian cancer. Science 224: 994–996

Rohl A N, Langer A M, Selikoff I J 1976 Consumer talcums and powders: mineral and chemical characterization. Journal of Toxicology and Environmental Health 2: 255–284

Rosenberg L, Shapiro S, Slone D, Kaufman D W, Helmrich S J, Miettinen O S et al 1982 Epithelial ovarian cancer and combination oral contraceptives. Journal of the American Medical Association 247: 3210–3212

Rosenshein N B 1983 Radioisotopes in the treatment of ovarian cancer. Clinics in Obstetrics and Gynecology 10: 279–295

Sarjadi S, Daunter B, Mackay E, Magon H, Khou S K 1980 A multiparametric approach to tumour markers detectable in serum in patients with carcinoma of the ovary or uterine cervix. Gynaecologic Oncology 10: 113

Schaburt J W 1960 Oophorectomy—is wanton removal justified by fact? Transactions of the College of Physicians of South Africa 4: 11

Schoenberg B S, Greenberg R A, Eisenberg H 1969 Occurrence of certain multiple primary cancers in females. Journal of the National Cancer Institute 43: 15–32

Schottenfeld D, Berg J W 1971 Incidence of multiple primary cancers. IV. Cancers of the female breast and genital organs. Journal of the National Cancer Institute 46: 161–170

Schottenfeld D, Berg J W, Vitsky B 1969 Incidence of multiple primary cancers. II. Index cancers arising in the stomach and lower digestive system. Journal of the National Cancer Institute 43: 77–86

Schwartz A L, Vasquez H, Selim M 1975 Serum lactic dehydrogenase and ovarian carcinoma (letter). American Journal of Obstetrics and Gynecology 123: 106

Schwartz P E 1981 Surgical management of ovarian cancer. Archives of Surgery 116: 99–106

Schwartz P E, Smith J P 1980 Second look operations in ovarian cancer. American Journal of Obstetrics and Gynecology 138: 1124

Schwartz P E, Keating G, Maclusky N, Naftolin F, Eisenfeld A 1982 Tamoxifen therapy for advanced ovarian cancer. Obstetrics and Gynecology 50: 583–588

Scully R E 1981 Definition of precursors in gynecologic cancer. Cancer 48: 531–537

Seppala M, Pihkoh H, Ruoslahti E 1975 CEA and AFP in malignant tumours of the female genital tract. Cancer 35: 1377

Shapiro S P, Nunez C 1983 Psammoma bodies in the cervicovaginal smear in association with a papillary tumour of the peritoneum. Obstetrics and Gynecology 61: 130–134

Sheid B, Lu T, Pedrinan L 1977 Plasma ribonuclease: a marker for the detection of ovarian cancer. Cancer 39: 2204

Sirsart A V, Talavdekar R V, Suraiya J N, Kullkami J N 1982 Studies on serum amylases in ovarian, prostatic and colonic cancer. Indian Journal of Cancer 19: 204

Smirz L R, Stehman F B, Ulbright T M, Sutton G P, Ehrlich C E 1985 Second look laparotomy after chemotherapy in the management of ovarian malignancy. American Journal of Obstetrics and Gynecology 152: 661–668

Smith J P, Day T G 1979 Review of ovarian cancer at the University of Texas Systems Cancer Center, MD Anderson Hospital and Tumor Institute. American Journal of Obstetrics and Gynecology 135: 984

Smith L H, Richard H O 1984 Detection of malignant ovarian neoplasms: a review of the literature. II. Laboratory detection. Obstetrical and Gynaecological Survey 39, 329–344

Smith W G, Day T G, Smith J P 1977 The use of laparoscopy to determine the results of chemotherapy for ovarian cancer. Journal of Reproductive Medicine 18: 257–260

Speert H 1949 Prophylaxis of ovarian cancer. Annals of Surgery 129: 468

Stall K E, Martin E W 1981 Plasma CEA levels in ovarian cancer patients: a chart review and survey of published data. Journal of Reproductive Medicine 26: 73

Stern J, Buscema J, Rosenshein N, Siegelman S 1981 Can computed tomography substitute for second look operations in ovarian carcinoma? Gynecologic Oncology 11: 82–88

Stuart G C E, Jeffries M, Stuart J L, Anderson R J 1982 The changing role of 'second look' laparotomy in the management of epithelial carcinoma of the ovary. American Journal of Obstetrics and Gynecology 142: 612–616

Takeuchi T, Fujiki H, Kaneya T 1981 Characterisation of amylase produced by tumours. Clinical Chemistry 27: 556

Taleman A, Haije W G, Baggerman L 1980 Serum AFP in patients with germ cell tumours of the gonads and extragonadal sites. Cancer 46: 380

Terz J J, Barber H R K, Brunschwiz A 1967 Incidence of carcinoma in the retained ovary. American Journal of Surgery 113: 511

Thigpen J T, Vance R B, Balducci L, Khansur T 1984 New drugs and experimental approaches in ovarian cancer treatment. Seminars in Oncology 11: 314–326

Thorp D 1950 Ovarian cancer subsequent to hysterectomy. Transactions of the Pacific Coast Obstetrics and Gynecology Society 18: 154

Tobias J S, Griffiths C T 1976 Management of ovarian carcinoma: current concepts and future prospects. New England Journal of Medicine 294: 877

Trichapoulos D, Papapostolou M, Polychromopouolou A 1981 Coffee and ovarian cancer. International Journal of Cancer 28: 691

Van Nagell J R, Kim E, Capser S 1980 Radioimmunoassay of primary and metastatic ovarian cancer using radiolabelled antibodies to carcinoembryonic antigen. Cancer Research 40: 502

Waalkhes T P, Rosenshein N B, Shaper J H, Ettinger D S, Wook B, Paone J F et al 1982 A feasibility study in the development of biological markers for ovarian cancer. Journal of Surgical Oncology 21: 207

Waterhouse J, Muir C, Correa P (eds) 1976 Cancer incidence in five continents, vol 2. IARC Scientific Publication No. 15, Lyons

Webb M J, Snyder J A, Williams T J, Decker D G 1983 Second look laparotomy in ovarian cancer. Gynecologic Oncology 14: 285–293

Weiss N S, Peterson A S 1978 Racial variation in the incidence of ovarian cancer in the United States. American Journal of Epidemiology 107: 91–95

Weiss N, Lyon J L, Liff J M, Vollmer W M, Dalny J R 1981 Incidence of ovarian cancer in relation to the use of oral contraceptives. International Journal of Cancer 28: 669–671

Weiss N S, Lyon J L, Kitshnamurthy S, Dietert S E, Liff J M, Dalny J R 1982 Noncontraceptive estrogen use and the occurrence of ovarian cancer. Journal of the National Cancer Institute 68: 95

Welander C, Alberts D 1977 Clonogenic assay studies of tumour cells from gynaecologic malignancies. In: Williams C, Whitehouse J (eds) Cancer investigation and management: female reproductive system. Wiley, Chichester, pp 79–94

Wharton J T, Herson J 1981 Surgery for common epithelial tumours of the ovary. Cancer 48: 582–589

Whitelaw R G 1959 Pathology and the conserved ovary. Journal of Obstetrics and Gynecology of the British Empire 66: 413

Wijnen J A, Rosensheim N B 1980 Surgery in ovarian cancer. Archives of Surgery 115: 863

Williams C J 1985 The usefulness of the human tumour stem cell assay. In: Bleeher N M (ed) Ovarian cancer. Springer-Verlag, Berlin, p 98

Woodruff J D 1979 The pathogenesis of ovarian neoplasia. Johns Hopkins Medical Journal 144: 117

Young R C, Chabner B A, Hubbard S P 1978 Prospective trial of melphalan (L-PAM) versus combination chemotherapy (Hexa-CAF) in ovarian adenocarcinoma. New England Journal of Medicine 299: 1261–1266

Young R C, Wharton J T, Decker D G 1979 Staging laparotomy in early ovarian cancer. Journal of the American Society of Clinical Oncologists 20: 399

Young R C, Howser D M, Myers C E 1981 Combination chemotherapy (CHex-UP) with intraperitoneal maintenance in advanced ovarian adenocarcinoma. Proceedings of the American Society of Clinical Oncologists 22: 465

Young R C, Decker D G, Wharton J T, Piver M S, Sudelar W F, Edwards B K et al 1983 Staging laparotomy in early ovarian cancer. Journal of the American Medical Association 250: 3072–3076

Zbroja-Sontag W 1983 Defence proteins and immune complexes in women with inflammatory and neoplastic lesions of the ovary. American Journal of Reproductive Immunology 4: 11

Index